Palliative Care Nursing

Quality Care to the End of Life

Marianne LaPorte Matzo, PhD, RN, GNP, CS, is a Professor of Nursing at New Hampshire Community Technical College in Manchester, New Hampshire and a Soros Scholar for the Project on Death in America. She was awarded a Doctorate in Gerontology from the University of Massachusetts-Boston and a Masters degree in Nursing from the Gerontological Nurse Practitioner Program at the University of Massachusetts-Lowell. The former Gerontology Project Director in the Department of Nursing at Saint Anselm College, Manchester, New Hampshire, she was also employed for eight years in the Massachusetts State Department of Mental Health. Dr. Matzo has presented educational programs both regionally and nationally on many topics related to Gerontological Nursing and Curriculum Development. Her work has been published in *Nurse Practitioner, Nurse Educator, Geriatric Nursing, Nursing Homes, Geriatric Psychiatry, The Journal of Gerontological Nursing* and *Gerontology and Geriatrics Education.*

Deborah Witt Sherman, PhD, RN, ANP, CS, is an assistant professor in the Division of Nursing at New York University where she is the program coordinator of the first nurse practitioner palliative care master's program in the United States. Dr. Sherman's background in critical care nursing, hospice nursing, and her certification as an adult nurse practitioner, as well as her research focus on populations with life-threatening and terminal illness, are foundational to her expertise and commitment to palliative care. In 1998, she was awarded the prestigious Project on Death in America Faculty Scholars Fellowship, funded by the Soros Foundation, to implement the Advanced Practice Palliative Care Master's Program at NYU, establish interdisciplinary palliative care initiatives with faculty from Mount Sinai School of Medicine, and participate as a nurse practitioner on the palliative care team of Mount Sinai Medical Center. Dr. Sherman is a member of the editorial boards of the *Journal of the New York State Nurses Association,* the *Journal of Applied Nursing Research,* and the *American Journal of Nursing.* She is also editor of the 1999 HIV/AIDS volume of *Nursing Clinics of North America,* a reviewer for the *Journal of Palliative Medicine* and for the EPERC project to educate physicians regarding end-of-life care. She serves on the advisory board and as faculty on the End-of-Life Nursing Education Consortium, whose aims are to educate nurses in palliative care across the country.

Palliative Care Nursing

Quality Care to the End of Life

Marianne LaPorte Matzo,
PhD, RN, GNP, CS
Deborah Witt Sherman,
PhD, RN, ANP, CS
Editors

 Springer Publishing Company

Springer Publishing Company, Inc.
536 Broadway
New York, NY 10012-3955

Acquisitions Editors: Sheri W. Sussman and Ruth Chasek
Production Editor: Jeanne W. Libby
Cover design by Susan Hauley

01 02 03 04/5 4 3

Cover photo, "Hudson Highlands Sundown," by Nick Zungoli. Reprinted with permission of Nick Zungoli and Exposures Gallery, www.exposures.com.

Library of Congress Cataloging-in-Publication Data

Palliative care nursing : quality care to the end of life / Marianne LaPorte Matzo and Deborah Witt Sherman, editors.
    p. cm.
    Includes bibliographical references and index.
    ISBN 0-8261-1384-2
    1. Terminal care. 2. Palliative treatment.   I. Matzo, Marianne.   II. Sherman, Deborah Witt.
RT87.T45 P343 2001
362.1'75—dc21   00-064094
                                                  CIP

Printed in Canada

Dedications

For LeaRose and Giuliana, the most precious gifts of my life, and to Roland, who shares and supports my life. I love and treasure all of you.   MLM

With deep love for my husband, Neal, and children, Ben, Rachel, and Joe, who are the wind beneath my wings.   DWS

As Project on Death in America Faculty Scholars we express our gratitude to George Soros and the members of the Board of Directors for their recognition of our nursing scholarship and their support of palliative care nursing education.   MLM & DWS

Contents

List of Education Plans
for Achieving Competencies

Contributors

Marilyn Bookbinder, PhD, RN
Director of Nursing Education and
  Quality Improvement
Pain, Medicine, and Palliative Care
Beth Israel Medical Center
New York, NY

Nessa Coyle, PhD(c), RN
Director of Pain and Palliative
  Care
Memorial Sloan-Kettering
  Cancer Center
New York, NY

**Suzanne K. Goetschius, MS, RN,
  GNP, CS**
Nurse Director, Elder Health
Fanny Allen Health Care
Colchester, VT

**Mary Layman Goldstein, RN, MS,
  OCN**
Clinical Nurse Specialist, Pain and
  Palliative Care Service
Memorial Sloan-Kettering
  Cancer Center
New York, NY

Mary K. Kazanowski, PhD, RN, CS
Professor
Saint Anselm College
Manchester, NH

Margaret Kiss, RN, MSN, AOCN
Memorial Sloan Kettering
  Cancer Center
New York, NY

Mary Jo Jacobs, RN, MSN, FNP
Northwestern Memorial Hospital
Palliative Care and Home Hospice
  Program
Chicago, IL

**Lisa M. Krammer, RN, MSN, ANP,
  AOCN**
Northwestern Memorial Hospital
Palliative Care and Home Hospice
  Program
Chicago, IL

Carla Mariano, EdD, RN
Associate Professor
Program Coordinator of the Ad-
  vanced Practice Holistic Nursing
  Program
New York University
New York, NY

**Jeanne Martinez, RN, MPH,
  CRNH**
Northwestern Memorial Hospital
Palliative Care and Home Hospice
  Program
Chicago, IL

**Kathleen O. Perrin, MS, RN,
    CCRN**
Associate Professor
Saint Anselm College
Manchester, NH

Mertie L. Potter, ND, ARNP, CS
Associate Professor
Saint Anselm College
Manchester, NH

Gloria C. Ramsey, RN, BSN, JD
Director, Legal and Ethical Aspects
    of Practice
New York University
New York, NY

Aileen Ring, RN, MSN
Northwestern Memorial Hospital
Palliative Care and Home Hospice
    Program
Chicago, IL

**Judith Kennedy Schwarz, PhD(c),
    RN, MS**
Doctoral Candidate
New York University
New York, NY

Mary Beth Williams, RN, MN
Northwestern Memorial Hospital
Palliative Care and Home Hospice
    Program
Chicago, IL

Foreword

Betty Rolling Ferrell

Quality nursing care provided to those facing life's end can be characterized by two words—competence and compassion. Pioneers in the emerging field of palliative care, such as Cicely Saunders, Florence Wald, and Jeanne Quint Beneliel, have emphasized that the recipients of our care deserve the most competent, expert, evidence-based care provided in a way that embodies compassion, respect for dignity, and an appreciation for the whole person and the family.

As an oncology nurse for the past 23 years, most of which time has been devoted to palliative care, I have come to understand a fundamental truth, which is that *nurses cannot practice what they do not know.* The provision of quality nursing care for those approaching death, exemplifying competence and compassion, will become a reality only when nursing education prepares students for that professional role.

Competent end-of-life care includes expert assessment skills, aggressive pain and symptom management, and the acquisition of knowledge, attitudes, and skills in a clinical area in which there is a rapid learning curve due to the increased focus on palliative care over the past decade. Pivotal events in just the past 5 years have included the Institute of Medicine's report on End of Life Care, the Supreme Court ruling on the right to die, the proliferation of hospice and palliative care programs, and a society faced with ethical dilemmas, such as withdrawal of life-sustaining treatment and assisted suicide. There is indeed, much to learn to gain competence in physical, psychological, social, and spiritual care of patients and families experiencing life-threatening, progressive illness. As the largest health care profession, nurses have long advocated for attention to quality of life. Achieving quality of life, even at the end of life, is contingent upon competent nursing care.

The management of one single symptom, such as dyspnea, requires expert knowledge of physiology, numerous pharmacological treatments, non-drug interventions and psychological support to ease the distress of patient and family experiencing this symptom. Terminal illness for most patients is not one symptom, but a multitude of physical and psychological symptoms. Nurses prepared at the undergraduate level and advanced practice nurses must, therefore, be prepared to address the complex needs of patients and families.

As if the challenge to promote competent palliative nursing care was not already a daunting task for educators, promoting compassion is more formidable a task. Fostering compassionate palliative nursing care begins with an evaluation of one's own death anxiety, given confrontation with mortality, as well as an assessment of one's faith and even the ultimate meaning of life and death. Advancing beyond self-evaluation to assuming the role of a compassionate caregiver requires the skills of active listening, comforting, reinforcing, or communicating bad news, and developing an intimate relationship between nurse and dying patient, which is intensely demanding yet ultimately rewarding. The greatest challenge for the nurse is often not all the "doing for" but the "being with."

Nursing has often been described as both an art and a science and this is so true in describing palliative nursing care. Compassionate care for the grieving patient or family, supporting a patient when first confronted with a terminal prognosis, being with a person confronting the reality of cancer recurrence, or instructing young parents on care of the body at the time of an infant death are art forms in the truest sense. These images are also reminders that palliative care occurs not only in hospice for elderly cancer patients, but rather across all settings including clinics, home care, long-term care, critical care units, and nurseries. Compassionate care provides a context for healing for patients and families of all ages, confronted with relatively sudden death or prolonged illness.

As a profession, nursing has an obligation to respond to the demands of society. The social demands of the year 2000 include an aging population, increasing chronic illness, a seriously burdened health care system, and very importantly—a society that has begun to face the reality that quality of life matters, even at the end of life. Just as activists in the 1960s and 1970s revolutionized childbirth by questioning how we are born, activists of the 1990s have begun to articulate an awareness of how we die, and are questioning the quality of care offered to individuals with advanced disease who are approaching death.

End-of-life care is not just "an elective." If the nursing profession is to embrace the challenges of society, it will be because we have moved the competence and compassion of palliative care to the status of a "required course" for nurses in all specialties and health care settings.

This text, *Palliative Care Nursing: Quality Care to the End of Life*, will be recognized as a foundation for nursing education. The authors, Drs. Marianne LaPorte Matzo and Deborah Witt Sherman, are recognized leaders in palliative nursing education. Through this text, they enable educators to teach compassionate and competent palliative care. The text addresses the essential nursing competencies proposed by the American Association of Colleges of Nursing (AACN) 1998 document entitled "Peaceful Death," and identifies the knowledge, attitudes, skills, undergraduate and graduate behavioral outcomes, and teaching/learning strategies related to each AACN nursing competency. Nurse educators and their students within undergraduate, graduate, and continuing education programs will find this to be a rich resource of not only the content of palliative care, but the methods by which this education can best be taught. The text is a comprehensive approach spanning the traditional to complementary treatments, care of the physical as well as the spiritual, and attention to patient, family, and nurse. The emphasis is on the nurse as a member of an interdisciplinary team and the need for attention to the cultural factors influencing care at the end of life.

Throughout the health care community there is a growing awareness of the wide gap between the reality of end-of-life care, and the kind of care each of us would seek for those we love. This book is a guide to preparing nurses to be the competent and compassionate professionals who can lead this transformation in care.

Preface

Palliative Care Nursing: Changing the Experience of Dying in America

Deborah Witt Sherman and Marianne LaPorte Matzo

Although death is an inevitable and natural human experience, it has been shrouded in mystery, contemplated in fear, and envisioned as an experience of great suffering. Yet, this has not always been the case. Our ancestors had a closer relationship with death, often welcoming its release from pain, recognizing the cycles of nature with a time to live and a time to die, and accepting death as a transition into a new life and a reward for one well-lived.

At the beginning of the 20th century, the focus of health care was on helping people to survive long enough to reach adulthood. Early health care interventions focused on improving sanitation, nutrition, and preventing injuries and the spread of disease. Without advanced medical technology and medications, death was a common occurrence. Although cure was not always possible, human caring was the critical element in achieving a peaceful and dignified death. Families accepted and even cherished the opportunities to care for their loved ones at the end of life and to provide an environment where physical, emotional, social, and spiritual needs could be met. The caregiving experience was a shared responsibility of the members of the community who each supported the dying and their families in meaningful ways. People died in the comfort of their own homes, close to their loved ones, with death as much a part of the collective consciousness as birth.

Toward the mid to late 20th century, advances in health care and the management of disease and illness created a mindset which challenged death, denied mortality, and fostered the belief that death was a medical failure. The care of the dying was shifted from family and community to experts in the health professions and occurred within medical institutions. Intervention efforts of the late 20th century focused on health and wellness, and developing health promotion strategies to insure a long, productive, and fulfilled life. Society embraced the value of self-responsibility and health care activism, and currently supports the pioneering of medical technology to eradicate inherited and acquired diseases. This health quest focuses on the continuance of life and well-being by conquering the deficits imposed by old age and disease in an effort to defy death.

Yet embedded in the unconsciousness of the human mind remains the recognition of personal mortality. For some, death is even welcomed as a relief from the complexities of their current existence. Since the advent of advanced medical technology, curative measures are considered a right of individuals, and their provision, a responsibility of health care professionals. Yet, one must question whether life-prolonging therapies are appropriate or whether an individual's right to a peaceful death supercedes medical interventions. Should technology countermand the natural laws of nature, or the will of God? Health care providers are beginning to acknowledge their responsibility to help patients weigh the risks versus benefits of potential interventions. The medicalization of death necessitates advocacy in protecting the values, beliefs, and traditions of individuals. It evokes an opportunity for individuals to reprioritize life's goals and contemplate the meaning of life, suffering, and death.

With the fastest growing section of the American population being those over 85, people are considering the implications of longevity not only within the context of individual well-being but within the context of societal health. An ethical dilemma faced by lay people and health professionals alike involves questions regarding "Is the *length* of life the ultimate value?" or "Is the *quality* of life the ultimate value?"

Very often the individuals posing and responding to these questions are those born after World War II, known as the baby boomers. Referencing past historical and familial experiences, these individuals have espoused the values and pursued the issues of human rights, responsibility, and control. With a proactive stance, the baby boomers have fought for the right to have a "natural" birth; sought control over what happens to their bodies and in their lives; and challenged complacency and the status quo. For many of these individuals who are now turning 50, their thoughts turn to their own mortality as they witness the death of their parents and even their peers. They reject the pain, suffering, loneliness, and isolation witnessed, and believe that they have a stake in, and responsibility for, changing the experience of dying in America.

The heightened consciousness of this generation of Americans has also been provoked by an awareness of societal changes. These include increasing cultural and spiritual diversity in the population; fragmentation and geographic dispersion of the family; and a shift in role responsibilities and expectations in families and work care settings due to economic demands. Changes within the health care delivery system, most notably the specialization of health care, emergence of managed care systems, and the resultant reimbursement restraints, have evolved over the last 2 decades. The outcome of these changes has been a heightened sense of vulnerability and risk for patients and families at the end of life.

The expectation by managed care systems of families to assume a major role in the care of family members with life-threatening or fatal illness creates overwhelming anxiety and insecurity, as well as physical and economic burdens on family caregivers. Familial burdens become community concerns and big business issues when work productivity and absenteeism impede economic advancement and prosperity. Clearly, the result has been significant societal dissatisfaction and disillusionment with health care, and an increasing physical, emotional, social, and even spiritual burden which negatively effects the quality of life of those receiving and providing care at the end of life.

The societal agenda has become one of developing mechanisms to deliver compassionate care to those with life-threatening illnesses. The relationships of patients with primary health care providers, once one of complete trust and acceptance of their authority, has been changed to that of a partnership. Individuals use the Internet to gain access to the latest health care information and demand an active role in determining their goals and plan of care. The rapid and diffuse exchange of information through the Internet and other information systems provides an opportunity for worldwide dialogue regarding end-of-life issues and palliative care. This has enhanced national and international initiatives to improve the care of the dying and their families.

Although medical technology has the ability to enhance quality of life until death, patients, families, and health care providers are weighing the benefits and burdens of recommended therapies. Quality of life will mean different things to different people but will typically refer to happiness or satisfaction with life. A person's perception of her quality of life relates to her personal, introspective evaluation of her life experiences and her ability to control all aspects of her life including illness. Important aspects of the quality of life as death approaches include physical concerns (pain and symptoms), psychological distress (depression and existential anxiety), level of functioning (physical, emotional, and social), spiritual well-being, social support, planning for preferences in care, and the health care provider-patient relationship (Fields & Cassell, 1997). Although the hospice movement, which began in the early 1970s, recognized and addressed quality of life at the end of life, the awakening of American's consciousness to the inevitability of death and end-of-life issues had not yet occurred. The stimulus was therefore lacking to mandate changes in end-of-life care in either mainstream medicine or nursing.

The health care consumer and health professionals now recognize the importance of making treatment judgments based on scientific evidence rather than on anecdotal reports. The SUPPORT study (SUPPORT, 1995) provided empirical evidence that across the country dying people were in moderate to severe pain at the end of life, were dying on ventilators in intensive care environments, and were dying with little to no recognition of their end-of-life wishes. Their health care providers also dismissed the need for collaborative relationships with patients, families, and other members of the health care team. In short, the report card on dying in America indicated failure. However, an awakening has begun, and the initiative known as "Palliative Care" is underway to improve quality of life and quality of dying for individuals and families facing life-threatening illness.

The result has been a major initiative across the United States to improve care at the end of life and promote a peaceful, respectful death. Funding to study and improve end-of-life care has totaled millions of dollars in recent years. This funding has been made possible by the Soros Foundation's Project on Death in America, which educates faculty scholars in end-of-life care, and supports both training and research initiatives. The Robert Wood Johnson Foundation funded the SUPPORT study and continues to take a national lead in educating health professionals in end-of-life care. Other initiatives are being supported by the United Hospital Fund, The Coalition to Improve the Care of the Dying, The Compassionate Care of the Dying, and the Institute of Medicine, to name a few. The movement to provide better care for the dying and their families has achieved greater momentum and coordination than any other professional initiative of recent times. This has most likely happened because, unlike other social initiatives, dying and death are universal experiences and all individuals have suffered in one way or another.

Palliative care is defined as a "philosophy of care that provides a combination of active and compassionate therapies intended to comfort and support patients and families who are living with life-threatening illness, being sensitive and respectful of their religious, cultural, and personal beliefs, values, and traditions" (Canadian Palliative Care Association, 1995). The current trend is toward the integration of hospice and palliative care and the inclusion of not only individuals with cancer or AIDS, but of patients with end-stage organ diseases, neuro-degenerative diseases, and dementia. Palliative care is offered from the time of diagnosis with advanced disease until death, and continues for families during the bereavement period. The challenge is to dispel the misunderstandings about hospice and palliative care as "no care" or having "nothing else to offer," and affirm hospice/

palliative care as the opportunity to provide "aggressive comfort and supportive care" which promotes quality of life and quality of dying throughout the illness/dying trajectory. Furthermore, the public and professional mindset must change from viewing death as failure to viewing death as a natural part of the life cycle and an opportunity for the continued actualization of one's potential. With this new mindset, the pattern of referral to hospice/palliative care will change from the last days of life to the time of initial diagnosis of advanced disease. With earlier referral, the members of the palliative care team (nurse, physician, social worker, and clergy/chaplain) would have the opportunity to more completely address the physical, psychological, social, and spiritual needs of patients and their families.

Nursing's history reveals the compassionate care of the dying and acknowledges that human caring exists beyond cure. As the largest number of health care professionals in the country, nurses have a tremendous potential to change the care of the dying and their families. With an understanding of human nature and education that addresses the holistic needs of individuals, families, and communities across the life span, nurses can play a leading role in palliative care. Nursing professionals can capitalize on the individual's desire for autonomy and control of his or her life, by reinforcing the importance and value of actively participating in the decisions at the end of life through advanced care planning. As nurses frame the discussion of dying and death within the context of hope and meaning, and as an opportunity for choices and continued achievement of goals, uncertainty is replaced with certainty, hopelessness is replaced with faith, and despair is replaced with empowerment. Dying and death have the possibility of then becoming one of the most meaningful and significant acts of life.

The value of the nurse's role in insuring the quality of life and the quality of dying is acknowledged and respected by all health disciplines. Nursing professionals are assuming leadership roles to insure that comprehensive, holistic end-of-life care is available to all patients and families experiencing life-threatening, progressive illness. With support from the Project on Death in America, the Robert Wood Johnson Foundation, and the Department of Health and Human Services, funding has been made available to educate nurses in palliative care. The intent is to integrate palliative care content into the curriculum of all undergraduate nursing programs (both associate and baccalaureate degree); to educate practicing nurses in palliative care through continuing education initiatives; and to prepare advanced practice nurses in palliative care to assume leadership positions in practice, education, and research.

Research has indicated that the education of health professionals in end-of-life care has been limited or nonexistent in both nursing and medicine. Given that competent and compassionate end-of-life care is a responsibility of all health professions, each discipline must determine strategies to educate their students and professionals in palliative care. As Project on Death in America Faculty Scholars, the editors have assumed the responsibility, in their roles as nurse practitioners, educators, and researchers, to work collaboratively with nursing colleagues in developing, implementing, and evaluating nursing initiatives in palliative care within the United States.

This book is written as a contribution to the initiatives of the nursing profession regarding palliative care. This work began in 1998 when the American Association of Colleges of Nursing (AACN) brought together palliative care experts and health care ethicists to develop undergraduate competency statements and curricular guidelines for end-of-life nursing care. The document entitled "Peaceful Death" outlines 15 end-of-life competencies and serves as the organizing framework for this book. Along with the new Oxford Textbook of Palliative Nursing, the Toolkit for Nursing Excellence at the End of Life (TNEEL), and the End of Life Nursing Education Consortium (ELNEC), this text provides the essential information to achieve best-practices in palliative care nursing.

For the purposes of this text, it should be noted that the nurse educated at the undergraduate level has been defined as one who is working on or who has completed an Associate or Baccalaureate Degree in Nursing, while the graduate level nurse has been defined as someone who is working on or has completed a Master's degree or Ph.D. in nursing. This text addresses the content, knowledge, attitudes, skills, undergraduate and graduate behavioral outcomes, and appropriate teaching/learning strategies to achieve the AACN End-of-Life nursing competencies. It is expected that the graduate level nurse will have already mastered the undergraduate behavioral outcomes that reflect the integration of his or her knowledge, attitudes, and skills. As such, this text is applicable to students, to educators, and to practicing nurses.

Nursing students enrolled in Advanced Practice Palliative Care Master's Programs, such as New York University's Palliative Care Nurse Practitioner Program and Post-Master's Certificate Program, or Ursuline College's Palliative Care Clinical Nurse Specialist Program, will also find this book an asset in providing care to patients with complex physical, emotional, social, and spiritual needs across health care settings. With knowledge of advanced pathophysiology, pharmacology, and physical assessment, advanced practice palliative care nurses can prescribe a vast array of pharmacological and nonpharmacological interventions discussed in this book to address the complex needs of patients and families at the end of life. Throughout the illness and dying trajectory, graduate nurses also assume leadership roles as members of interdisciplinary palliative care teams, develop standards of care, clinical guidelines, and health care policies. They educate and mentor undergraduate-prepared nursing colleagues and participate in research related to the end of life. The information presented in this text will therefore serve as a foundation to advanced palliative care competencies.

It is important to realize that students and practicing nurses bring to palliative care nursing their own spiritual and cultural beliefs and values, and their personal and professional experiences with life-threatening illness, dying, and death. The acquisition of knowledge is therefore only one aspect of education in palliative care nursing. Faculty should also assist students in recognizing their own feelings, needs, and issues so that they can be aware of their assumptions and biases, and be open and accepting of human diversity. An emphasis in education must therefore also be on self-care, self-healing, and the resolution of issues of loss and grief and mutual support. This is extremely important as nurses and other team members bear witness to the suffering of others, experience the loss of those for whom they deeply cared, and address their own fears of vulnerability and mortality. In contrast to the demands of palliative care are the rewards that include intimately sharing in the lives of fellow human beings at their most vulnerable times, witnessing intense moments of support and love, and often learning from patients how to die with grace and dignity. These are the opportunities that transcend the traditional experiences in both nursing and medicine.

Although nursing espouses a holistic approach to care, the constraints of time and resources have mandated a focus on addressing the physical needs of patients with less attention to spiritual, social, and emotional concerns. However, in the face of life-threatening illness and the end of life, spiritual, social, and psychological needs of patients and families move to the forefront and provide an individualized context, which guides the goals and plan of care. As such, the authors have made a conscious decision regarding the presentation of palliative care content in this text.

This text is organized to emphasize the importance of a holistic perspective and an understanding of the patient and family as individuals with diverse spiritual and cultural needs and expectations. The first section of the text will address the more abstract spiritual and cultural needs of patients, families, and health care providers, with an emphasis on the value of complementary holistic modalities in promoting health, wholeness, and wellness even as death approaches. In the second section, societal aspects of end-of-life care are discussed, followed by the psychological aspects of dying. The text concludes with a discussion of the physical aspects of death and dying, specifically pain and symptom management and the needs and experiences of individuals who are actively dying. The authors believe that decisions regarding physical interventions at the end of life must be addressed based on knowledge of the spiritual, social, and psychological beliefs, values, expectations, and wishes of the patient and family.

Palliative care nursing therefore offers an exquisite blend of holistic, humanistic caring coupled with aggressive management of pain and symptoms associated with advanced disease. Educational and research initiatives will transform the care offered to patients and families at the end of life and improve their quality of life until death. Through collaborative interdisciplinary care, patients and families can regain a sense of trust and security knowing that a peaceful, respectful death is their right. Society may come to acknowledge dying and death without fear. The envisioned possibilities are of dying as an opportunity for continued growth and transcendence. Palliative care nursing will change the experience of dying in America.

REFERENCES

Author (1995). *Canadian palliative care association: Palliative care: Towards a consensus in standardized principles of practice.* Ontario, Canada.

Fields, M., & Cassell, C. (1997). *Approaching death: Improving care at the end of life.* Washington, DC: National Academy Press.

SUPPORT Principal Investigators. (1995). A controlled trial to improve care for seriously ill hospitalized patients. *Journal of the American Medical Association,* 274(20), 1591–1598.

PART 1

Holistic Aspects
of Palliative Care

April 12, 1999

Today, I admitted Candy Harris to our home-care agency. Candy is a 42-year-old woman who up until a month ago worked as a nurse with developmentally delayed children. She has been married to Ron for the last 20 years; a picture taken of them at their Senior Prom sits on a bookshelf. They have two children ages 5 and 8 and live in a new neighborhood development. She seemed so sad when I arrived, but I would be, too, if I were in her situation. I find admissions like this so difficult; she is close to my age and we are so similar in other ways.

She tells me the history of her disease in a very matter-of-fact way. For the 9 months prior to her diagnosis, Candy had noticed increased flatus that had not gotten better, despite alterations in her diet. For the 2 months prior she said that she had little appetite, but still had gained 5 pounds. She felt bloated all of the time and the waistbands of her clothes were tight. Her mother started menopause in her early 40s and died at age 56 of breast/ovarian cancer. Candy thought that her symptoms were related to the early start of menopause and so decided to visit her nurse practitioner for a physical exam and pap smear.

Given Candy's symptoms and her positive family history of cancer, the nurse practitioner ordered an abdominal CT scan in addition to a complete physical work-up. An ovarian mass was detected and Candy was scheduled for a laparotomy. Stage III ovarian cancer was diagnosed. The surgeon was able to use cytoreduction to decrease the tumor volume to < 2 cm in diameter and the oncologist suggested platinum-based combination chemotherapy. She was in shock that all of this was happening to her so fast. The children were really too young to completely understand what was going on and her husband insisted that they were going to "fight this."

Candy has just finished her third cycle of chemotherapy. She is very weak and in need of home health care support. Candy was sitting in a chair in the living room when I arrived. Her hair had all fallen out and her eyes were red, as though she had been crying, and she was holding a rosary in her hand. One section of the wall was covered with get well cards; she referred to this area as her "prayer wall." As I was assessing her, she burst into tears and told me that she thinks "God is punishing her for something" and that this is why she has cancer. This was not the first time that I have heard this from a patient. Believing in the importance of atoning for her sins, Candy has been attending mass whenever she has the strength, praying the rosary regularly, and asking the church congregation to pray for her. She has gone to confession and received the "Sacrament of the Sick." She also admitted that she wanted to "cover all of her bases" and that she has turned to holistic interventions in addition to her chemotherapy so that her body, mind, and soul will also heal. After her initial diagnosis she researched complementary interventions for cancer and started on a macrobiotic diet with additional B12 and D vitamins.

Candy receives Reiki twice a week and is seeing a therapist weekly. She said that she and her husband use mental imagery and relaxation techniques to imagine her body defenses as a powerful source to annihilate the cancer cells. Candy said that she has so much to live for, that she has a lot of good friends, a loving husband, and great kids. She really doesn't know what she has "done wrong" but she asks for God's forgiveness and hopes to get on with her life.

As a nurse, I marvel at her will to live and her determination to beat this disease. She seems to draw her strength from her religion and her relationships. Her strength is an inspiration to all who care for her.

1

Spiritually and Culturally Competent Palliative Care

Deborah Witt Sherman

AACN Competency

#4: Recognize one's own attitudes, feelings, values, and expectations about death and the individual, cultural, and spiritual diversity existing in these beliefs and customs.

> Death is not the ultimate tragedy of life. The ultimate tragedy is depersonalization—dying in an alien and sterile environment, separated from the spiritual nourishment that comes from being able to reach out to a loving hand, separated from a desire to experience the things that make life worth living, separated from hope.
>
> —Cousins, 1979

Spirituality and culture are among the most important factors that structure human experience, values, behaviors, and illness patterns. Life-threatening illness is a crisis on many levels—physical, psychological, familial, social, and spiritual (Doka & Morgan, 1993). Given the uniqueness and individuality of each person, even people of the same religion or culture may have different backgrounds, experiences, needs, concerns, and interpretation of illness. In addition to the individuality of the person, the nature of the life-threatening illness may be different and the person may be at different points in adapting to the reality of their disease. Spiritual and cultural concerns may permeate the illness experience or may arise at any point across the illness/dying trajectory. For patients and families experiencing life-threatening illness, the concerns may be of suffering which may take multiple forms relative to the mind-body-spirit.

It is now recognized that the uncertain and long-term nature of many life-threatening illnesses poses the potential for pain, alterations in body image, and confrontation with death, which may lead to spiritual distress. The renewed focus on incorporating spiritual care into nursing practice is congruent with nursings' commitment to holistic practice and the renewed valuing of human experiences that defy scientific description and explanation (O'Neill & Kenny, 1998). Within the past few years, research has shown that religious beliefs and spiritual practices affect the meaning of illness, physical and emotional well-being, coping with illness, and health care decisions, particularly for individuals facing life-threatening illness (Koenig, 1999).

Every culture has a worldview or construct of reality that defines the individual within that reality. A patient's cultural background is therefore fundamental in defining and creating their reality and determining their purpose in life (Ersek, Kagawa-Singer, Barnes, Blackhall, & Koenig, 1998). One's culture gives an individual the beliefs and values that support a sense of identity and security, as well as providing a prescription for behaviors about how one is to conduct life and approach death.

A transformation of identity begins when an individual is diagnosed with a terminal illness. Cultural rituals provide the sacred elements that support patients and families during times of illness and transition. Specific rituals assist individuals and families in coping with death, which is the final transition in life. The rituals of death change the identity of the patient from the living to the dead, and the identify of the family member, such as from spouse to widow or widower (Kagawa-Singer, 1998).

Spiritual and cultural competence are central tenets of palliative care. As a philosophy of care, palliative care combines active and compassionate therapies to support and comfort individuals and families who are living with life-threatening illness. Palliative care strives to meet the physical, psychological, social, and spiritual expectations and needs, while remaining sensitive to personal, cultural, and religious beliefs and practices (Ferris & Cummings, 1995). Undergraduate prepared nurses and advanced practice nurses must become spiritually and culturally competent in the care they offer across the illness/dying trajectory. Such care is critical to enhancing the quality of life and quality of dying and supporting the intrinsic dignity of patients and their family.

THE SPIRITUAL NATURE OF THE PERSON

Spirituality is often the lens through which people interpret their world and their reality, as they search to understand themselves, their needs, and their relationships to self, others, nature, and God. The word spirituality derives from the Latin word spiritus, which refers to breath, air, and wind. The spirit connotes "whatever is at the center of all aspects of one's life or that which gives life to a person" (Dombeck, 1995, p. 38). Spirituality has also been described as our inner being (Carson, 1989), or as the integrating life force which allows human beings to transcend their physical nature (Conrad, 1985). Moberg (1984) conceptualized spiritual well-being as encompassing both vertical and horizontal dimensions that involve transcendence. The vertical dimension refers to our sense of well-being in relation to God, while the horizontal dimension refers to a sense of purpose in life and life satisfaction.

Recognition of the spiritual nature of human beings was reflected in the early writings of Florence Nightingale, who viewed spirituality as a dimension of human nature and the highest level of human consciousness. Nightingale espoused that human beings must use God-given powers to discover and apply the universal laws to relieve pain and suffering on physical, emotional, social, and spiritual levels (Macrae, 1999). She felt that religion was a means of expressing and developing spirituality, but that it is possible to develop spirituality outside of organized religion (Macrae, 1999). Believing that God's plan is to raise mankind from imperfection to perfection, which cannot be completed in one lifetime, Nightingale viewed death as a new mode of existence that allows for continued development (Macrae, 1999).

The concept of spirituality includes references to the spirit, the soul, spiritual perspectives, spiritual needs, and spiritual well-being and is viewed as more basic than and different from religion (Burkhardt, 1989). Spirituality is a broader concept than religion, although religion is one form of expression of spirituality as is prayer or meditation (Puchalski, 1998a). The quest for meaning in life and transcendence has been typically conducted within the framework of organized religion. S. Ryan (1997), a chaplain, proposes that every human being has five fundamental spiritual needs: 1) the need to find meaning in life, particularly at times of illness; 2) the need for a relationship with a transcendent other, through which we find meaning and purpose in life; 3) the need to change whatever causes us to suffer or be unhappy; 4) the need for hope no matter how difficult life can be; and 5) the need for others who will care for us and are willing to co-journey with us.

In recent years, the meaning of spirituality has changed as individuals searched for personal and transpersonal meaning outside the confines of organized religion (Wink, 1999). Moore (1992) identifies the spiritual quest as a process of "resacralization" of the self and the world surrounding us. The goal is to embark on a personal journey in discovering the transcendent in everyday life and in all human relationships. According to Moore, the outcome of the spiritual quest is not to find some higher, inner-order truth, but rather the ability to inject magic, mystery, and sacredness into every moment of our lives and in everything one does.

Individuals with life-threatening illness may question the purpose of their lives as they suffer and seek to transcend their suffering. Arnold (1989) believes that spirituality embodies the ultimate virtues of life in the form of hope, courage, faith, love, acceptance, and a meaningful encounter with death. Understanding the nourishment of the spirit either by prayer, religious commitment, personal faith, or relationships with others, health professionals can be a source of support or solace in achieving spiritual well-being, and healing. The word "heal" comes from the old English word Halen which means not only to restore by way of cure, but "to make whole or sound" (Urdang, 1972, p. 609). To heal can therefore mean to "restore a person to spiritual wholeness."

Fricchione (1999) believes that the crisis of physical illness leads to adaptive tasks and the testing of coping skills that will determine the outcome of the crisis. As a physician, he has learned from his patients that the worst part of illness is often the fear of separation and loss of attachment. Illness creates an intermediate area between separation and attachment, a point where spirituality in medicine and nursing may be examined and nurtured (Fricchione, 1999).

For individuals who are dying, the task work often involves spiritual energy and hope. At this time, the task may be to find a source of spiritual energy or reaffirm one's spiritual focus (Corr, Nabe, & Corr, 1997). Spiritual energy may come from a personal God, or an individual value system. Doka (1993) identified three principal spiritual tasks for those who are dying: 1) to find meaning in life; 2) to die in a way that is consistent with one's self-identity; and 3) to find hope that extends beyond the grave. This hope may go beyond the hope of cure to the hope of symbolic immortality, as one lives on genetically through one's children, or is remembered through one's artwork, music, writing, or contributions to the community.

In caring for patients with life-threatening illness or those who are actively dying, nurses need to recognize that spiritual concern or distress can effect physical well-being. An individual's beliefs and values can significantly affect how they cope with illness and its treatment. In assessing spiritual well-being, the questions explored may include:

- Are they suffering in physical, emotional, social, or spiritual ways?;
- Do they see purpose in life as they suffer?;

- Are they able to transcend their suffering and see something, or someone beyond that?;
- Are they at peace, hopeful, or do they despair?; and
- Do personal beliefs help them to cope with anxiety about death, their pain, and achieving peace? (Puchalski, 1998a).

People who are dying need to make peace not only with death, but also with life. Rather than encouraging people to fight death to the end, health professionals can provide an opportunity for them to bring closure to their lives; to complete unfinished goals; to forgive those they had conflicts with, and be forgiven; to make peace with themselves and with God; to say goodbye, and to die with dignity. Therefore, "remembering, assessing, searching for meaning, forgiving, reconciling, loving, and hoping are all part of the spiritual journey especially active during the time of dying" (Puchalski, 1998a, p. 38). According to McGregor (1999), the healing work of the soul in illness, dying, and bereavement happens when illness becomes an opportunity for connection, personal growth, and the finding of meaning; and when dying becomes an opportunity for growth, resolution, and transcendence for oneself and others.

SUFFERING AS A HUMAN CONDITION

Suffering is a part of life and the human condition, with suffering either personally experienced in a physical, emotional, social, or spiritual way, or experienced as witnesses to another's suffering. Cassell (1982) defines suffering as "the state of severe distress associated with events that threaten the intactness of a person" (p. 639). Suffering can be defined as the endurance of or submission to affliction, pain, or loss. Suffering is usually psychological, as a result of distressing circumstances that arise in the process of living, but can also be the effects of physical pain. Cassell (1982) believes that many aspects of a person can be sources of, or affected by suffering such as personality, character, the past, relationships, life experiences, roles, one's rights and responsibilities, family, and cultural background.

According to Kahn and Steeves (1996), suffering is a private lived experience of a whole person, unique to each individual. As such, suffering cannot be assumed present or absent in any given clinical condition or situation since suffering is dependent on the meaning of the event or loss. The experience of suffering is also both intrapersonal and interpersonal since it involves the person's own coping with suffering and the caring of others (Kahn & Steeves, 1996). Although we may not find answers as to why we suffer, as a part of the human family, we build relationships, communities, and society to reach out to one another to relieve suffering and sustain us in our struggle (McGann, 1997).

Suffering varies with the type of disease, type of personality, and the relationship between these factors. "The loss of physical integrity and the impending destruction of the unity of one's person can cause profound suffering" (DeBellis et al., 1986, p. 6). Within the context of illness, suffering can occur because of unfavorable prognoses, loss of function, disability, the complexity of treatment, failure to achieve relief of symptoms, expense of treatment, and the effects of disease on all social relationships and economic security (DeBellis et al., 1986).

Although suffering and pain are often referred to interchangeably, they are not identical. In some cases they are mutually present, when in other cases, one exists without the other. The transition from pain to suffering can occur when pain is unrelieved and out of control or when the source of pain is unknown. The persistence of pain and uncertainty can therefore exponentially increase suffering. Yet, suffering can continue even when pain is controlled. At the end of life, suffering may be exacerbated because of protracted or chronic illness, multiple simultaneous diseases and co-morbid conditions, recurrent disease, and awareness of mortality. Since suffering has to do with a personal understanding of the physical, emotional, and spiritual self and their interrelationships, we learn about suffering only by the ways in which an individual expresses an awareness of the threats to their personal wholeness (Smith, 1996).

Coyle (1995) gives examples of suffering, such as when patients experience despair, loneliness, and vulnerability; feel trapped by fear and bewilderment; experience loss and worry about treatment decisions; worry about being a burden; have financial concerns; experience abandonment; or fear dying yet are weary of life, and experience pain or the loss of hope. Families suffer as they assume the responsibilities of caregiving; watch the patient's deterioration; become exhausted; neglect their own needs; experience uncertainty about goals of care and anxiety about the place of care. The suffering of family members also occurs because of fear of the dying process, and the experience of losses of life as it was, the person they knew, and of hope, as well as guilt in wanting death to come soon.

RECIPROCAL SUFFERING OF PATIENTS AND FAMILY

Within the context of life-threatening illness, suffering, in the form of physical, emotional, social, and spiritual distress, often becomes an experience not only of the patient, but of their family caregivers, as the suffering of one amplifies the distress of the other (Foley, 1995). Family members, like patients themselves, are in transition from living with the disease to anticipating the death of their loved one from the disease (Davies, Reimer, & Marten, 1994). Families fear that death will occur in their absence, and may therefore refuse to leave the patient's side for even a moment. There is also a strong compulsion to attend to the patient's every need with disregard for their own needs (Klein, 1998). As the patient's illness progresses, the needs of the family also intensify and change with both patients and family caregivers potentially experiencing a significant compromise in the quality of their lives (Sherman, 1998).

Although family members may express the rewards of caring for terminally ill relatives, such care can have major psychosocial and physical effects, including heightened symptoms of depression, anxiety, psychosomatic symptoms, restrictions of roles and activities, strain in relationships, and poor physical health (Higginson, 1998). As witnesses to patient's pain and suffering, family caregivers may also experience a sense of powerlessness, and are often frightened and confused by the dramatic physical and emotional changes they perceive in their loved one as the disease progresses (Loscalzo & Zabora, 1998).

There are also many conflicting emotions and adjustment tasks, including conflict among feelings of loss, sadness, guilt, difficulty in knowing how to talk with the person who is dying, and worry about dying and death (Beeney, Butow, & Dunn, 1997). Furthermore, the family caregiver must adapt to changes in family roles and responsibilities, while attempting to meet the increased emotional needs of other family members and performing standard family functions (Doyle, 1994). Given that 25% of caregivers lose their job due to caregiver responsibilities and nearly one-third of families lose their major source of income or their savings, families also experience significant financial burdens (Lederberg, 1998). This may lead to feelings of anger, jealousy, and an increase in the family caregiver's own needs because of their heightened psychological distress. In addition, there is often the loss of social mobility, as well as social abandonment by friends, all of which negatively impact on the quality of life of family caregivers (Lederberg, 1998).

From a spiritual perspective, family members may question the meaning of the illness and suffering. They often spend considerable time reviewing painful aspects of the past with feelings of regret for disagreements, conflicts, or failures and a wish that relationships with the patient and with each other were somehow different. With each family member's unique experience of the stress, families may find it difficult to come together to effectively cope with the imposed life changes (Sherman, 1998). In their search for meaning, patients and families affirm spiritual values, change life priorities, and examine how the experience of illness has contributed to their personal growth.

Like their dying loved one, they live day to day to make the most of the present as they prepare for death on practical, cognitive, emotional, and spiritual levels (Davies et al., 1994). The hope is that through palliative nursing care, both patients and family members can transcend their reciprocal suffering and experience growth as they face the challenges of life-threatening or terminal illness (Sherman, 1998).

THE CARE OF THOSE WHO ARE SUFFERING

Cassell (1982) believes that the ways to relieve suffering are first, through the assignment of meaning to the injurious condition or event; and second, through transcendence, which is the most powerful way of restoring an individual's personhood to wholeness. Watson (1986) proposes four generic meanings of suffering, which include: correction in which an individual is being corrected of their wrongdoing; *affirmation* in which a person is affirmed of their right doing and the ability to be a role model for others; *naturalism* in which the individual is experiencing general human destiny; and *altruism* in which an individual's suffering will have benefit to others. In caring for those who are suffering, health professionals may help individuals come to a healthy, maintainable higher meaning to their suffering. From a theological perspective, Smith (1996) discusses the religious response to suffering and the possibility of transcendence of suffering through intellectual, ethical, and experiential dimensions of religion. The intellectual dimension involves the realization of some transcendent meaning, which connects the suffering person with some greater reality and delivers the individual from the threat of meaninglessness raised by illness and pain. The ethical dimension of religious life provides a perspective regarding how to interpret and respond to suffering. Suffering may be seen as a test of virtue or fidelity to God, a test of the worth of religious commitment, or as an opportunity of personal transformation. Within the experiential dimension of religion, the life of oneself and others, and of the relationship of these lives to each other and God are contemplated. The religious experience of suffering may therefore enable an individual to provide redemptive relationships with others, including God, and experience transcendence.

In caring for the suffering, Spross (1996) believes that the role of the nurse is one of coaching. "Coaching is an interpersonal intervention that requires the therapeutic use of the self—one's mind, past experience, words, heart, and hand—to comfort those who suffer" (Spross, 1996, p. 201). In coaching, the nurse:

- Establishes a trusting partnership;
- Assesses those who are at risk for suffering or who are vulnerable;

- Reassures patients that although their suffering may not disappear, they will not be abandoned;
- Identifies factors that may be eliminated or modified to alleviate suffering; and
- Intervenes to facilitate expression of feelings, find meaning in suffering, and help patients and families redefine the quality of life.

Spross (1996) states that the ability to alleviate suffering or find meaning in the experiences of suffering depends on the intrapersonal and interpersonal qualities of the nurse. The nurse must be self-accepting, secure in his/her own self-concept, and feel confident in strengthening others. As coach, the nurse values others and communicates that the individuals' feelings, goals, and opinions are respected, while conveying that the person is trustworthy, responsible, capable of self-direction, and able to identify relevant goals and find meaning in life.

Watson (1986) believes that nurses and other health professionals can relieve suffering in six ways: First, by being a companion to sufferers by identifying the pain of their losses, and exploring the circumstance and extent of the loss. Second, by listening for statements of meaning from sufferers and allowing the person's natural instincts and energy to surface the issue of higher meaning. Third, by valuing any self-disclosure on meaning a sufferer offers, by analyzing the meaning of the statements and learning what the statement reveals about the sufferer's view of himself. Fourth, by encouraging the sufferer's interpretation of their own experience. Fifth, by validating the sufferer's interpretation of their own experience while clarifying the meaning, seeking further definition of the meaning, and offering alternatives for reframing the meaning. Lastly, the nurse can identify supportive resources and hope for the sufferer to extend his identity and meaning in the future.

In alleviating the suffering of others, Bird (1986) offers seven principles to be considered within the context of nursing practice:

1. Remember that institutions don't dehumanize patients, staff members do.
2. Assume responsibility for morale whenever you are in the chain of command.
3. Be a whole person yourself with a healthy sense of humor and attitude.
4. Do not add clinical ineptitude to the further suffering of patients.
5. Be empathetic rather than sympathetic to patient's needs; otherwise human suffering can emotionally devastate one.
6. Offer holistic care and well-chosen words to allay suffering.

7. Determine to touch the life of at least one patient daily with some depth.

Halifax (1999) believes that health care providers, patients, and families can go to the root of their own suffering and transform the suffering into inherent wisdom. As a Buddhist, she reminds health professionals to come to the caregiving relationship with loving kindness, compassion by being in touch with one's own and other's suffering, joy in the well-being of others, and equanimity.

SPIRITUAL AND RELIGIOUS PERSPECTIVES ON DEATH

Losses in life often challenge our faith and philosophical systems. Those who experience loss and grief may differ regarding religious and spiritual perspectives from which they seek answers, search for meaning, and to which they turn for ritual, comfort, and support (Doka & Davidson, 1998). Understanding the ways that spirituality or religiosity facilitates or complicates the adjustment to loss and grief is a critical task to those involved in palliative care.

DEATH FROM A JEWISH PERSPECTIVE

The focus of those of the Jewish faith is on life and its preservation and in fostering and establishing religion in the life of people on earth, rather than focusing on the world beyond. The Jewish faith offers consolation in death by affirmation of life. Sickness and death are viewed neither as punishment nor reward. Death is not considered evil but rather inevitable and natural, as it comes from God and should not be feared. Jewish teachings are that the soul exists before the body comes into existence and continues to live on after the body is dead. Although the Orthodox believe in resurrection, this belief may be figurative rather than literal (Grollman, 1993).

Jewish death practices help the bereaved to realize that the loved one is dead and to gradually fill the void in a constructive way. The memory of the deceased must be perpetuated. Although Jews are usually buried, cremations are also done. A religious rite is the rendering of mourners' clothes, signified by the cutting of a black ribbon which is pinned to the mourners clothing in the funeral chapel or cemetery. This signifies the loss of a loved one. The Jewish funeral is a rite of separation, in which the casket actualizes the experience. The Rabbi recites prayers expressive of the spirit of Judaism and the memory of the deceased. Shiva refers to the seven days of intensive mourning beginning right after the funeral. The bereaved remain at home and condolence calls are made to pay respects to the family. The Shiva candle burns for seven days and the family prepares the meal of consolation, known as Seudat Havra-ah. Following Shiva comes the 30 days of Sloshim. During this time normal activities are resumed but entertainment is avoided. If a parent dies, the mourning continues for an entire year. The mourner's prayer is called the Kaddish, which is recited during the weekly Sabbath as a pledge to dedicate one's life to God, acknowledge the reality of death, and affirm life. The anniversary of the death is called Yahrzeit. The Kaddish prayer is recited and Yahrzeit candles are again kindled (Grollman, 1993).

DEATH FROM A ROMAN CATHOLIC PERSPECTIVE

In Catholicism, it is believed that Jesus experienced suffering, grief, and death. Jesus' death and the death of all others are viewed as a part of God's divine providence. As sinners, human beings experience the tragedy of death, yet are beneficiaries of its forgiveness and liberation. Although sins are forgiven, individuals must pay a debt by punishment. In Catholicism, resurrection is integral to death. Catholics believe that Christ died and rose from the dead, and that faith will allow them to see death as an entry into life with God. The sacrament of Anointing the Sick provides bodily and spiritual renewal and has replaced the term the Last Rites, which was viewed as a harbinger of death.

Since the second Vatican Council, the Catholic contemporary view places emphasis on risen life. There is a move from a preoccupation with sin and death toward an orientation of blessing for a Christian life. Christians follow Jesus into the mystery of death in order to find a life like his own (Miller, 1993). The funeral becomes one of Thanksgiving and consolation; the funeral mass is offered on behalf of the deceased, aiding them to the other side of death, and giving the bereaved the consolation of hope. It is believed that Christ accompanies the dying person to heaven and that dying is an act of faith in God (Miller, 1993).

DEATH FROM A PROTESTANT PERSPECTIVE

In Protestantism, spirituality is viewed as a dimension of humanness, a process of interaction, and an awareness of relationship. Spirituality cannot be lived in the abstract but rather is lived through one's religion, which is regarded as a cultural institution (Klass, 1993). God is viewed as a single being, who spoke to his people through the bible; God protects but also judges. Each Protestant has a direct and personal relationship with God unmediated by priest or sacrament. The church is viewed as a voluntary association of believers. The Protestant community is the local congregation or particular denomination supporting interpersonal relationships, yet is often split along racial, ethnic, and social class lines (Klass, 1993). Death is a challenge because it raises the problem of evil and the problem of meaningfulness of suffering. Suffering and overcoming evil are the core of Protestant teaching. For Protestants, the focus is salvation, which depends on the moral quality of life on earth. Heaven is known in hope, but not as a guarantee. The belief in an afterlife is through experiences of memory and sense of presence and shared community. Although Jesus is a model for physical, emotional, social, and spiritual suffering, the individual faces the cosmos alone. The issue is not how the individual can participate in Jesus' suffering, but rather the individual accepting the gift of God's grace in Jesus' death (Klass, 1993).

DEATH FROM EASTERN PERSPECTIVES

Hinduism originated in India, with belief in the cycles of being born and dying in an infinite series of lives or successive creations. Hinduism teaches the belief in karma, which is that every act of a human being, even an internal act, such as desire, has an effect on who that person becomes. One becomes virtuous by good actions and bad by bad actions (Ryan, 1993). A Supreme Being exists in the individual's soul and is the ultimate all.

The second Eastern perspective from India is Buddhism in which there is also the belief in karma and rebirth. Buddhists believe that life changes and death occurs. Buddha taught that a way to overcome ignorance and attain truth is through the path to enlightenment or changed state of awareness called Nirvana. Buddhists believe that the way to Nirvana is through meditation. Others believe that Nirvana can be attained through faith.

A third Eastern tradition is that of Confucianism, which has its origins in China and which stresses the importance of improving human relationships. The proper relationship between the living and dead is one of continuous remembrance and affection, through which one attains social immortality. The value of rituals is that they relate the living with the dead. Memory of parents and ancestors are kept through regular remembrance rituals, which also provide a vehicle for the expression of the human emotions of grief and affection.

A fourth Eastern perspective is that of Taoism, which also has its origins in China. In Taoism, there is a focus on nature and remedying society's disorder and lack of harmony. Nature is looked toward to discover the principles of life. Life is viewed as the companion of death, and death is viewed as the beginning of life and part of the living-dying process. Taoism offers a way of transcending the limits of the world, as there are ceaseless transformations where the person is not lost. The yin and yang are the basis for all natural change. The light half is the yang, which is characterized as masculine, active, hot, bright, dry, and hard. The dark half is the yin, which is characterized as feminine, passive, cold, dark, wet, and soft. They are viewed as complementary forces that transform into the other. There is no light without dark, evil without good, or life without death (Ryan, 1993).

Many Asian patients, Chinese, Japanese, Koreans, have an Eastern perspective in which formal behaviors are valued. It is believed that to rebel against death reveals a fundamental lack of understanding about life. Therefore, sadness and grief are kept private. Such behavior sets a good example and contributes to one's good reputation (Ryan, 1993). Patients may seek comfort in images, such as Buddha, Krishna or the Divine Mother, or in repeating holy mantras. Those from an Eastern perspective believe that a person's final dying thoughts may determine one's rebirth.

SPIRITUAL ISSUES IN DEATH AND DYING FOR THOSE WHO HAVE NO CONVENTIONAL RELIGIOUS BELIEFS

Religion has traditionally provided a context from which to understand and interpret death. However, individuals who are not religious can still find comfort and meaning through spirituality and by stepping back from the material world (Orion, 1993). Individuals with no conventional religious beliefs often interpret life based on a sense of being a part of a larger whole and from a scientific worldview. There is belief that an individual's life has a beginning and an ending, but the life process is indefinite. Whether the process is defined in terms of social or biological continuity, the brevity of life does not suggest insignificance. A particular life is short and seemingly inconsequential but assumes value and importance as a significant element in the entire ongoing process. Even brief life is viewed as a contribution to the life process.

Those without conventional religious beliefs often consider the present as the real world and take full responsibility for their decisions. There is the belief that immortality occurs by biological immortality such as living on in the genetic pool of one's descendants, or living on in the memories of others or one's contributions to the world (Orion, 1993). The focus is on actualizing human potential. From the naturalistic perspective, death is not avoided or denied. Death is viewed as real, final, and inevitable and a mark of man's solidarity with nature and the evolutionary process. Naturalism leads an effort to place the death of an individual in a framework of the process of living and dying, emergence, and extinction. In this framework, death is:

- A working out of the natural law by which all living things die;
- The absorption of the differentiated person in the natural process;
- A contribution to the evolutionary process;
- Cessation of life's potential for negative and positive contributions; and
- Reabsorption into new ways in nature (Orion, 1993).

Fear of death can be overcome by remembering that everything dies, but existence goes on. When death is seen as part of the natural order or part of the universal condition, it can be tolerated more easily. Life and death are continuous parts of the whole (Orion, 1993).

RESEARCH REGARDING SPIRITUALITY

Over the last 10 years, there has been increasing interest in the relationship between spirituality, religion, and health care. A Gallup Poll Survey (1990) showed that religion, an expression of spirituality, plays a central role in the life of Americans. Ninety-five percent of those Americans espoused a belief in God, with 57% praying daily, and 42% attending a weekly worship service. A more recent Gallup Poll (1997) showed that people overwhelmingly want their spiritual needs addressed at the end of life and felt that health professionals, physicians, and nurses, should speak with patients about their spiritual concerns. A national survey of 1,200 adults (Nathan Cummings Foundation, 1999) explored the relationships between the dying process and spiritual needs. Respondents expressed a need for companionship and spiritual support, particularly in the form of human contact, and to have the opportunity to pray alone or have someone pray for or with them. Eighty-one percent of the respondents stated the importance of receiving comfort, particularly from family and close friends, with only 36% finding comfort in the support of clergy, or from doctors or nurses. Those who sought support from clergy were more often female, older than 65 years, having less than a college education, and incomes under $40,000.

The relationship between the frequency and characteristics of religious coping and depression was examined by Koenig et al. (1992). Based on a sample of 850 hospitalized elderly men, the results indicated that 20%

reported the use of religion for coping and 56% gave a rating of 7.5 or higher on a scale of 0–10 of the importance of religion as a method of coping. Religious coping was inversely, but weakly related to depression scores ($r = .16$, $p < 001$).

The relationship between death anxiety, age, and intrinsic religiosity was examined by Thorson and Powell (1992) based on a sample of 345 individuals from diverse settings. The results indicated that intrinsic religiosity, or one's sense of personal connection, was positively related with age ($r = .27$, $p < .001$), while death anxiety was negatively correlated with age ($r = -.27$, $p < .001$). There was no difference in religiosity by gender, however, females were slightly more death anxious than males ($r = .10$, $p < .05$).

Poloma and Pendleton (1989) studied the effects of various types of prayer on quality of life by conducting a random telephone survey of 560 individuals. Using multiple regression analysis, prayer experience was positively related to quality of life, existential well-being, happiness, and religious satisfaction. Meditative prayer was positively associated with existential well-being and religious satisfaction. Colloquial prayer, of thanking God, was positively associated with happiness, each below the 0.5 level of statistical significance.

Based on a sample of 600 severely ill hospitalized patients, aged 55 and over, Koenig (1998) found that spiritual coping via connection with God and receiving religious support, was associated with less depression, greater compliance with care, and better quality of life. Roberts (1997) reported that for women coping with gynecologic cancer that religion had a serious place in their lives (76%), helped them sustain their hopes (91%), and supported their sense of worth (41%). According to Kaldjian (1998), patients who are HIV-positive expressed less fear of death when they read the bible frequently, attended church regularly, and saw God as playing a central role in their life.

QUALITY NURSING CARE: ADDRESSING THE SPIRITUAL NEEDS OF PATIENTS AND THEIR FAMILIES

SPIRITUAL CAREGIVING

Munley (1983) believes that spiritual caregiving is the human capacity to enter the world of others and respond with feeling, which touched them at a level that is deeper than doctrinal differences. Spiritual care involves the nurse's presence, compassion, hopefulness, and recognition that life, although it may no longer be productive, remains fruitful and an opportunity to connect with others in a very meaningful way. Being present to terminally ill patients and their families means listening in the broadest sense of the word, and conveying unconditional acceptance and compassion. According to Puchalski (1998a), individuals with life-threatening illness often ask such questions as: What gives meaning in my life?; Why is this thing happening to me?; How will I survive this loss?; and What will happen to me when life ends?

Although nurses may not be able to cure the disease and restore physical integrity, through compassionate care, they can promote hope and promote patients' healing. As an ongoing process, healing continues within the context of the person's life pattern of religious beliefs and practices and provides the opportunity for renewal and rebirth in relationship to oneself and with a higher being. Patients may also enrich nurses' lives as they allow nurses to enter their lives and share in their journey at extremely intimate and vulnerable times.

Integrating religion and spirituality into nursing care is therefore important because: 1) nursing is concerned with the whole person, body-mind-spirit; 2) many, although not all, patients are religious or spiritual; 3) many patients want to address spiritual issues; 4) and religious commitment is associated with relief from physical, emotional suffering, and enhanced quality of life (Matthews, 1999). Matthews also proposes that spirituality and religion are of benefit because they construct a coherent worldview to help individuals to interpret life experiences and suffering, help individuals develop meaning and purpose in life and connectedness with others, and engender serenity and transcendence, thereby buffering stress.

According to Doka and Morgan (1993), the spiritual care offered to patients and families should be based on the following principles:

- Each person has a spiritual dimension which must be considered along with mental, emotional, and physical dimensions;
- A spiritual orientation influences mental, emotional, and physical responses to dying and bereavement;
- When facing a terminal illness, death and bereavement may be a stimulus for spiritual growth;
- No single approach to spiritual care is satisfactory for all individuals given the diversity of individuals from different cultures;
- Spirituality is expressed and enhanced in formal and informal, religious and secular ways, including symbols, rituals, practices, patterns, gestures, art forms, prayers, and meditation which should be accessible and available;
- Care should be taken to offer settings, which will accommodate individual preferences as well as communal experiences;

- Health care systems should support spiritual care in their written statements of philosophy, and resources of time, money, and staff;
- Patients and caregivers should feel free to express humor and to laugh as this provides medicine for the soul; and
- A caring environment should be in place to promote spiritual work at any time.

ASSESSMENT OF SPIRITUAL WELL-BEING

An awareness and appreciation of a patient's and family's spiritual orientation is essential to holistic care. Although patients may have a strong religious affiliation, this may either support or hinder spiritual exploration and the acknowledgment of spiritual issues. It is important to know if the patients' and family's religious affiliation is a source of strength and support and was used to meet needs in the past. It is also important to understand if an individual's religious beliefs are a source of fear and distress, particularly if the individual fears judgment. The spiritual pain of an individual is often evident by the manifestation of sorrow and grief, isolation from self and others, sense of meaninglessness and emptiness, fear and avoidance of the future, hopelessness and despair, and anger and bitterness towards God (Matthews, 1999).

Although it is not the nurses' responsibility to solve all spiritual problems or provide the answers, the nurse can create an environment, which nurtures the patients' exploration of spiritual needs and concerns and supports them in their search for answers. This can be done by asking basic questions, such as "How are your spirits?," "Can you share with me your spiritual journey?," "How do you define your spirit?," or "What nourishes your spirit?" (O'Connor, 1993). These questions often reveal the patients' spiritual orientation and validate their spiritual nature.

By taking a spiritual history, nurses learn about the patient's beliefs or what is important to them. You can ask them questions during the history and address spirituality at each follow-up visit, as spirituality is an ongoing issue. In conducting such a history, it is important for the nurse not to impose his or her values, but to listen nonjudgmentally. However, nurses often recognize that awareness of one's own spiritual and religious values may assist in providing a supportive environment for the patient. With support, the sufferer is not isolated by pain, but may be brought closer to the source of meaning and to the community that share the meaning. This leads to transpersonal transcendence (O'Connor, 1993).

Assessment of valuable spiritual interventions preferred by the patient and family may range from religious rituals such as prayer, communion, and blessing of the sick to secular observances such as sunsets, music, or poetry (O'Connor, 1993). Nurses may also question, "How did you relieve your spiritual pain in the past?" It must be recognized that spiritual pain, like physical pain, may change in intensity over time, and that the time of dying may raise spiritual issues, but not necessarily spiritual pain (O'Connor, 1993). Nurses should also listen to not only verbal, but also nonverbal messages that may indicate the patient's feelings, needs, or spiritual pain. In some circumstances, spiritual pain can be eased, yet in other circumstances, spiritual pain may be viewed by patients as a way to salvation, making them more worthy of heaven or the afterlife, or as a way of coming closer to God.

In taking a spiritual history, Puchalski (1998b) suggests that the acronym FICA be used: "F" standing for faith or beliefs; "I" referring to the importance and influence of spirituality or religiosity in one's life; "C" signifying participation in a spiritual or religious community; and "A" asking if they would like the health professional to address spiritual issues. Specific questions in the spiritual history may therefore include:

F: Faith: What is your faith or belief? Do you consider yourself spiritual or religious? Does religious faith or spirituality play an important part in your life? What things give you meaning in life?

I: Influence: How does your religious faith or spirituality influence the way you think about health or the way that you take care of yourself?

C: Community: Are you a part of a spiritual or religious community or congregation? Is this of support to you?

A: Address: Would you like me to address any religious or spiritual issues and concerns with you? (Puchalski, 1998b).

SPIRITUAL INTERVENTIONS AND CARE

Nurses can alleviate spiritual distress by inquiring about religious beliefs and practices, encouraging such religious practices, traditions, and rituals, praying with or for the patient, providing spiritual support, or referring the patient to the clergy or chaplain. In the past, nurses often called exclusively on clergy to facilitate resolution of spiritual issues and crises, however, the emerging focus on holistic care has reinforced the role of nurses as providers of spiritual care (O'Neill & Kenny, 1998). However, collaborative relationship with the clergy, as members of the interdisciplinary team, can provide the best possible support for patients experiencing spiritual distress and lead to the development of a spiritual plan of care to help them cope with whatever is happening in their lives. Direct spiritual care may involve crisis intervention, pastoral visitation, group facilitation, prayer and worship, ministry to families, ministry to staff, and ethical consultations (Driscoll, 1999). Ongoing spiritual care, across health care settings, may involve pastoral counseling/therapy, spiritual direction, parish or congregational connection, and linkages with community resources.

In providing spiritual care, all practitioners, be they health care practitioners or spiritual care practitioners, can provide a listening presence and assist people in articulating their spirituality in either religious or nonreligious language. Health professionals must not assume that since a patient expresses a religious affiliation, that spiritual care is being given. Active listening and presence should therefore be spiritual interventions for all patients. Patients should be encouraged to tell their life stories, with the possibilities of recognizing the meaning and purpose of their lives. Spiritual care may also involve empowering people to draw upon their strengths to overcome feelings of isolation and loneliness, and a sense of pain, suffering, and powerlessness. Matthews (1999) suggests that nurses can connect spiritually with patients by getting on the "WEB" which means:

W: *Welcome* by demonstrating acceptance that "you're welcome here" and providing reassurance and concern regardless of faith background or for those without a particular faith. It also involves inviting the patient to discuss important issues of faith and belief as exemplified by such statements as "Please feel free to talk about whatever is of most importance to you or of concern to you, including matters of faith."

E: *Encouragement* reinforces to persons of faith the value of continuing healthy religious beliefs and practices. A nurse may say, "I see that you joined the prayer group. I've noticed that patients who participate in these groups often feel less isolated and more at peace." Encouragement of others to consider spiritual practices can be discussed within the context of the scientific literature, which shows the benefits of spiritual and religious practices in promoting well-being and quality of life. The nurse may say, "Many studies now show the benefits of spiritual practices. Would this be something you would like to pursue." If a patient expresses a wish to pray, the nurse may offer to pray with or for the patient.

B: *Blessings* refer to the expression of blessings in a faith-sensitive manner. The nurse may say "Blessings to you," "God bless you," or "Shalom."

To anoint patients with peace, nurses can also give the gift of music as they sing a gentle, loving song to their patients. As part of deathbed healing, music thanatologists play the harp, which is a contemplative practice, and the medicine of attunement. Music at the end of life can alleviate pain and suffering. The rhythm of the music mirrors the natural rhythms of the patient's body, their breathing or heart rate, allowing the person to unbind from their physical body. Music offered by others is another form of physical and spiritual presence, which supports the dying person as they begin their journey (Schroeder-Sheker, 1999).

EDUCATING NURSES AND PHYSICIANS REGARDING SPIRITUALITY

Puchalski and Larson (1998) have identified key components to educating nurses and physicians regarding spirituality. They include:

- Demonstrating the completion of a spiritual history/assessment as part of the routine history;
- Role playing as a way of learning to discuss spiritual/religious beliefs and values in a respectful, nonjudgmental way;
- Critiquing the research regarding the role of spirituality in health care;
- Discussing illustrative cases where patient's beliefs negatively affected their health and potential spiritual interventions;
- Discussing the role of clergy as members of the interdisciplinary team in palliative care; and
- Conducting a value clarification exercise for students to identify their own spiritual values.
- Role play compassionate and effective communication regarding spiritual issues and needs of patients from diverse cultures; or role play conducting values clarification with patients and family members.
- Review religious traditions and aspects that may affect health care choices.

LIFE AND DEATH ACROSS CULTURES

There is increasing cultural diversity within American society, which challenges nurses and other health professionals to look through different eyes in providing holistic care (Showalter, 1998). "Culture is defined as a way of life. While culture is often identified with ethnicity, it's a far broader concept which encompasses spirituality and class" (Doka & Davidson, 1998, p. 4). Although there may be many cultural similarities and universal aspects to life, family, love, hope, funeral customs, grieving, and caring, cultural diversity exists. Such diversity refers to differences between people based on treasured beliefs, shared teachings, norms, customs, language and meaning that influence the individuals and families response to illness, treatment, death, and bereavement (Showalter, 1998).

Members of the palliative care team bring their own cultural perspectives and life experiences to the caregiving setting. Hospice/palliative care nurses must be culturally sensitive and responsive, providing care in a culturally appropriate manner. Although nurses and other health professionals acknowledge death as a common human experience, there is often a failure to recognize that loss, grief, death, and bereavement occur within a cultural context. Across cultures, people differ in their beliefs and attitudes about life, illness, and death; in what they feel; what evokes emotions; the implications of those feelings; and the ways of expressing and dealing with emotions (Rosenblatt, 1993). With such acknowledgment comes the opportunity to support the bereaved and channel the grief through specific cultural rituals.

With a broad understanding of the meaning and function of cultural beliefs and practices, nurses are able to provide appropriate and culturally sensitive interventions to support patients and families in times of loss and transition. Ethnic and cultural differences are often influential in "the methods of coping with life-threatening illness, the perception of pain, the support of the dying, the behavioral manifestations of grief, mourning styles, and funeral customs" (DeSpelder & Strickland, 1999, p. 108). Various cultures have different beliefs about dying and the relationship of the deceased with their loved ones. Many cultures maintain a strong bond between the living and the dead, who are the voice of the ancestors. Most cultures do not shun their dead, but honor them and hold ceremonies to celebrate their life. In some cultures, the dead performs services for the living as interpreters and intermediaries. Dependent on the culture, calling the name of the dead may be avoided so as not to disturb the dead or may stem from a desire to minimize grief (DeSpelder & Strickland, 1999). However, in other cultures, names have special meaning and value in honoring the deceased.

In some cultures, there is a circular pattern of life and death with multiple deaths and rebirths. For Native Americans and some sects of Buddhism, in death there is a parallel world where the dead can affect the lives of the living. In many cultures, there is ancestor worship where the deceased communicate with the family through daily rituals. However, in some cultures there is an abrupt and final disengagement with the deceased with sanctions against speaking the deceased's name which may keep them from moving to the land of the dead, and maintain their ghostly presence on earth (Kagawa-Singer, 1998). In the majority of cultures, funeral rites help ensure the successful journey of the soul into the realm of the dead, and are of benefit to the living.

CULTURAL PERSPECTIVES REGARDING ILLNESS AND DEATH

NATIVE AMERICAN PERSPECTIVES

For Native Americans, death is viewed as a part of a natural process. Time is not considered linear but a recurring cycle. Native Americans are mainly interested in how this cycle affects people in this life and only have a vague notion of another existence after death. A death song is sung which represents the summary of a person's life and acknowledgment of death. The dead are considered guardian spirits. After death, the spirit lingers near the site of the death for several days. Native Americans use a funeral pyre and adorn the corpse with flowers, feathers, and skins. For 6 months to a year, the name of the deceased is not called to confirm their separation from the living. In the Cocopa tribe, violent grief is expressed until cremation when they invite the spirits to join them in celebration. In the Hopi tribe, death is kept at a distance because it threatens order and control. The expression of grief remains limited and funerals are attended by few and held privately. For Native Americans, hallucinations, in which they see and converse with the dead, are regarded as a part of mourning (DeSpelder & Strickland, 1999).

AFRICAN AND AFRICAN AMERICAN PERSPECTIVES

Within the African culture, death is integrated into the totality of life. Ancestor worship involves the communion with the living dead through memories and the deceased are remembered by name. When the deceased are no longer remembered by people alive, they becomes part of the anonymous dead, but by this time their spirit has been reborn in a new child. Within the African community, death elicits a response from all members. Funeral ceremonies serve three purposes: 1) to separate the dead from the bereaved family; 2) as an opportunity to redistribute the roles of the deceased to living persons, and 3) acknowledgement that the dead joins the ancestors and the living return to the community in a way that reflects their changed status.

African Americans have their own perspectives given the oppression of slavery. The focus during the time of slavery was on a better life after death and many African Americans converted to Christianity. Slavery and racism had impact on the way suffering was perceived when compared to the white majority. Common themes of justice and respect have reinforced the importance of self-determination. Undesired deaths from cancer, AIDS, suicide, and violence are higher in African American communities than in general society. Given that African Americans do not benefit from modern medical technology to the same degree as the White population, they have a lower life expectancy and higher death rate. This has created a distrust of the medical system and a lack of interest of African Americans in Hospice care (DeSpelder & Strickland, 1999). There is also a low rate of organ donations after death.

For African Americans, the church has been important in maintaining their spirit, and Black preachers are viewed as the shepherds of their flock. There is a strong belief in family and the valuing of each other as brothers and sisters which is a source of mutual aid and support. Family is therefore central to the care of the terminally ill. Patients rely on family, friends, church associates, and neighbors for support. Black families have a more adoptive, absorptive sense of community with an unfavorable response to outside help. Given a strong sense of family loyalty, they are reluctant to hospitalize family members and prefer keeping the ill person at home (DeSpelder & Strickland, 1999).

African Americans regard funerals as important and the number of people who attend the funeral and the appearance of the casket reflect the value of the deceased. In the African American culture, the deceased is touched, but not kissed, and families are unlikely to visit the grave. Visits from family and friends are important to the bereaved with a strong expression of emotion and unrestrained grief (DeSpelder & Strickland, 1999).

HISPANIC PERSPECTIVES: MEXICAN AND PUERTO RICAN

Within the Mexican culture, it is believed that the dying should be protected from knowing their prognosis, as death is viewed as an adversity. Puerto Rican women show extreme grief or hysteria, while men show little or no grief. Death is often confronted with a humorous sarcasm and is viewed as an equalizer (DeSpelder & Strickland, 1999). Mexican Americans are likely to call the priest for the sacrament of the sick, and the bereaved may take shifts being with the deceased person. There is strong support of family as a unit. The funeral is the single most important family ceremony, and goes on for several days, as there is the belief that it takes time to grieve. Individuals are prohibited from speaking ill of the person who died and the bereaved visit the grave frequently. The day of the dead is celebrated in November and coincides with All Saint's Day, the feast of the commemoration of the dead. It is a time of celebration with special foods, music, and the decoration of graves. It is believed that the dead return to the world of the living for this special celebration, and families are scorned if they neglect their responsibilities. The bereaved are discouraged against crying too many tears, as excessive grief may make the pathway traveled on by the dead slippery, and burden them in the journey (DeSpelder & Strickland, 1999).

ASIAN PERSPECTIVES

In Asian cultures, there is great respect for the ancestors, as they are part of the biological and social past. Funeral and memorial rituals transform the ancestors into sources of blessings for the living (DeSpelder & Strickland, 1999). The dead share joys of the achievements of the living and may be given credit for the success. In the Japanese culture, there are strict funeral rituals and the family is not likely to touch the deceased's body. Ancestors are venerated by installing an ancestral shrine in the home called a budsudan or household alter. On the 49th day after death, the deceased is transformed into a benevolent ancestor after having the spirit linger in the home during this time. The rituals of the first 49 days accomplish what Western society would call grief work (Klass & Goss, 1998). The body is cremated and ashes and bones are put in an urn and buried in the family grave (haka) following a funeral service. Buddhist scripture is read and the deceased is given a Buddhist name indicating that the material aspect of the individual is gone. The name (kaimyo) is inscribed in the budsudan. Memorial ceremonies are held on the 100th day after death, first and third anniversary, and at fixed intervals thereafter. The O-bon marks the annual celebration of the return of the ancestral spirits to their families. Japanese attitudes and practices support the idea that survivors seldom sever their bonds with deceased loved ones, but rather the inner representations of the dead continue to have an active role in the bereaved's ongoing life (Klass & Goss, 1998).

Chinese Americans blend the traditions of Confucianism and Taoism. Confucianism emphasizes the value of familial relationships of parents and their children and living life according to strong ethical principles. Taoism stresses the balance of yin (female energies) and yang (male energies) and the relationship with the five elements of earth, water, wood, fire, and metal to achieve immortality (Klass & Goss, 1998). The Chinese culture believes that the most important obligation in life is to bury the dead and honor the ancestors with religious rites. Chinese Americans hold funerals in funeral homes and the women are more demonstrative in their grieving (Klass & Goss, 1998). Mourners pick up wrapped candy as they leave the funeral, which wards off bad luck for those who have come in close proximity to the dead. White clothes are often worn, however bright colored clothes are worn to celebrate the life of the elderly. Most Chinese Americans practice burial rather than cremation. The procession back from the grave symbolizes the movement of the bereaved back to life without the deceased. After the funeral, all mourners attend a banquet feast. Post-funeral ceremonies continue 3 days after death when the family burns paper money and leaves food at the gravesite. These rituals occur again on the 21st, 35th, and 49th days after the death, which reinforces the bond between the living and the dead ancestors.

CULTURAL VALUES UNDERLYING ADVANCE DIRECTIVES AND MEDICAL DECISION MAKING AT THE END OF LIFE

As a nation primarily of immigrants, nurses and other health care providers must be able to respond to the cultural diversity of their patients to avoid misunderstanding and miscommunication. When working with culturally diverse groups, conflicts can arise when health professionals automatically apply European American cultural concepts, inherent in the use of advance directives, to other sociocultural groups. The interrelated values that underlie end of life decision making and the use of advance directives include patient autonomy, informed decision making, truth telling, and control over the dying process. Autonomy infers that a patient has the inherent right to make treatment decisions and to be an active participant in their care; informed decision making requires patient access to all information regarding their diagnosis, prognosis, and treatment options; truth telling involves open and honest discussions of all information; and control over their own life and death involves respecting patient's decisions regarding how to lead their lives and how they plan for their own deaths (Ersek et al., 1998).

In a review of the literature regarding multicultural considerations in the use of advance directives, Ersek et al. (1998) reported that in many non–European American cultures, interdependence among family and community members is valued more than autonomy, particularly with respect to decision making. The family is therefore the smallest unit of identity and decision making. Families plan, manage, and participate in all aspects of patient care as a basic duty. In many non-European American cultures full disclosure and truth telling is prohibited because the information is believed to burden and harm the individual. Family members therefore receive the threatening information and the family protects the patients from emotional distress, allowing the patient to maintain some hope. Other cultures view full disclosure of information as disrespectful and rude. For non-European American cultures, controlling of life and death is unnatural and inappropriate; the belief is that death is a part of the life cycle and natural. The social and political history of the people may also influence their sense of trust or mistrust of the health care system and issues of power, as well as influencing decision making. For example, given their history of discrimination, African Americans are reluctant to prepare advance directives fearing that they will be denied access to desired care at the end of life.

RESEARCH REGARDING CULTURE AND END OF LIFE ISSUES

Based on a study of 800 older individuals from four ethnic groups, specifically European Americans, African Americans, Korean Americans, and Mexican Americans, Blackhall, Murphy, Frank, Michel, and Azen (1995) examined the relationship between ethnicity and attitudes toward patient autonomy. The finding indicated that Korean Americans and Mexican Americans were significantly less likely than European Americans and African Americans to believe that a patient should be told their diagnosis of metastatic cancer and were less likely to believe that the patient should make decisions about the use of life-supporting technology. Korean and Mexican Americans believe that the family should make the decisions to use life support, holding a family centered model of decision making rather than a patient autonomy model favored by European Americans and African Americans.

With regard to attitudes toward life-sustaining treatments, Caralis, Davis, Wright, and Marcial (1993) found that non-Hispanic whites were more likely to agree to withhold life-sustaining treatments in various clinical scenarios than were Hispanics and African Americans. Klessig (1992) found that European Americans were also less likely to start life support under hopeless and terminal conditions than African Americans, Chinese Americans, Filipino Americans, Korean Americans, and Mexican Americans.

QUALITY NURSING CARE: ADDRESSING THE CULTURAL NEEDS OF PATIENTS AND THEIR FAMILIES

NURSES' CULTURAL SELF-AWARENESS AND DEVELOPMENT OF CULTURAL COMPETENCY

The key to accommodating cultural diversity is for nurses to understand their own values, beliefs, and customs related to the celebration of life, and coping with illness and death. Irish, Lundquist, and Nelsen (1993) suggest that health professionals assess the degree in which they are proactive in their attitudes and activities toward diversity by asking themselves the following questions:

- Have I actively sought information to enhance my own awareness and understanding of multicultural diversity?;
- Have I consciously pondered my own attitudes and behaviors as they either enhance or hinder my relationships with others?;
- Have I evaluated my use of terms or phrases that may be perceived by others as degrading or hurtful?;
- Have I suggested or initiated workshops or discussions about multicultural diversity?;
- Have I openly disagreed with racial, cultural, or religious jokes, comments, or slurs?;
- Have I utilized in my work setting appropriate occasions to discuss the multicultural climate in the organizations with my colleagues and with institutional administration?; and
- Have I complained to the author when I see a broadcast, advertisement, or newspaper article that is racially, culturally, or religiously biased? (p. 45).

Furthermore, DeSpelder (1998) suggests that health care professionals develop end of life cultural competence, when they reflect on their own attitudes, beliefs, and practices toward dying and death. Nurses may explore for themselves:

- Their own beliefs about death and what influenced these attitudes;
- How significant religion is in their attitudes toward death;
- What kind of death would they prefer;
- If diagnosed with a terminal illness, who would they want to tell;
- What efforts should be made to keep a seriously ill person alive;
- How would they want their body to be disposed; and
- What is their experience of participating in rituals to remember the dead?

By awareness of one's own feelings, attitudes, preferences and biases, nurses can be more in-touch with themselves, acknowledging their right to their own beliefs, but not allowing those values and beliefs to take precedence over those expressed by patients and families. For nurses to effectively care for patients from diverse cultural groups, nurses must also be willing to learn about the cultures of their patients and presuppositions. The first step is to find educational sources that provide information about the various cultures, yet recognizing that there are individual differences even among individuals of the same culture because of differences in social stratum, personal experiences with illness and death, and individual preferences and values. By asking someone of a particular culture to help them understand the taboos and meanings of experiences and events, nurses can actively learn about other cultures. Nurses must also recognize that losses have different meanings from person to person and culture to culture and that losses may be viewed as major or minor.

CULTURAL ASSESSMENT AND INTERVENTIONS

Developing cultural competency also requires that nurses listen carefully and gather cultural information. The patient's background may provide clues about a person's beliefs; however, these are only assumptions unless validated by asking the patient about their beliefs, needs, expectations, and wishes. Knowledge about a person's cultural group should serve only as a starting point or guideline in assessing individual beliefs and behaviors (Kagawa-Singer, 1998; Lipson, Dibble, & Minarik, 1996). In an attempt to assess patient and family attitudes and values, Ersek et al. (1998) suggest that several areas be addressed:

- Assess the language used by patients and families in discussing illness and disease, including the extent of openness about diagnosis, prognosis, and treatments;
- Determine who is making the decisions, such as the individual patient, the family, or another social unit;
- Consider gender and power issues within relationships and with regard to decision making;
- Solicit the patient's and family's views about the appropriate timing and location of death;
- Assess the degree of fatalism or activism in accepting or controlling care and death;
- Assess religious/spiritual beliefs and practices, while focusing on the meaning of illness, suffering, and death, and belief in an afterlife;
- Assess how hope is maintained by the patient and family and how hope is culturally maintained;
- Consider sociopolitical and historical factors that influence beliefs about health, health care, and death; and
- Solicit information about sources of support within the community.

In providing culturally sensitive care, DeSpelder (1998) also suggests that health professionals listen for and mirror the language patterns based on an individual's culture. Small differences in language, such as saying passed away or passed on can indicate much about the speaker's experience. For example, passed away may describe the deceased from the survivor's perspective, while passed on may imply a belief in a life after death. Nurses can also attend to the cultural needs of their patients by gathering information about distinctive rituals, practices, and beliefs, particularly an understanding of what is meaningful to the individual person. This assessment involves listening, observing, and asking about unfamiliar practices of patients and families. Furthermore, nurses can determine the strengths an individual draws on when encountering death, dying, or bereavement, such as internal resources provided by the individual's belief system or past experiences, and external resources, such as the comfort provided by cultural customs (DeSpelder & Strickland, 1999).

As nurses interact with patients and families from diverse cultures, they have the experiential opportunity to learn about cultural values, expectations, and needs regarding illness, dying, and death. In caring for patients and families at the end of life, nurses can enhance the quality of life and quality of dying by promoting a respectful and peaceful death through the recognition of their spiritual and cultural needs.

THE NURSES' NEED FOR SELF-REFLECTION AND SELF-HEALING IN PALLIATIVE CARE

Doka and Morgan (1993) describe the caregivers' assumptions and principles of spiritual care. First, nurses represent diverse spiritual or cultural backgrounds and like patients, have the right to expect respect for their belief systems. Second, nurses should be offered opportunities to explore their own values and attitudes about life and death, and their meaning and purpose in life. Third, nurses should be aware that they have the potential for providing spiritual care, and should be encouraged to offer spiritual care to dying patients and their families, as needed. Fourth, nurses, as all caregivers, should be flexible and realistic in setting spiritual goals. Fifth, ongoing care of the dying and bereaved may cause a severe drain of energy and uncover old and new spiritual issues for the caregiver. Spiritual growth and renewal is, therefore, a necessary part of staff support, and a personal priority for each caregiver.

Indeed, in caring for dying patients and bereaved families, nurses may have experiences that create a grief response of their own because they have lost someone in whom they have invested themselves emotionally. Nurses' grief response, like their patients, will be influenced by their spiritual and cultural values and beliefs. If accumulated grief is not worked through, the nurse is vulnerable to all manifestations of unresolved grief as is any other individual who has had a loss, but failed to complete the grief work (Rando, 1984). Nurses, therefore, need to resolve their own feelings of loss, with their spiritual convictions supported, sense of failure alleviated, and emotional strength replenished (Rando, 1984).

In coping with the stress of caring for the dying, Rando (1984) believes that nurses progress through five stages: 1) focusing on professional knowledge and factual information; 2) experiencing the trauma of the patient's illness, often accompanied by guilt and frustration as they confront their patient's impending death; 3) moving through the pain and coming to an acceptance of the reality of death; 4) identifying the pain and suffering with sensitivity, but freeing themselves from the incapacitating effects; and 5) relating compassionately with the dying person in full acceptance of impending death. In caring for patients in palliative care, nurses must develop an awareness of their own emotional, physical, or spiritual limits, and develop an awareness of their own energy levels. By realizing the need for self-care, acknowledging their own feelings about dying and death, and the stresses in caring for the dying that are most troublesome to them individually, nurses can prevent caregiver burnout (Rando, 1984).

In developing such an awareness and supporting nurses' spiritual well-being, nurse educators may ask their students or nursing colleagues the following questions:

- What expectations do you have about yourself in caring for the dying and bereaved?
- What would define success in your work?
- What are the three most difficult aspects of your work in caring for patients with life-threatening illness?
- What are you doing to help yourself cope with stress, and replenish yourself to avoid becoming overstressed?

Within the context of end of life care, and given that spirituality has emerged as a vital component of health, it becomes necessary for nurses to acknowledge their own spiritual beliefs and values, and to deal with their own spiritual issues. In caring for people at the end of life, nurses must remain in tune with their own spiritual needs, healing thyself as well as others. To do so, Halifax (1999) suggests a contemplative exercise for nurses to remain centered, renewed, and whole as they care for others. Sitting in a relaxed position, with eyes closed and aware of the rhythm of your breath, the nurse focuses on the following five phrases, which are slowly repeated twice. The nurse then allows the phrase to pass into the background of her/his awareness, moving attention to the breath and to the next phrase. The phrases are as follows:

- May I offer my care and presence unconditionally, knowing that it may be met with gratitude, indifference, anger, or anguish;

- May I offer love knowing that I cannot control the course of life's suffering or death;
- May I remain in ease and let go of my expectations;
- May I view my own suffering with compassion just as I do the suffering of others;
- May I be aware that my suffering does not limit my good heart;
- May I forgive myself for things left undone;
- May I forgive all who have hurt me;
- May those whom I have hurt forgive me;
- May all beings and I live and die in peace.

Spiritually and culturally competent care, therefore, requires self-reflection and self-care of nurses. Replenishing one's own vessel in spiritually and culturally renewing ways is important in supporting nurses' caregiving potential. For only by doing so, will nurses come to the beside with the strong healing presence and true compassion needed to alleviate the suffering of patients and their families.

CONCLUSION

Illness and dying are occurrences that take us to the very core of our being. Although they are intensely personal experiences, they occur within the context of our spiritual and cultural traditions. Spirituality and culture can therefore not be separated from who we are, as they are often the very source of our nourishment and physical, emotional, social, and spiritual well-being. Through sensitive and competent spiritual and cultural care, nurses can protect patients and families from the ultimate tragedy of depersonalization. They will be able to sustain them in a personalized environment that recognizes their individual needs, reduces their fears, and offers them hope and dignity. Sulmasy (1997) believes that "when patients collapse spiritually in the face of illness, a clinician with the right perspective will understand much more acutely how desperate their plight really is and will treat the wounds of such patients with even more liberal applications of the wine of fervent zeal and the oil of compassion" (p. 52).

Education Plan 1.1 Plan for Achieving Competencies: Spiritually and Culturally Competent Palliative Care

Knowledge Needed	Attitude	Skills	Undergraduate Behavioral Outcomes	Graduate Behavioral Outcomes	Teaching/Learning Strategies
Spirituality and culture as factors that structure responses to life-threatening illness.	*Affirm nurses' commitment to holistic practice. *Emphasize the value of spirituality and culture in providing end of life care.	*Act in accordance with the patients' and families' spiritual and cultural values and wishes.	*Incorporate spiritual and cultural care in nursing practice.	*Role model and expect of others spiritually and culturally competent care for patients and families.	*Write a position paper about the role of spirituality and culture in providing nursing care.
The Spiritual Nature of the Person	*Value and support the spirituality of human beings. *Appreciate the needs of the dying to make peace with life and death.		*Provide spiritually competent care to patients and families experiencing life-threatening illness by considering spiritual well-being.	*Create an environment in which the spiritual nature of people is recognized, valued, and supported. *Assist patients and families to find a source of spiritual energy or reaffirm students'/nurses'/ nurses' spiritual focus.	*Based on the spiritual assessment of a particular patient and family, develop a spiritual plan of care. Review the plan of care clergy/ chaplain.

Education Plan 1.1 *(continued)*

Knowledge Needed	Attitude	Skills	Undergraduate Behavioral Outcomes	Graduate Behavioral Outcomes	Teaching/Learning Strategies
Suffering as a Human Condition —Reciprocal suffering of patients and family; —Care of those who are suffering.	*Acknowledge suffering as a multidimensional experience. *Recognize that suffering may be personal or experienced as witnessed to another's suffering. *Appreciate that suffering and pain are not identical. *Consider the effect of suffering on health and quality of life of patients, families, and health care providers.	*Demonstrate therapeutic use of self in alleviating suffering.	*Assist patients and family to identify the meaning of suffering and refer to members of other disciplines as appropriate.	*Assess the impact of suffering on patient, family, health care providers, and community. *Implement the role of nurse as a coach in caring for those who are suffering. *Support patients and family in achieving some transcendent meaning to their suffering.	*Based on a case study, identify the dimensions of suffering and nursing strategies to alleviate suffering.

Education Plan 1.1 *(continued)*

Knowledge Needed	Attitude	Skills	Undergraduate Behavioral Outcomes	Graduate Behavioral Outcomes	Teaching/Learning Strategies
Spiritual and religious perspectives of death: —Jewish —Roman Catholic —Protestant —Eastern —No conventional religious beliefs —Research regarding spirituality	*Appreciate varying spiritual and religious perspectives of death. *Value research in informing spiritual care.	*Demonstrate sensitivity to spiritual and religious beliefs and customs.	*Develop a plan of care with the patient and family that addresses their spiritual and religious perspectives on death and associated needs. *Critique and utilize research in guiding spiritual caregiving.	*Address conflicts that result from differences in spiritual and religious perspectives on death of patients, families, and health care providers. *Participate in conducting research regarding spirituality and health-related outcomes.	*Role play as a way of learning about different spiritual/religious beliefs and values in a nonjudgmental way. Self-critique attitudes and interaction followed by feedback from faculty and peers. *Critique five research articles related to spiritual or religious beliefs and health care issues. Synthesize the findings and discuss the implications for nursing practice.

Education Plan 1.1 *(continued)*

Knowledge Needed	Attitude	Skills	Undergraduate Behavioral Outcomes	Graduate Behavioral Outcomes	Teaching/Learning Strategies
					*Distribute 3 × 5 cards and ask the students what happens at the time of death on side one and how that belief serves them on side two of the card. Ask the students to pass the card to another student. They are to take on the belief of the other student as their own. They are now asked how this new belief may benefit them.

Education Plan 1.1 *(continued)*

Knowledge Needed	Attitude	Skills	Undergraduate Behavioral Outcomes	Graduate Behavioral Outcomes	Teaching/Learning Strategies
Quality Nursing Care: Addressing Spiritual Needs of Patients and Families: —Spiritual caregiving —Spiritual assessment —Spiritual interventions and care —Educating nurses and physicians regarding spirituality.	*Recognize students'/nurses' own spiritual and religious beliefs and values. *Value nurses' presence, compassion, and hopefulness in providing quality spiritual care. *Appreciate the role of chaplains and clergy in offering spiritual care.	*Convey unconditional acceptance of patients and families of diverse spiritual and religious beliefs and backgrounds. *Demonstrate the completion of a spiritual history/assessment.	*Create an environment that nurtures the patient's exploration of spiritual needs and concerns. *Address patients' and families' spiritual and religious needs through presencing, active listening, unconditional regard, and support of meaningful rituals.	*Identify patients and family who are at risk for spiritual distress. *Develop a comprehensive plan of care to alleviate spiritual suffering. *Educate other health care in providing spiritually competent care.	*Write a position statement identifying students'/nurses' personal beliefs and assumptions as it relates to spirituality or religiosity. *Conduct a values clarification exercise for students/nurses to identify their own spiritual values. *Discuss the role of clergy as members of the interdisciplinary team in post-conference or seminar. *Discuss illustrative cases where patient's spirituality or religiosity negatively affected their health outcomes and potential spiritual interventions.

Education Plan 1.1 *(continued)*

Knowledge Needed	Attitude	Skills	Undergraduate Behavioral Outcomes	Graduate Behavioral Outcomes	Teaching/Learning Strategies
Cultural Perspectives Regarding Illness and Death: —Native American; —African and African American; —Hispanic; —Asian; —Cultural values underlying advanced directives and medical decision making; —Research regarding culture and end of life issues.	*Appreciate varying cultural perspectives of death. *Value research in informing cultural care.	*Demonstrate sensitivity to cultural beliefs and customs.	*Develop a plan of care with the patient and family that addresses their cultural perspectives on death and cultural needs. *Critique and utilize research in guiding culturally competent care.	*Address conflicts that result from differences in cultural perspectives on death of patients, families, and health care providers. *Participate in conducting research regarding culture and health-related outcomes.	*Have students interview two individuals of diverse cultural backgrounds and compare beliefs, values, expectations and traditions related to illness and death. Compare the information obtained from information written in textbooks or journal articles. Share findings in class. *Critique five research articles related to cultural beliefs and health care issues. Synthesize the findings and discuss the implications for nursing practice.

39

Education Plan 1.1 *(continued)*

Knowledge Needed	Attitude	Skills	Undergraduate Behavioral Outcomes	Graduate Behavioral Outcomes	Teaching/Learning Strategies
Quality Nursing Care: Addressing the Cultural Needs of Patients and their Families —Nurses' Cultural Self-Awareness and Development of Cultural Competency —Cultural Assessment and Interventions.	*Recognize students'/nurses' own cultural beliefs and values.	*Convey unconditional acceptance of patients and families of various cultural backgrounds. *Demonstrate the completion of a cultural assessment.	*Create an environment which supports cultural beliefs, values, traditions, and rituals.	*Develop a comprehensive plan of care which takes into account cultural values, needs, and expectation. *Educate other health care providers in providing culturally competent care.	*In post-conference or seminar, encourage students to express feelings of appreciation regarding their own cultural heritage while introducing the topic of ethnocentrism in connection with the value of cultural diversity. *Have students identify who was significant in teaching or transmitting to them their cultural identity and discuss the impact of their identity on their present life. *Have students identify how members of their cultural group approach personal or emotional problems.

Education Plan 1.1 *(continued)*

Knowledge Needed	Attitude	Skills	Undergraduate Behavioral Outcomes	Graduate Behavioral Outcomes	Teaching/Learning Strategies
					*In the clinical setting, conduct a cultural assessment of a patient/family and report findings in post-conference or seminar. *In post-conference or seminar, create and discuss a list of behaviors or comments which may be viewed as culturally insensitive based on past, personal, or professional experiences. *Role play compassionate and effective communication regarding cultural issues relevant to palliative care.

Education Plan 1.1 *(continued)*

Knowledge Needed	Attitude	Skills	Undergraduate Behavioral Outcomes	Graduate Behavioral Outcomes	Teaching/Learning Strategies
Nurses' Needs for Self-Reflection and Self-Healing in Palliative Care.	*Affirm nurses' right to be respected for their belief systems. *Acknowledge students'/nurses' personal potential for providing spiritual and cultural care. *Appreciate the potential drain of energy and resurfacing of personal spiritual issues related to caregiving.		*Develop an awareness of students'/nurses' own spiritual, emotional, and physical limits. *Establish a personal plan of care for maintaining health and promoting personal and professional growth.	*Assess colleagues at risk for caregiving burnout. *Advocate for systems that support student's/nurses' self-care and personal and professional growth.	*Write a personal plan of care to address the students'/nurses' physical, emotional, social, and spiritual needs, and strategies to promote personal and professional growth within the next 6 months. *Create a suggestion box and contribute one recommended change, which would support the nurses' caregiving potential within the educational setting.

Education Plan 1.1 *(continued)*

Knowledge Needed	Attitude	Skills	Undergraduate Behavioral Outcomes	Graduate Behavioral Outcomes	Teaching/Learning Strategies
					*Discuss in the classroom, post-conference or seminar ways in which students/nurses have been able to provide spiritual care and the responses of the individual and family. *Beginning with a 5-minute relaxation exercise, have students/nurses write a poem asking a transcendent life force for support. Have each student/nurse read their poem, twice slowly.

REFERENCES

Arnold, E. (1989). Burnout as a spiritual issue: Rediscovering meaning in nursing practice. In V. Carson (Eds.), *Spiritual dimensions of nursing practice* (pp. 320–353). Philadelphia: W. B. Saunders Company.

Beeney, L., Butow, P., & Dunn, S. (1997). Normal adjustment to cancer: Characteristics and assessment. In R. K. Portenoy & E. Bruera (Eds.), *Topics in palliative care: Volume 1* (pp. 213–244). New York: Oxford University Press.

Bird, L. (1986). Suffering, thanatology, and whole-person medicine. In R. DeBellis, E. Marcus, A. Kutscher, C. Smith Torres, V. Barrett, & M. Siegel (Eds.), *Suffering: Psychological and social aspects in loss, grief, and care* (pp. 31–39). New York: Haworth Press.

Blackhall, L., Murphy, S., Frank, G., Michel, V., & Azen, S. (1995). Ethnicity and attitudes toward patient autonomy. *JAMA, 274*(10), 820–825.

Burkhardt, M. A. (1989). Spirituality: An analysis of the concept. *Holistic Nursing Practice, 3*(3), 69–75.

Caralis, P. V., Davis, B., Wright, K., & Marcial, E. (1993). The influence of ethnicity and race on attitudes towards advance directives, life-prolonging treatments, and euthanasia. *Journal of Clinical Ethics, 4*, 155–165.

Carson, V. B. (1989). *Spiritual dimensions of nursing practice.* Philadelphia: W. B. Saunders Company.

Cassell, E. (1982). The nature of suffering and the goals of medicine. *New England Journal of Medicine, 306*, 639–645.

Conrad, N. L. (1985). Spiritual support for the dying. *Nursing Clinics of North America, 20*(2), 415–425.

Corr, C., Nabe, C., & Corr, D. (1997). *Death and dying; life and living.* California: Brooks/Cole Publishing Company.

Cousins, N. (1979). *Anatomy of an illness.* New York: Norton.

Coyle, N. (1995). Suffering in the first person. In B. R. Fernell (Ed.), *Suffering.* Boston: Jones & Bartlett.

Davies, B., Reimer, J., & Marten, N. (1994). Family functioning and its implications for palliative care. *Journal of Palliative Care, 10*, 35–36.

DeBellis, R., Marcus, E., Kutscher, A., Smith Torres, C., Barrett, V., & Siegel, M. (1986). *Suffering: Psychological and social aspects in loss, grief, and care.* New York: The Haworth Press.

DeSpelder, L. (1998). Developing cultural competency. In K. Doka & J. Davidson (Eds.), *Living with grief* (pp. 97–106). Washington, DC: Hospice Foundation in America.

DeSpelder, L., & Strickland, A. (1999). *The last dance: Encountering death and dying.* California: Mayfield Publishing Company.

Doka, K. (1993). The spiritual needs of the dying. In K. Doka & J. Morgan (Eds.), *Death and spirituality* (pp. 143–150). Amityville, NY: Baywood Publishing Company.

Doka, K., & Davidson, J. (1998). *Living with grief.* Philadelphia, PA: Hospice Foundation of America.

Doka, K., & Morgan, J. (1993). *Death and spirituality.* Amityville, NY: Baywood Publishing Company.

Dombeck, M. B. (1995). Dream telling: A means of spiritual awareness. *Holistic Nursing Practice, 9*(2), 37–47.

Doyle, D. (1994). *Caring for a dying relative: A guide for families.* New York: Oxford University Press.

Driscoll, J. (1999). *Chaplain-physician partnerships.* Paper presented at the Harvard University, Spirituality and Healing Conference, Denver, Colorado.

Ersek, M., Kagawa-Singer, M., Barnes, D., Blackhall, L., & Koenig, B. (1998). Multicultural considerations in the use of advance directives. *Oncology Nursing Forum, 25*(10), 1683–1689.

Ferris, F., & Cummings, I. (1995). *Palliative care: Towards a consensus in standardized principles of practice.* Ottawa, ON: Canadian Palliative Care Association.

Foley, K. (1995). Pain, physician-assisted suicide, and euthanasia. *Pain Forum, 4,* 163–176.

Fricchione, G. L. (1999). *Spirituality and healing at the bedside.* Paper presented at the Harvard University, Spirituality and Healing Conference, Denver, Colorado.

Gallop, G. (1990). *Religion in America.* Princeton, New Jersey: Princeton Religion and Research Center.

Gallop, G. (1997). *Spiritual beliefs and the dying process. A national survey conducted for the Nathan Cummings Foundation and the Fetzer Institute.* New York: The Nathan Cummings Foundation.

Grollman, E. (1993). Death in Jewish thought. In K. Doka & J. Morgan (Eds.), *Death and spirituality* (pp. 21–32). Amityville, NY: Baywood Publishing Company.

Halifax, J. (1999). *Being with dying: Contemplations on death and dying.* Presentation at the Art of Dying III Conference: Spiritual, Scientific and Practical Approaches to Living and Dying by the New York Open Center and Tibet House New York, New York.

Higginson, I. J. (1998). Introduction: Defining the unit of care: Who are we supporting and how? In E. Bruera & R. K. Portenoy (Eds.), *Topics in palliative care: Volume 2* (pp. 205–207). New York: Oxford University Press.

Irish, D., Lundquist, K., & Nelsen, V. (1993). *Ethnic variations in dying, death, and grief.* Philadelphia, PA: Taylor & Francis.

Kagawa-Singer, M. (1998). The cultural context of death rituals and mourning practices. *Oncology Nursing Forum, 25*(10), 1752–1756.

Kahn, D. L., & Steeves, R. (1996). An understanding of suffering grounded in clinical practice and research. In B. R. Ferrel (Eds.), *Suffering* (pp. 3–27). Sudbury, MA: Jones and Bartlett Publishers.

Kaldjian, L. C. (1998). End of life decisions in HIV-positive patients: The role of spiritual beliefs. *AIDS, 12*(1), 103–107.

Klass, D. (1993). Spirituality, Protestantism, and death. In K. Doka & J. Morgan (Eds.), *Death and spirituality* (pp. 51–73). Amityville, NY: Baywood Publishing Company.

Klass, D., & Goss, R. (1998). Asian ways of grief. In K. Doka & J. Davidson (Eds.), *Living with grief* (pp. 13–26). Philadelphia, PA: The Hospice Foundation.

Klein, S. J. (1998). *Heavenly hurts: Surviving AIDS-related deaths and losses.* New York: Baywood Publishing Company.

Klessig, J. (1992). The effects of values and culture on life support decisions. *Western Journal of Medicine, 163,* 316–322.

Koenig, H. G. (1998). Religious coping and health status in medically ill hospitalized older adults. *Journal of Nervous Mental Disease, 186*(9), 513–518.

Koenig, H. G. (1999). *The healing power of faith: When serious illness strikes.* Paper presented at the Harvard University, Spirituality and Healing Conference, Denver, Colorado.

Koenig, H. G., Cohen, H. J., Blazer, D., Pieper, C., Meador, K., Shelp, G., Goli, V., & DiPasquale, B. (1992). Religious coping and depression among hospitalized elderly medically ill men. *American Journal of Psychiatry, 149*(12), 1693–1700.

Lederberg, M. (1998). The family of the cancer patient. In J. Holland (Eds.), *Psychooncology* (pp. 981–993). New York: Oxford University Press.

Lipson, J., Dibble, S., & Minarik, P. A. (1996). *Culture and nursing care: A pocket guide.* St. Louis: Mosby.

Loscalzo, M., & Zabora, J. (1998). Care of the cancer patient: Response of family and staff. In E. Bruera & R. K. Portenoy (Eds.), *Topics in palliative care: Volume 2* (pp. 209–246). New York: Oxford University Press.

Macrae, J. (1999). *Nursing with emphasis on Florence Nightingale.* Paper presented at the Harvard University, Spirituality and Healing Conference, Denver, Colorado.

Matthews, D. (1999). *The faith factor: Is religion good for your health.* Paper presented at the Harvard University, Spirituality and Healing Conference, Denver, Colorado.

McGann, J. (1997). *Comfort my people: Finding peace as life ends.* Rockville Center, New York: The Long Island Catholic.

McGreggor, B. (1999). *Spirituality and healing in children.* Paper presented at the Harvard University, Spirituality and Healing Conference, Denver, Colorado.

Miller, E. (1993). A Roman Catholic view of death. In K. Doka & J. Morgan (Eds.), *Death and spirituality* (pp. 33–49). Amityville, NY: Baywood Publishing Company.

Moberg, D. O. (1984). Subjective measures for spiritual well-being. *Review of Religious Research, 25*(4), 351–364.

Moore, T. (1992). *Care of the soul: A guide for cultivating depth and sacredness in everyday life.* New York: Harper-Collins.

Munley, A. (1983). *The hospice alternative.* New York: Basic Books.

Nathan Cummings Foundation. (1999). Spiritual beliefs and the dying process: Key findings. [Online: http://www.ncf.org/ncf/publications/reports/fetzer/fetzer_keyfindings.html]

O'Connor, P. (1993). A clinical paradigm for exploring spiritual concerns. In K. Doka & J. Morgan (Eds.), *Death and spirituality* (pp. 133–150). Amityville, NY: Baywood Publishing Company.

O'Neill, D., & Kenny, E. (1998). Spirituality and chronic illness. *Image: Journal of Nursing Scholarship, 30*(3), 275–279.

Orion, P. (1993). Spiritual issues in death and dying for those who do not have conventional religious beliefs. In K. Doka & J. Morgan (Eds.), *Death and spirituality* (pp. 93–112). Amityville, NY: Baywood Publishing Company.

Poloma, M. M., & Pendleton, B. F. (1989). Exploring types of prayer and quality of life. *Review of Religious Research, 31*(1), 46–53.

Puchalski, C. (1998a). Facing death with dignity. *The World and I, 3,* 34–39.

Puchalski, C. (1998b). FICA: A spiritual assessment. Unpublished manuscript.

Puchalski, C., & Larson, D. (1998). Developing curricula in spirituality and medicine. *Academic Medicine, 73*(9), 970–974.

Rando, T. (1984). *Grief, dying, and death: Clinical interventions for caregivers.* Illinois: Research Press Company.

Roberts, J. A. (1997). Coping with gynecologic cancer. *American Journal of Obstetrics and Gynecology, 176*(1), 166–172.

Rosenblatt, P. (1993). Cross-cultural variation in the experience, expression, and understanding of grief. In D. Irish, K. Lundquist, & V. Nelsen (Eds.), *Ethnic variations in dying, death and grief* (pp. 13–19). Philadelphia, PA: Taylor & Francis.

Ryan, D. (1993). Death: Eastern perspectives. In K. Doka & J. Morgan (Eds.), *Death and spirituality* (pp. 75–92). Amityville, NY: Baywood Publishing Company.

Ryan, S. (1997). Chaplains are more than what chaplains do. *Visions, 7,* 8–9.

Schroeder-Sheker, T. (1999). *I die awake: The luminous wound.* Presentation at the Art of Dying III Conference: Spiritual, Scientific and Practical Approaches to Living and Dying by the New York Open Center and Tibet House New York, New York.

Sherman, D. W. (1998). Reciprocal suffering: The need to improve family caregiver's quality of life through palliative care. *Journal of Palliative Medicine, 1*(4), 357–366.

Showalter, S. (1998). Looking through different eyes: Beyond cultural diversity. In K. Doka & J. Davidson (Eds.), *Living with grief* (pp. 71–82). Washington, DC: Hospice Foundation of America.

Smith, R. (1996). Theological perspectives. In B. R. Ferrel (Ed.), *Suffering* (pp. 159–171). Sudbury, MA: Jones and Bartlett Publishers.

Spross, J. (1996). Coaching and suffering: The role of the nurse in helping people face illness. In B. R. Ferrel (Ed.), *Suffering* (pp. 173–208). Sudbury, MA: Jones and Bartlett Publishers.

Sulmasy, D. (1997). *The healer's calling: A spirituality for physicians and other health care professionals.* New York: Paulist Press.

Thorson, J. A., & Powell, F. C. (1992). Meanings of death and intrinsic religiosity. *Journal of Clinical Psychology, 46*(4), 379–391.

Urdang, L. (1972). *The Random House college dictionary.* New York: Random House.

Watson, J. (1986). Suffering and the quest for meaning. In R. DeBellis, E. Marcus, A. Kutscher, C. Smith Torres, V. Barrett, & M. Siegel (Eds.), *Suffering: Psychological and social aspects in loss, grief, and care* (pp. 175–187). New York: Haworth Press.

Wink, P. (1999). Addressing end of life issues: Spirituality and inner life. *Generations, 23*(1), 75–80.

2

Holistic Integrative Therapies in Palliative Care

Carla Mariano

AACN Competency

#9: Evaluate the impact of traditional, complementary, and technological therapies on patient-centered outcomes.

> The greatest discovery of any generation is that human beings can alter their lives by altering the attitudes of their minds.
>
> —Albert Schweitzer

This chapter introduces the reader to a variety of Holistic Modalities used in nursing practice today. The modalities are defined and shown where they are most useful. In addition, this chapter includes a selection on exercises that can be readily used by nurses and incorporated into their practice. It also includes resources where more information on each of these modalities can be obtained. In the education of nurses, it is particularly important for nursing faculty to incorporate these healing modalities into the curriculum for both undergraduate and graduate level students.

Holism focuses on unity, mutuality, meaning, and the interrelationship of all beings, events, and things. The words heal and health comes from haelan, which means to be or become whole. Holism emphasizes the basic wholeness and integrity of the individual. It views the body, mind, and spirit as inseparable and interdependent. All behaviors, including health, illness, and dying are manifestations of the life process of the whole person (Quinn, 1985).

Holistic nursing care draws on nursing knowledge, theories, expertise, and intuition as nurses and clients become therapeutic partners in a shared evolving process toward healing. Holistic care—

- Believes that people can grow and learn from health, illness, and dying;
- Promotes clients' active participation in their own health care, wellness, and healing;
- Uses appropriate interventions in the context of the client's total needs;
- Works to alleviate clients' physical signs and symptoms; and
- Concentrates on the underlying meanings of symptoms and illness events, and changes in the clients' life patterns and perceptions (Mariano, 1998).

There are numerous modalities used in the provision of holistic care. Some of these, that are particularly useful in end-of-life care, are discussed in a subsequent section of this chapter. Nurses can practice holistic care in any setting where healing occurs.

"*Healing the dying* sounds like an oxymoron. . . . But to heal is not necessarily to cure. . . . To heal is to bring various levels of oneself—cellular, physical, intrapersonal, interpersonal, societal, spiritual, perhaps even cosmic—into new relationship with each other" (Olson, 1997a, p. 3). The nurse must assess the relationship of the individual who is dying with self, others, a higher power, and provide appropriate interventions to assist in the development or maintenance of new or right relationships.

"Dying *healed* means that a person has finished the business of life, said good-goodbyes, and reached life's goals. An individual knows who he is, and has a sense of integration of self and life" (Olson, 1997a, p. 3). S/he realizes that one's life was unique and one's death matters to someone. One looks inward and realizes that life's difficulties have created a certain wisdom. Significant others have had time to grieve and plan for changes, and comfort and peace are attained. Control of the dying process is maintained as long as possible by the individual and as much as possible as the person is willing. Dying is seen as a stage of life. It is part of a larger philosophy and perception in which both life and death have meaning.

As mentioned previously, healing the dying necessitates regard for relationships and connectedness. We speak of transcendence when implying a sense of connectedness between self and a greater reality. Transcendence "integrates self with past and future, giving meaning to life. It is a set of introspective activities that reflect concern for others or for meaning" (Olson, 1997b, p. 128). Many of the integrative modalities described in this chapter facilitate self-transcendence. As noted by Olson (1997b), positive outcomes for the self-transcendent person, even when nearing death, include less depression, neglect, and hopelessness: a greater sense of well-being and ability to cope with grief and death; and the ability to live and find meaning in the present and connect with a higher power.

This caring relationship emphasizes quality rather than length of life. Healing the dying includes palliative care, and focuses on relationships of all kinds. There is the provision for opportunities and choices where the dying client can live life to its fullest, and at some point comfortably forgive, let go, release, and experience a peaceful death.

The nurse is in a partnership with the dying client, sharing rather than denying the experience. The focus of nursing care is on providing sacred space and the milieu for a calm and peaceful death. The nurse works with the client to foster hope and cultivate an appreciation of the seemingly irrelevant things in life. Learning to appreciate simple occurrences such as a sunset or the joys of life can cultivate a more positive view of life and one's present experience. Enhancing avenues of support, be they professional, social (family and friends), and support groups can often facilitate grieving and increase a sense of meaning in illness. Developing unrecognized inner strengths and resources is of great importance to the person who is dying or grieving.

As the Chinese symbol for crisis indicates, crisis offers an opportunity for growth and a different perspective. Grief can serve as a building block for personal growth and healing. Asking the dying person about spiritual needs gives the client an occasion to verbalize unmet needs. All of this requires skill, knowledge, compassion, caring, and anticipation/organization on the part of the nurse, as well as a willingness to face one's own impermanence and mortality. It also necessitates caring for one's self.

SPECIFIC HOLISTIC HEALING MODALITIES

Holism is the theoretical and philosophical foundation for alternative/ complementary integrative healing modalities. There are numerous such modalities used in health care today. This chapter will cover only a few of those that are most useful in end of life care. Many of these modalities can be effectively used by both the nurse as well as the client, such as, centering, relaxation, imagery, meditation, and prayer. Others are described in use with clients, such as, sense therapies, reminiscence and life review, touch, and Reiki. In addition to their calming influence and physiological benefits, these techniques also may alter the perception of pain.

CENTERING

Centering is a process by which one quiets the mind and focuses one's thoughts. It calms the mind and allows the practitioner to access inmost resources that are powerful forces in healing. Krieger (1997) notes that "Being on-center does not mean being still, immobile, rigid. . . . In centering, we are quiet and 'listen' to another language. Our attention goes to the heart region, where we find our own center of peace and know it as an attribute of our true self. We find that this sense of deep serenity is reminiscent to the truer peace we find in untrammeled nature and, with a thrill of personal discovery, realize that it is through such profound natural experiences that we can be at-one with the universe" (p. 22). Centering is a shift in consciousness, an integrated sense of being. Bodily movements become quieted, and yet one is in an actively conscious state. There is a sense of inner equilibrium and well-being. Perception deepens and one is less aware of the chaos of the moment or day and the mind's chatter. Practice in the act of centering (closing eyes, quieting one's mind and activities, focusing on one's center or inner peace) leads to intuition and inner wisdom (Krieger, 1997).

By remaining on-center, the nurse is able to convey to the client an awareness, a sensitivity, an empathy and deep sense of peace and regard that often creates a relaxation response in the client. One must give oneself permission to center, as the environment is always calling us to be present for it rather than ourselves. But when one is centered and personally present, compassion becomes real and this state is needed for those who would heal. One important exercise that the nurse can practice is to center before entering into each client encounter—detaching from any prior encounter, to approach each client with awareness and with, as Carl Rogers states, "unconditional positive regard" (Laurant & Shlien, 1984).

RELAXATION

Relaxation is a state where there is an absence of physical, mental, and emotional tension. A pleasant sensation and the lack of stressful or uncomfortable thoughts also accompany it. It is often referred to as the opposite of the "fight or flight" response. "Relaxation makes it possible to quiet the body/mind and focus inward. One learns to retreat mentally from one's surroundings, still thoughts, relax muscles, and maintain the state of relaxation . . . to reap the benefits of decreased tension, anxiety, and pain. Regardless of the approach [use of meditation, yoga, muscle and breathing exercises, hypnosis, prayer, and other forms of stress management], the end result is a movement of the person toward balance and healing" (Kolkmeier, 1995b, p. 575).

Relaxation has three aims (Payne, 1998): 1) As a prevention to protect body organs from unnecessary stress and wear; 2) As a treatment to alleviate stress in numerous conditions, for example, hypertension, tension headache, insomnia, asthma, immune deficiency, panic, pain; and 3) As a coping skill to calm the mind and to help thinking to become more clear and effective. Positive information in memory also becomes more accessible when a person is relaxed.

There are numerous benefits to the relaxed state, including lowered blood pressure, decreased heat rate, increased body temperature, decreased anxiety associated with painful situations, easing muscle tension pain such as in contractures, a general sense of intense calm, decreasing fatigue, but also helping the client to sleep, increasing the effects of medications, improvements in side effects of cancer therapy and AIDS therapy, assisting in preparation for surgery or other treatments, and helping to dissociate from pain (Payne, 1998).

Payne (1998), Kolkmeier (1995b), and Barrett and Kolkmeier (1997) provide excellent guidelines for the nurse in preparing the client for relaxation and actual scripts to guide one through various relaxation exercises. Table 2.1 includes guidelines or key points for relaxation.

IMAGERY

Imagery influences an individual's attitudes, feelings, behaviors, and anxiety which can either lead to a sense of hopelessness or promote a perception of well-being that assists in changing opinions about disease, treatment, and healing potential. "Imagery [is the] internal experience of memories, dreams, fantasies, and visions—sometimes involving one, several, or all the senses [sight, hearing, touch, smell, taste]—that serve as the bridge for connecting body, mind, and spirit" (Dossey, 1995b, p. 610). Guided imagery and interactive guided imagery (having the client directly interact with the image) are techniques to access the imagination through a guide. There are numerous types of imagery: receptive imagery (inner knowing or "bubble-up" images); active imagery (a focus on the conscious formation of an image); correct biological imagery (recognizing the impact of negative im-

TABLE 2.1 Guidelines for Relaxation

Be familiar with the relaxation exercise before introducing it to the client

Encourage use of familiar relaxation techniques that the client knows

Assess the client's level of tension, level of readiness to learn to relax, pain, anxiety, fear, and perception of reality or history of depersonalization

Ask the client what it means for him/her to be relaxed

Assess the client's ability to remain comfortably in one position for 10–20 minutes

Decrease as much environmental stimuli as possible

Assist the client to develop a positive expectation of what is to occur. Describe the potential benefits of relaxation and enlist cooperation

Reduce the opportunity for self-blame if the session does not go as expected

Have the client close their eyes

Use a tone of voice that is quiet and calm, conversational at first, and decreasing in volume as the session goes on

Use either tapes or a live voice. Music can provide background if desired

Guide the client through a basic breathing exercise (see Exercises section)

Phrase all suggestions in a positive form, e.g., "*Let go* of your tension," "Feel the tightness *melting* away," "*Loosen and soften* your muscles," "Allow the tension to *drift* away;"

Clients may experience a release of emotion as they relax such as tears, vomiting, or faster and more shallow breathing. Gently ask if the client can put words to those feelings. Allow time for expression before continuing

At the completion of the session, bring the client gradually back into reality by taking deep breaths, moving hands and feet, and stretching if able

Have the client evaluate the experience

Engage the client's cooperation in continuing practice until the next session.

A basic breathing exercise and relaxation exercise that can be used with the client or by the nurse is found in the *Exercise* section of this chapter.

ages on physiology and creating positive correct biological images); symbolic imagery (images emerging from both the unconscious and conscious which shape attitudes, belief systems, and cultural experiences, often mythic symbols; process imagery (a step-by-step rehearsal of any procedure, treatment, surgery, or other event prior to its occurrence); end-state imagery (rehearsal of an image of being in a final, healed state) general healing imagery (images that have a personal healing significance such as a wise person, an animal, the sun, etc.); packaged imagery (another person's images such as commercial tapes); and customized imagery (images specific to an individual) (Dossey, 1995b).

Guided imagery has many applications in end of life care, including relaxation, stress reduction, pain relief, symptom management, grief work, and assisting clients to comprehend meaning in their illness experience. Not only is it useful in mobilizing latent, innate healing abilities of the client by intensifying the impact of healing messages that the autonomic nervous system sends to the immune system and other bodily functions, it also is very useful in the self-care of the nurse. It has been found helpful in relieving chronic pain and headaches, stimulating healing, tolerating medical procedures, exploring emotions that may have caused illness, solving difficult problems, and envisioning and planning for the future.

It is usually helpful for the nurse to have training in the use of interactive guided imagery because of possible overwhelming effects with this type of imagery (Rossman, 1999). Otherwise, as Dossey (1995b) notes, imagery scripts are more effective when one learns the speaking skills of voice modulation, specific word emphasis, and the use of pauses. Guidelines for the nurse to use in teaching the client the imagery process are presented in Table 2.2.

MEDITATION

Meditation is a quiet turning inward. It is the practice of focusing one's attention internally to achieve clearer consciousness and inner stillness.

TABLE 2.2   Guidelines to Imagery

Help the client to identify the problem or goal of imagery

Develop a basic understanding of the physiology involved in the healing process

Begin with a few minutes of relaxation, meditation, or paying attention to the breath exercise

Assist the client to develop images of:
—the problem
—inner healing resources (beliefs, coping strategies, etc.)
—external healing resources (medications, treatments, family, etc.)

End with images of the desired state of well-being

A basic imagery exercise that nurses can use with clients is under the *Exercises* section of this chapter.

There are numerous methods and schools of meditation, all having an individual interpretation of the practice. However, all methods believe in emptying the mind and letting go of the mind's chatter that preoccupies us.

Meditation originated in the eastern tradition and is integral to Hinduism, Taoism, and Buddhism and is both a state of mind and a method. The state is one where the mind is quiet and listening to itself. The practitioner is relaxed but alert. The method involves the focusing of attention on something such as the breath, an image, a word, or action such as Tai chi or Qigong. There is a sustained concentration but it should be effortless.

The objective of meditation is to detach the mediator from external events as well as one's own mental activity. If thoughts enter the mind, rather than examining them, the mediator allows them to drift away. There is no criticism or judgment, but an attitude of a beginner's mind; a mind which is open and receptive, clear of attachment to any thoughts. The mind is emptied of all thought except awareness of the image, word, or breath. "Passive concentration" keeps the mediator in a state of heightened awareness and alertness rather than drowsiness, and intently focused on the present moment. There should be no blame, guilt, or recrimination if the mediator loses focus or if the mind wanders; but instructed to simply return the mind to its original focus. Reentry into the normal waking state should be gentle and relaxed. Meditation requires practice on a regular schedule, usually once or twice daily to achieve maximal results.

There are various reasons for practicing meditation: to find peace, achieve awareness and enlightenment, find oneself, and to experience true reality, and enhance a sense of well-being. Research has demonstrated that relaxed forms of meditation decrease heart rate and blood pressure, increase breathing volume, but decreasing the number of breaths per minute (Gatchel & Maddrey, 1998; Hall, 1997). It is believed that meditation activates the right cerebral hemisphere and the parasympathetic nervous system, thereby quieting the nerves and allowing intuitive, wordless thinking to occur. Advantages of meditation cited by Payne (1998) are listed in Table 2.3.

SENSE THERAPIES

Sense therapies use the senses to treat physical and psychological problems and to adjust chemical or other imbalances within the body. These can include behavioral vision therapy, eye movement, desensitization, flower remedies, hydrotherapy, and light therapy. Two therapies will be explored under sense therapies: Music therapy and music-thanatology, and aromatherapy.

TABLE 2.3   Advantages of Meditation[a]

A better understanding of the self and increased receptivity to insights arising from one's deeper being. Practicing meditation can bring the experience of self for the dying; where the individual may attain calm and often a sense of purpose.

A new sense of relaxation and inner peace.

A clearer mind and improved concentration.

More harmony with and within the self.

As a result of the detachment an acceptance that many unpleasant emotional responses are short-lived sensations created by one's thoughts.

An emphasis on living in the present and valuing the here and now.

[a]A simple meditation that can be practiced by the nurse or with a client is in the *Exercises* section of this chapter.

Music Therapy and Music Thanatology

Guzzetta (1995) defines music therapy as the "behavioral science concerned with the systematic application of music to produce relaxation and desired changes in emotions, behavior, and physiology" (p. 670). The elements of music, sound, rhythm, hearing, melody, harmony, and movement are part of people's primary experiences. Listening to, creating, or moving to music assists people to improve, change, or better integrate aspects of themselves. Music has a power that cannot be expressed in verbal language.

There are references to the therapeutic powers of music in philosophy, art, and literature throughout the ages. Music is used in healing ceremonies throughout the world. Our own experiences demonstrates the psychological effect that music has on us. Despite varying musical tastes, certain types of music create specific moods, for example, a march, ominous music, lively music at sports events, quiet relaxing music in waiting rooms, or a mother's singing and rocking her baby in times of distress (McCraty, Barrios-Choplin, Atkinson, & Tomasino, 1998).

Music therapy can reduce bio-psychological stress, pain, anxiety, and isolation. It assists clients to reach a deep state of relaxation, develop self-awareness and creativity, improve learning, clarify personal values, and cope with a variety of psychophysiological problems. It also provides clients with integrated body/mind episodes and encourages them to become active participants in their own healing. Appropriate music produces the relaxation response, often removing a client's inner restlessness and quieting ceaseless thinking. It is used as a healing technique to quiet the mind and bring about inner relaxation (Guzzetta, 1995; McBride, Graydon, Sidani, & Hall, 1999).

Because music therapy focuses on process and not outcome, one need not have any musical skills or talents to derive benefits. Frank-Schwebel (1999) recommends that clients be induced to a relaxed state through breathing, suggestive imagery, or a relaxation exercise. Music selected by the client or the nurse is played, and the client is invited to explore images, sensations, emotions, memories, and visions brought on by the music. No one type of music works well for all individuals in all situations. A variety of soothing selections (popular, new age, classical, country, opera, folk, jazz, choral hymns, etc.) should be available because one cannot always predict a client's particular preference or response to the music. Often the client experiences an altered state of consciousness, which is usually very relaxing. After the listening, the client is brought back to reality to discuss the experience. In some instances, the client chooses the music and moves or paints to the music.

The nurse should assess the following factors in preparing to use music therapy (Guzzetta, 1995) as presented in Table 2.4.

Music has the greatest effect when the client is appropriately prepared. Find a quiet environment and have the client assume a comfortable position. Suggest that s/he maintain a passive attitude, neither forcing nor resisting the experience and remind the client to focus all concentration on the music.

Music Thanatology

Music thanatology, founded by Therese Schroeder-Sheker (1994), is a relatively new field that addresses the needs of the dying by assisting the client to complete the transition between life and death. Specially trained therapists, using harp, voice, and chanting, assist the client in leave-taking during the

TABLE 2.4   Assessment for Music Therapy

The client's music history and music preferences.

The client's identification of music that make him/her happy, excited, sad, or relaxed.

The client's identification of music that is distasteful and make him/her tense.

Assessment of the importance of music in the client's life.

The frequency of music playing in the client's life.

Previous participation in relaxation/imagery techniques combined with music.

The client's mood—this will determine the type of music to be played.

last hours of life by reinforcing peace, acceptance, and a calm anticipation of death. Schroeder-Sheker (1994) describes music-thanatology as a "palliative medical modality employing prescriptive music to tend the complex physical and spiritual needs of the dying . . . music thanatology is concerned with the possibility of a blessed death and the gift that conscious dying can bring to the fullness of life" (p. 83). This music is live (not taped), dynamic, and prescriptive. It is individual to each patient and each death, much like childbirth. According to Schroeder-Sheker, music-thanatology has been found to be most effective in deaths from cancer, AIDS, burns, and slowly degenerative diseases.

Schroeder-Sheker identifies six foundational assumptions of music thanatology which include:

- A recognition of dying as a spiritual process and as an opportunity for growth;
- The musical deathbed vigil, often called "musical-sacramental-midwifery," is a contemplative practice requiring serious inner work and integration of the physical, emotional, mental, and spiritual aspects of the caregiver;
- Death is not an enemy and it is not a failure. It is a critical chapter of human biography;
- The way in which each person dies is equally as important as the way in which that person lived. Beauty, reverence, dignity, and intimacy are central to life and especially so for death. The infirmary music can bring things to the surface in a nonthreatening way or serve the role of meditation. Music is a flow weaving body, soul, and spirit together;
- This work is a vocation, not merely a career. It requires clear intention and attention at each deathbed vigil;
- Death and dying should be returned to the human, personal realm rather than denying or ignoring loss and leave-taking, thus reducing them to legal or corporate medical matters.

Music thanatology focuses on music for the dying versus music for the living. The dying person should not spend energy, only receive energy. "The entire surface of the skin can become an extension of the ear, thus enabling the patient to absorb infirmary music, creating the possibility for even deeper emotional, mental, and spiritual reception. . . . The sole focus is to help the person move toward completion and to unbind from anything that prevents, impedes, or clouds a tranquil passage" (Schroeder-Sheker, 1994, pp. 93–94).

Aromatherapy

Aromatherapy is an offshoot of herbal medicine "in which aromatic plant extracts are inhaled or applied to the skin as a means of treating illness and promoting beneficial changes in mood and outlook. Though aromatherapy and herbal medicine use many of the same plants, in aromatherapy the plants are distilled into oils of exceptional potency" (Allison, 1999a, p. 86). The benefit of these oils comes from their influence on the limbic system that coordinates mind and body activity. This system is very sensitive to odors and encodes them into associations and memories, which when awakened, alter basic physical functions such as heart rate, blood pressure, breathing, and hormone level. When these oils are rubbed into the skin or inhaled, they set off a reaction leading to rapid and significant alterations in memory, heart rate, and other bodily mechanisms. Some boost energy, some promote relaxation, and others have pharmaceutical effects. However, no treatment should ever involve more than a few drops of oil.

There are hundreds of plants used for aromatherapy. Some of the more common ones that are useful in the care of the dying include: chamomile used to overcome anxiety, anger, tension, stress, and insomnia; lavender used for exhaustion and depression; marjoram used for those who are physically debilitated; neroli used for countering depression, anxiety, nervous tension, and fearfulness; peppermint and rosewood for treating nausea; and chamomile, camphor fennel, lavender, peppermint, and rose for relieving vomiting (Duke, 1997). Aromatherapy also is used in the relief of pain (lavender and capsicum) and is most useful in the enhancement of mood, increase in vitality, and relaxation (Robins, 1999). These plants and oils can be found in natural or health food stores.

Reminiscence and Life Review

Life review or reminiscence therapy is the remembering of significant past events that enable one to reintegrate past issues and experiences in the present for the purpose of achieving a sense of meaning and ego integrity (Dossey, 1995a). The concept has been most frequently used with the elderly but is just as effective with those nearing the end of life. Reminiscence is a natural phenomenon. It is the process of recounting of past events to someone else or can be a more complex process of transpersonal focusing and inward reflection. The level of complexity depends on the wish of the client and the training of the nurse. Life review can be oral, including audio and video recordings, or written. Journal and letter writing can also be useful techniques in life review. Photographs and personal items often provide the opportunity for reminiscence and give information about the client that assists the nurse in providing personal and meaningful care.

Because life review is a process of "unfolding and opening" (Kolkmeier, 1995a), the intervention cannot be hurried. A life review can be one or many sessions. Olsen (1997a) provides a guide for a structured life review that usually includes six to eight sessions:

- Use open-ended questions. Ask about childhood and earliest memories and be sure to be supportive if the client recalls sad events;
- Again, using open-ended questions, proceed through their life history by asking about adolescence, family and home, adulthood, and later life;
- Have a summary session inquiring about the following: "Generally, what kind of life do you think you have had? What would you do over again?"

To promote the process, Kolkmeier (1995a) suggests that the nurse encourage self-expression, involve significant others, keep the information confidential, be sure the client has sufficient physical strength and a desire for sharing, listen carefully, use touch as appropriate, and allow the client periods of silence to reflect. Life review provides integration, a feeling that this life was individual and unique. The client may verbalize sadness as well as achievement, but the objective is to allow a person to see the meaning in their life.

JOURNAL WRITING

Keeping a log or journal is a very healing technique to use for individuals experiencing life-threatening illness and during the grieving process. It allows the person to express innermost feelings and thoughts without fear of criticism. It is often helpful for those who are uncomfortable or unable to articulate how they feel or what they are going through. The healing emanates from the actual writing and expression, and not from an analysis of the content of the journal. The writing may be totally private or shared with others. Many clients do not think of this technique and the nurse may suggest it. Roach and Nieto (1997) offer some suggested topics for journal writing:

- special thoughts of the dying person or about the deceased
- feelings that were never expressed
- saying good-bye
- ways that grief or dying has helped me grow
- positive aspects of the past, present, and future

There are numerous topics for journal writing or the client can just write thoughts and feelings as they occur. The individual may find comfort in writing when difficult times occur, for example, unanticipated news about diagnosis or prognosis, dealing with family members, or writing to God, a loved one, or one's disease. Often the journal becomes one's own record of grieving. It often serves as a chronicle of personal growth, insights, and wisdom gleaned from the experience of dying or loss.

TOUCH

In the later stages of life, individuals are often deprived of tender and nurturing physical contact such as being touched in a way that is healing, nourishing, relaxing, and pleasurable. Touch is essential to one's quality of existence. It provides comfort, warmth, and renewed vitality—a sense of security and assurance that we are not alone. Reasons for the lack of touch of the dying include fear, discomfort, stereotypes about dying people, and a sense of one's own vulnerability. However, the benefits of touch on individuals are many. There is an increase of circulation and mobility (e.g., range of motion or hand grasp); the experience of being nurtured and cared for; a boost in self-esteem; an increased motivation to receive and give attention to self and others; energy and emotional release; a sense memory triggering relaxation response; relief from loneliness and isolation; decreased feelings of abandonment and deprivation; verbal interaction; and calming reassurance and support (Giasson & Bouchard, 1998).

There are many forms of touch considered to be holistic/integrative modalities (Dossey, 1995a; Allison, 1999a; Credit, Hartunian, & Nowak, 1998). These include but are not limited to:

Accupressure—the application of pressure, using fingers, thumbs, palms, or elbows to specific sites along the body's energy meridians to stimulate, disperse, and regulate the body's healing energy for the purpose of relieving tension and reestablishing the flow of energy along the meridian lines.

Body therapy—a general term used for approaches (e.g., Alexander technique, chiropractic, Rolfing, shiatsu, Feldenkrais, etc.) that use hands-on techniques to manipulate and balance the musculoskeletal system to facilitate healing, increase energy, relieve pain, and promote relaxation and well-being.

Foot reflexology—the application of pressure to specific reflex areas on the feet corresponding to other parts of the body to locate and correct problems in the body.

Massage—the practice of kneading or otherwise manipulating a person's muscles and other soft tissue with the intent of inducing physical and psychological relaxation, improvement of circulation, relief of pain and sore muscles, and improving that individual's well-being. Procedural massage is done to diagnose, monitor, or treat the illness itself, focusing on the end result of curing the illness or preventing further complications.

Therapeutic touch—(TT) developed by Dolores Krieger and Dora Kunz. This is a specific modality of centering intention while the practitioner moves the hands through the client's energy field for the purpose of assessment and treatment. It is based on the philosophy that universal life energy flows through and around us, and any interruption in this free flow of energy leads to illness. The goal is to balance and repattern the body's energy so that it flows most efficiently to promote health and prevent disease. The TT practitioner scans the client's energy flow, replenishing it where necessary, releasing congestion, removing obstructions, and restoring order and balance in the ill system. This approach is also an effective complementary care approach for facilitation of the body's natural restorative processes thereby accelerating healing, promoting relaxation, reducing pain and anxiety, and treating chronic conditions (Krieger, 1997).

Janet Macrae (1987), a well-known TT practitioner states, "Since therapeutic Touch is an interaction, it has the potential to heal the practitioner as well as the patient. . . . You can also use the principles of TT to assist in healing yourself . . . the use of mental imagery can facilitate both the energy transfer and the rebalancing of the [practitioner's] field. If you have pain or discomfort somewhere: 1) Sit quietly and center yourself; 2) Visualize the healing energy (as light, if you wish) coming down from above and flowing through you; 3) Visualize the energy clearing away the pain or discomfort (as light shines through a dark area)" (pp. 79–80).

Compassionate touch—developed by Nelson (1994) specifically for hands-on care given to the elderly, the ill, and the dying. It is described as a "gentle, sensitive, and non-intrusive program of massage, attentive touch, and supportive comfort care for those individuals who are temporarily or permanently less active. . . . It also includes individuals of any age who are actively beginning the mysterious life transition that we call death" (p. 1). It is a hands-on technique stemming not from the hands but from the heart. It combines massage and attentive touch with active listening, reflective communication, relaxation, imagery, and breathing awareness exercises. It focuses not only on the physical condition of the client, but also on the psychosocial, emotional, and spiritual needs as well.

According to Nelson (1994), "compassion for another implies a feeling of unconditional regard for that other; it also implies a genuine, sincere interest in that person's well-being. The compassionate heart shares in, and is affected by the suffering of another. . . . The compassionate individual is able to put aside his or her own concerns for a time in order to give attention to someone else. Some say compassion is love in action" (p. 1). Compassionate touch is not something we give, it is a way of being. It is a way of providing contact, reassurance, relief, and comfort for those who may be frightened, depressed, out of control, abandoned, overwhelmed, confused, or in despair. It is a means of relating to others rather than a prescribed set of techniques to be practiced on others. It is a spontaneous event of relationship that unfolds moment to moment. Compassionate Touch can be administered by anyone who feels inspired to reach out toward a fellow human being in need.

Reiki—based on Buddhist teachings using hands-on touch to support and intensify energy in the physical, emotional, intellectual, and spiritual areas. "Universal and individual energy are aligned and balanced through the application of gentle hands-on touch to energy pathways of the body" (Abrams, 1999, p. 133). Those who use Reiki attribute it to reducing stress and stress-related illnesses including acute and chronic conditions, helping in debilitating disease because it bolsters the immune system by increasing energy, and contributing to a general sense of overall well-being in the client.

The philosophy of Reiki contends that a person is vitalized by a vital energy that comes from the universal life force. One becomes ill when the energy flow is interrupted or stopped. Everyone has access to this life force. Opening pathways for energy flow is the prime objective of Reiki. Learners of Reiki must themselves receive an attunement by an expert Reiki master in an initiation ceremony so they are attuned to the energy transfer process.

Reiki bodywork is not massage. The touch is gentle and "aims not to manipulate tissue, but rather to transmit universal life force to the recipient. The practitioner uses both hands, palms down, fingers held together, and proceeds in a pattern over the recipient's body. After the front surface has been treated, the client turns and treatment continues on the back. Each positioning of the hands is maintained for 3–5 minutes without any movement of the fingers or change in the initial gentle touch" (Abrams, 1999 p. 136).

Reiki bodywork is very individualized and the client's perception of the energy transfer is unique to each person. Most find it rejuvenating and relaxing. The effects may be felt immediately or several days later. Following attunement/initiation of the caregiver, Reiki can be used as a method of self-healing as well as caring for others.

As can be seen, there are numerous holistic healing modalities that can be used during end of life care.

THE HEALING JOURNEY AT THE END OF LIFE

Individuals become aware of their own deaths in phases, and this awareness can lead to consciousness in dying. Olson (1997a) and Dossey (1995a) identify some tasks for dying consciously, specifically,

1. "*Live fully* until death comes and to direct or participate in the death process [treatment decisions, determinations about the kinds of care] until one is comfortable with accepting the ministrations of others" (Olson, 1997b, p. 128).

2. *Plan* to say good-bye to family and friends, finish things one wanted to do, make final decisions, regarding: Last Will and Testament, estate, organ donation, etcetera. Consider what an ideal death would be like. Who do you want with you, or do you want to be alone? Who are the important people in your life and have you told them? Are there rituals you want at your death, for example, memorial service, cremation, etcetera? What kind of ceremony do you want? Are there certain treasures that you want particular people to have? Are there particular prayers, poems, or music you want read or played?

3. *Participate* in emotional and spiritual tasks such as forgiving oneself and others, feeling that life mattered and the world is different because I was here, and knowing and accepting love as one changes. Forgiving self and others necessitates recognizing that we are responsible for what we are holding onto; confessing one's story to self and others, looking for the good points in ourselves and others; making amends where possible; looking to a higher power for help; and considering what we have learned (Borysenko, 1990). Forgiving others and ourselves helps one recognize unconditional love, connect more with the source of our joy instead of focusing on loss, sadness, and pain. Unconditional love helps release one from fear and anxiety.

4. *Rehearse* the dying process, through an awareness of dying learn to diminish the fear of death, and to "let go of this life" when it is time to do so. Imagery, relaxation, meditation, and prayer scripts on learning forgiveness in peace, letting go, opening the heart, forgiving self and others, releasing pain and grief, conscious dying, moving into the light, and closure can facilitate the detachment from pain and grief, the establishment of comfort and peace, and the achievement of closure. Dossey (1995a) is an excellent source for some of these scripts. However, the nurse should have some practice experience prior to their use with clients.

SELF-CARE FOR THE HEALER

Working with the dying and their families can create much stress for the nurse. It is sometimes referred to as "death overload." Olson (1997a) notes that caregivers of dying persons often reexamine their own belief systems and may suffer an existential crisis of faith. Health professionals grieve the loss of their clients, and when the losses come too quickly, they may not complete the grieving process before the next death. This may lead to feelings of guilt, anger, irritability, frustration, helplessness, inadequacy, sleeplessness, and depression. Problems may arise in interaction with clients, family members, and other staff. Olson (1997a) further notes consequences when staff are not dealing well with the deaths of clients:

- "avoiding patients
- poor clinical judgment
- unrealistic expectations
- staff absences
- outbursts of anger
- lack of anticipatory planning
- staff conflict
- scapegoating
- interdisciplinary power struggles
- staff fatigue
- ambivalence toward patients." (p. 207)

These problems can affect an individual or an entire team. Therefore it is imperative that health professionals learn self-care techniques (Tinnerman, 1999). Roach and Nieto (1997) in discussing bereavement care and the role of nurse healers identify five self-care areas and questions that need to be explored when working with the dying and their families, which include:

1. Spiritual Self Care—Is spirituality important in my life; what is my relationship with God or a higher power; why am I here and what is my purpose; what is my relationship to the universe?
2. Emotional Self Care—Can I identify my emotions; how do I deal with them; am I usually in control; can I discuss my emotions; am I open to others and do I respect the feelings of others or do I jump to conclusions; when do my emotions get out of control?
3. Physical Self Care—What areas of my lifestyle are unhealthy or do I have a healthy lifestyle; what can I do to improve my lifestyle?
4. Mental Self Care—Am I knowledgeable and do I continually increase my knowledge; am I satisfied with the status quo or am I open to new ideas; what am I doing to stimulate my mind?
5. Relationships Self Care—Am I open and honest with myself and others; do I have satisfying relationships with others; am I willing to accept the thoughts and feelings of others even though they are different from my own or am I judgmental; must I have all the control or can I share it; do I have a balance between work, home, and leisure? (pp. 171–175)

Worden (1982) identified four tasks of mourning that are equally applicable to staff. Accepting the reality of the loss, although painful, is necessary for healing to occur. It may sometimes feel that the nurse in end of life care is in chronic grieving because of the number of dying clients. But denying the emotional pain, especially of a favored patient, only slows or inhibits the healing process from occurring.

Experiencing the pain of the loss, including anger, depression, and guilt, although more obvious in the significant others, also occurs in the staff. Healing support of each other involves encouraging expression of feelings and emotions such as sadness, anger, guilt, resentment, and pain. Validating the normalcy of the feelings and emotions is also important. One should identify coping strategies that might work or are not working; forgive self and others; and remember shared experiences with the deceased client.

Rediscovering meaning is a period of yearning, searching, and discovery. One yearns for the lost person(s) or assumed state of ordinariness, searches for some type of normalcy to reenter the everyday living or working situation, and then discovers the meaning of the loss or losses. Meaning to each of us is individual, unique, and personal. But if one can find meaning, s/he seems to adjust more easily. Some find meaning in religion, some in support or supportive groups, and some in going inward. Some may never find the answer to the question, "Why did they have to die or why am I surrounded by so much death?" However, even if these questions are not answered, one may find a new meaning to life—to the present and to the future.

Reinvesting in life or work is somewhat like hope (Roach & Nieto, 1997). One realizes that there is a purpose to this type of work, that the future can be full and good. There is a letting go of remorse and fear of the future, a sense of empowerment and a sense of one's place in the world. With letting go, the nurse is free to remember the meaningful times with clients, and the lessons learned. Although many techniques described above help in reinvesting in work, it also is useful for one to engage in an area of interest outside of work, enroll in a class, take a trip, do special things for oneself, or review one's job goals and setting. Reinvesting in work doesn't necessarily mean that everything is solved; however, it can be the motivation for growth. This growth can be expressed as feeling more intensely, empathizing more completely, caring more fully, and developing more sensitivity to and compassion for others.

As noted earlier, those who care for the terminally ill are at risk for stress associated with many losses. There is also opportunity for a career leading to joy, a sense of personal and professional proficiency, and a capability of living life to the fullest. Olson (1997b) identifies three aspects of developing growth when working with the dying. Identifying one's motivation for practicing end of life care is important. Is it unresolved personal issues; a professional challenge beyond the physical that involves a search for meaning and peace; a desire to witness the growth of each individual as one comes to terms with mortality and the nature of life; a spiritual calling; a joy in physical care that involves a variety of techniques including complementary modalities such as breathing, TT, and/or relaxation? Whatever the motivation, exploring this question leads the nurse in end of life care to a certain insight and wisdom.

Coping techniques include those strategies used to change the negative effects of stress. It can be forgiving self and others, maintaining health through good nutrition, weight control, regular exercise, adequate sleep, and sufficient resources to maintain oneself in a healthy state. Other kinds of physical activities include massage, diaphragmatic breathing, and distraction. Time needs to be scheduled so that the staff can focus on themselves. An example of diaphragmatic breathing is found in the *Exercises* section of this chapter. Those who use this technique regularly can do so on cue, even at the bedside of a dying patient. Distraction includes humor, a massage break, lunch out, a day off or just a break. One needs these distractions to rest and refresh one's spirit. Scheduling things that are not reminders of patients, death, or dying are important aspects in addition to grieving and remembering.

Developing the spiritual self includes knowing that one's life has meaning, and confronting one's mortality. These are key aspects in caring for the dying and their significant others. "*Healing the Dying* means healing oneself by forming connections with the Universe and all that it is. It means a path one can count on, a way one travels with confidence" (Olson, 1997b, p. 218). Searching for meaning necessitates learning to listen, quieting the mind's chatter, hearing the whisper of the inner self, and connecting to one's spirituality. A sense of connection with meaningfulness and purpose can be with an organized religion, with a group, or the path can be an inner process. There are many ways to develop an ability to listen to the inner self: meditation, creating an environment that supports peace, for example, nature or sound; reading literature about the development of a spiritual path; setting a regular time to practice; keeping a journal; sharing one's spiritual journey with like-minded people; and enjoying life. Whatever the technique, there is a growing sense of unity and purpose in being. One belongs here, one has a mission and a purpose.

This chapter has presented some of the more common alternative/ complementary/integrative healing modalities that are and can be used by nurses and by students of nursing. It should be noted that centering, relaxation, imagery, meditation, reminiscence, and life review and journal writing are basic and can be practiced by nurses and students with little or no experience. The sense therapies, touch therapies, and Reiki bodywork necessitate further study which are offered through a few Master's degree programs and workshops. Whenever one learns these therapies, it is imperative that nurses practicing end of life care be familiar with healing modalities and their beneficial effects for clients during the dying process.

EXERCISES

PASSIVE RELAXATION[1]

Procedure for participants who are lying down:

- With your eyes closed, let your attention focus on your breathing . . . notice how gentle, slow, and regular it is becoming . . . imagine each breath out carrying your tensions away, leaving you more relaxed than you were before . . . if you want to, take one deep breath . . . then allow your breathing to settle into its own rhythm . . . easy, calm, and even . . . and forget about it.
- I'm going to ask you to take a trip around the body, checking that all the muscle groups are as relaxed as possible and letting go any tension that might still remain. If outside thoughts creep in, hold them in a bubble and let them flow away. I'll begin with the feet.
- Bring your attention to your toes . . . are they lying still? If they are curled or stretched out in some way not entirely comfortable, wiggle them gently. As they come to rest, feel all the tensions leaving them . . . feel them sinking down, heavy and motionless.
- Let your feet roll out at the ankles. This is the most relaxed position for them. Let all the tension flow out of them . . . enjoy the sensation of just letting them go.
- Moving on to the lower legs: feel the tension leaving the calf muscles and the shins. As the tension goes, so they feel heavier . . . so they feel warm and pleasantly tingling.
- The thighs next: to be fully relaxed they need to be slightly rolling outwards . . . feel the relaxing effect of this position . . . make sure you have released all tension, and feel your thighs resting heavily on the surface you are resting on.
- Focus for a moment on the sensation of sagging heaviness throughout your legs . . . let the muscles shed their last remaining hint of tension and settle into a deep relaxation.

------

[1]Source: Payne, R. (1998). *Relaxation techniques a practical handbook for the health care professional.* New York: Churchill Livingston.

- And now, think of your hips. Let them settle into the surface you are lying on . . . recognize any tension that linger in the muscles . . . then relax it away . . . let it go on relaxing a bit further than you thought possible.
- Settle your spine into the rug or mattress . . . become aware of how it is resting on a surface. Let it sink down, making contact whenever it wants to . . . all tension draining out of it.
- Let your abdominal muscles lose their tension. Let them go soft and loose. Feel them spreading as they give their last vestige of tension . . . notice how your relaxed abdomen rises and falls with your breathing . . . rises as the air is drawn in and falls as the air is expelled . . . abdominal breathing is relaxed breathing.
- Move up to your chest and shoulders, to muscles which are prone to carry tension . . . feel them letting go . . . feel them spreading . . . feel them easing into the surface, limp and heavy . . . feel them drooping down towards your feet . . . imagine them shedding their burdens . . . and as the space between your shoulders and your neck opens out, imagine your neck a bit longer than it was before.

Now, direct your thoughts to the muscles of your left arm. Check that it lies limply on a surface. Notice the feeling of relaxation and allow this feeling to sweep down to your wrist and hand. Think of the fingers, are they curved and still? . . . neither drawn up nor stretched out . . . neither opened nor closed, but gently resting . . . totally relaxed. As you breathe out, let the arm relax a little bit more . . . let it lie heavy and loose . . . so heavy and loose that if someone were to pick it up, then let it go, it would flop down again like the arm of a rag doll.

- Repeat the last paragraph with the muscles of the right arm.
- Your neck muscles have no need to work with your head supported, so let them go . . . enjoy the feeling of "letting go" in muscles which work so hard the rest of the time to keep your head upright. If you find any tension in the neck, release it and let this process of releasing continue, even below the surface . . . feel how pleasant it is when you let go the tension in these muscles.
- Bring your attention now to your face, to the many small muscles whose job it is to manage your expressions. At the moment there's no need to have any expression at all on your face, so allow your muscles to feel relaxed . . . imagine how your face is when you are asleep . . . calm and motionless . . .
- Now, think about the jaw . . . and as you do, allow it to drop slightly so that your teeth are separated . . . feel it relaxing with your lips gently

touching. Check that your tongue is still, and lying in the middle of your mouth, soft and shapeless. Relax your throat so that all tension leaves it and the muscles feel smooth and resting.

- With no expression on your face, your cheeks are relaxed and soft. If you think of your nose, it is just to register the passage of cool air traveling up your nostrils while the warmer air passes down . . . breathe tension out with the warm air . . . breathe stillness in with cool air.
- Check that your forehead is smooth . . . not furrowed in any direction . . . and as you release its remaining tension, imagine it being a little higher and a little wider than it was before . . . continue this feeling into your scalp and behind your ears . . . feel a sense of calm as you do this.
- Let your thoughts focus on your eyes as they lie behind gently closed lids. Think of them resting in their sockets, floating rather than fixed . . . and as they come to rest, so do your thoughts.
- Spend a few minutes continuing to relax, deepening the effect of the above sequences . . .
- You now have relaxed all the major muscle groups in your body. Think about them now as a whole . . . a totally relaxed whole . . . soothed by your gentle breathing rhythm, feel the peacefulness of this idea . . .
- Images may drift in and out of your mind . . . see them as thoughts passing through. Feel yourself letting go of them. Say to yourself: "I am feeling calm, I am feeling peaceful." Let your mind conjure up a sense of contentment.

IMAGERY

- The instructor picks one of the following: a sunny beach, a river bank, or a scented garden. If trainees suffer from hay fever the first item is the best choice. Imagery is best used after a short relaxation exercise.

A Sunny Beach

- See yourself lying on the hot sand of a sunny beach within an enclosed bay. It is sheltered from storms and protected from ocean currents. It is safe. You watch the light dancing on the water; you smell the sea air as it fills your nostrils; you hear the gulls calling above the sound of waves; you feel the warm sun on your skin. The grains of dry sand run through your fingers, forming little bumps and hollows beneath your hand.

A River Bank

- Imagine you are lying in the soft, juicy long grass of early summer. You are in a green meadow that rolls down to the river. Scents rise up from the wild flowers, seeping over you in waves. The sun is warm but a gentle breeze softens its intensity. Closing your eyes you become aware of the sound of water flowing, of birds calling and of leaves rustling.

A Scented Garden

- Picture yourself lying on a newly mown lawn with the sun beating down on the moist cuttings, drawing out their fragrance. Reach out and feel the coolness of the damp grass. Through your half-closed eyelids you can see the tops of the trees swaying against the sky. Light breezes carry the scent of honeysuckle.

Following one of these short passages of visualization, trainees can relax for a few minutes, before the session is brought to an end.

RELAXATION[2]

I'd like for you to be as comfortable as you possibly can. Take a couple of deep breaths. Inhale deeply. Exhale very slowly and very completely. Focus on your breathing. Again, inhale very deeply and exhale very slowly. Become aware of your ability to relax your muscles. Allow every muscle in your body to be as relaxed as possible, starting with the feet. Allow the feet to become very, very comfortable. Relax the feet completely. As the muscles relax you may notice a tingly sensation in the soles and toes of the feet. This simply indicates that the muscles are relaxing.

Be aware as this sensation of relaxation begins to move upward from the feet to the ankles. This sensation of relaxation flows from the ankles to the calves of the legs. The muscles of the calves release the tension and relax. The calves become very comfortable as the tension is released.

This comfortable, relaxed sensation moves from the calves to the upper legs and thighs. These muscles also relax and become very comfortable. Feel the muscles on the sides of the legs, the outside of the legs, the inner legs, and on the top of the legs become very comfortable and relaxed.

The sensation of relaxation moves up towards the buttocks and toward the pelvic area. Occasionally you may feel a muscle twitch. This is just

---

[2]Source: Roach, S., & Nieto, B. (1997). *Healing and the grief process.* New York: Delmar Publications.

another sign that relaxation is occurring. The tension of the muscles of the buttocks, pelvic area, and the lower abdomen is released. The internal organs relax and the muscles that surround them feel completely tension free.

The sensation of relaxation moves up the body to the upper abdomen, to the chest, and from the lower back toward the upper back. The muscles are relaxing from the chest and the upper back to the shoulders.

This relaxation extends to the neck and the throat. Feel the tension draining from the back of the neck. Tension is draining away from the back of the neck and the back of the head. As tension drains away a sense of relaxation settles in. These feelings are so comfortable and so pleasant. Feel the muscles of the throat, the jaw, and across the bridge of the nose relaxing.

The tension in the arms is released and these muscles feel relaxed. Relaxation spreads to the hands and the fingers as the tension is released.

From the feet, to the head, to the arms, to the fingertips, the whole body is completely and totally relaxed. Take a few moments to savor this comfortable state of total relaxation of body and mind.

CLOSURE

- Allow time for the client to appreciate this restful state of complete relaxation.
- After a few minutes instruct the client to bring his attention back to the present. At times the nurse may want to count slowly from one to ten as the client progressively returns to a more wakeful state.

MEDITATION[3]

Using a Mantra

1. Select a word to focus on.

   - A neutral word such as "one."
   - A Sanskrit mantra such as "Om Shanti," "Sri Ram," "So-Hum."
   - A word or phrase that has some special significance within your personal belief system. In his recent book, *Beyond the Relaxation Response*, Benson (1985) describes how a word or phrase of special

---

[3]Source: Edmund J. Bourne. (1995). *The Anxiety & Phobia Workbook*, Second Edition, Copyright © 1995 by New Harbinger Publications, Inc. All rights reserved.

personal significance (such as "I am at peace" or "Let go let God") deepens the effects of meditation.

2. Repeat this word or phrase, ideally on each exhalation.
3. As any thoughts come to mind, just let them pass over and through you and gently bring your attention back to the repetitive word or phrase.

Continuing Breaths

1. As you sit quietly, focus on the inflow and outflow of your breath. Each time you breath out, count the breath. You can count up to 10 and start over again, or keep counting as high as you like, or you can use Benson's method of repeating "one" on each exhalation.
2. Each time your focus wanders, bring it back to your breathing and counting. If you get caught in an internal monologue or fantasy, don't worry about it or judge yourself. Just relax and return to the count again.
3. If you lose track of the count, start over at one or at a round number like 50 or 100.
4. After practicing breath-counting meditation for a while, you may want to let go of the counting and just focus on the inflow and outflow of your breathing.

Whichever form of meditation you try, you might want to start out with short periods of 5 to 10 minutes and gradually lengthen them to 20 to 30 minutes over a period of 2 to 3 weeks. Most people find that it takes persistent and disciplined effort over a period of several months to become proficient at meditating. Even though meditation is the most demanding of relaxation techniques to learn, it is for many people the most rewarding. Research has found that among all relaxation techniques, meditation is the one people are most likely to persist in doing regularly.

If you are truly interested in establishing a meditation practice, you may want to find a class, group, or teacher to study with. This will make it easier for you to continue your practice.

SCRIPT FOR BREATHING FOR RELAXATION AND HEALTH[4]

- Close your eyes . . . Focus your mind on your breath . . . just follow the air as it goes in . . . and as it goes out.

------

[4]Source: Julie T. Lusk, *30 Scripts for Relaxation, Imagery and Inner Healing,* Vol. 1 © Julie T. Lusk, Volumes 1 and 2 are available from Whole Persons Associates, 210 W. Michigan, Duluth, Minnesota, 55802, 800–247-6789. Julie T. Lusk is also the author of *Refreshing Journeys,* a

- Feel it as it comes in . . . and as it goes out . . . If your mind begins to wander, just bring it back to your breath.
- Feel your stomach rise . . . your ribs expand . . . and your collarbone rise . . . Breathe in naturally and slowly.
- On your next exhalation, release all the air from your lungs without straining . . . Let it all go . . . Let it all out . . . Prepare your lungs to receive fresh oxygen.
- Now take in a full, deep breath and let the air go to the bottom of your lungs . . . Feel your stomach rise . . . your chest expand, and the collarbone area fill.
- Now empty your lungs from top to bottom . . . Let all the air out . . . Compress your stomach to squeeze out all the stale air and carbon dioxide. Squeeze out every bit of air . . . Let it all go.
- Take in another deep breath . . . As you breathe in, your diaphragm expands and massages all the internal organs in the abdominal region . . . aiding your digestion.
- Breathe out . . . Relax . . . Feel the knots in your stomach untie . . . Let go.
- Breath in . . . Your diaphragm is stimulating your vagus nerve, slowing down the beating of your heart . . . relaxing you.
- Breath out . . . Let it all go . . . relax . . . relax more and more . . . Breathing heals you . . . calms you . . . soothes you.
- Breathe in again, fully and completely. Oxygen is entering your bloodstream, nourishing all your organs and cells . . . protecting you.
- Breath out . . . Release all the poisons and toxins with your breath . . . Your breathing is cleansing you . . . healing you.
- Breathe in.
- Now imagine exhaling confusion . . . and inhaling clarity.
- Imagine exhaling darkness . . . and inhaling light.
- Imagine exhaling hatred . . . and inhaling love.
- Exhaling anxiety . . . and inhaling peace.
- Exhaling selfishness . . . and inhaling generosity.
- Exhaling guilt . . . and inhaling forgiveness.
- Exhaling weakness . . . and inhaling courage.
- Breathe in through your nose and sigh out through your mouth. Let the air stay out of your lungs as long as it is comfortable, and then take another breath.
- Let your breath return to its normal and natural pace. Continue to breath in slowly, smoothly, and deeply . . . Your breathing is steady, easy, silent.

---

relaxation audiotape available from Whole Persons Associates, and the *Desktop Yoga*™, available from Perigee Books, 1-800-631-8751.

- Each time you exhale . . . allow yourself to feel peaceful . . . calm . . . and completely relaxed . . . If your mind wanders, bring your attention back to your breath.
- Stretch and open your eyes, feeling refreshed and rejuvenated, alert, and full alive.

Repeat the above instructions until everyone is alert.

WHITE LIGHT OF HEALING ENERGY IMAGERY[5]

Begin to imagine that there is a sphere of white light of healing energy about 4 inches above your head. The white light is now touching the top of your head. Begin to feel this light as it flows from the top of your head and allow it to flow down through the entire inside of the body.

The healing light has filled the inside of your head . . . and it now flows down your shoulders, back, down your arms, and into your fingertips. The white light is now flowing into your chest . . . around your sides . . . into your middle and lower back . . . below your waist . . . around your sides flowing into your abdomen . . . into your buttocks . . . and into your pelvis. The light now flows down your thighs . . . to your lower legs . . . and to your feet.

The white light has now completely filled the inside of your body. There is now a wonderful abundance of this healing light . . . and it begins to bubble up and flow back out through the top of your head . . . down the outside of your body . . . coating the entire outside of your body. The more you allow it to flow throughout your body . . . the more abundant it is. Send the healing white light to specific areas that need extra attention, such as places of discomfort or disease.

INNER GUIDE IMAGERY[6]

As you begin to feel even more relaxed now . . . going to a greater depth of inner being . . . more relaxed . . . more secure and safe . . . let yourself become aware of the presence of not being alone. With you right now is a guide . . . who is wise and concerned with your well-being. Let yourself begin

---

[5]Source: Barbara Montgomery Dossey, "Imagery," *Holistic Nursing: A Handbook for Practice,* 2nd ed. Barbara Montgomery Dossey, Lynn Keegan, Cathie E. Guzetta, & L. Kolkmeier, Eds. Gaithersburg, MD: Aspen Publishers, Inc., © 1995.

[6]Source: Adapted from Barbara Montgomery Dossey, "Imagery: Awakening the Inner Healer," in Barbara Montgomery Dossey, Lynn Keegan, Cathie E. Guzzeetta, and Leslie Gooding Kolkmeier, *Holistic Nursing: A Handbook for Practice,* 2nd ed., Gaithersburg, MD: Aspen Publishers, Inc., © 1995.

to see this wise being with whom you can share your fears or your joys. You have trust in this wise guide.

If you do not see anyone, let yourself be aware of hearing or feeling this wise being, noticing the presence of care and concern. In whatever way seems best for you . . . proceed to make contact with the wise inner guide. Let yourself establish contact with your guide now . . . in any way that comes. Your guide may appear to you in any form, such as a person, an animal, or inner presence/peace . . . or as an image of the very wisest part of you.

Notice the love and wisdom with which you are surrounded. This wisdom and love are present for you now . . . Let yourself ask for advice . . . about anything that is important for you just now. Be receptive to what emerges . . . Let yourself receive some new information. This inner guide may have a special message to share with you . . . Listen with openness and pure intention to receive.

Allow yourself to look at any issue in your life. It may be a symptom, a choice, or decision . . . Tell your wise guide anything that you wish . . . Listen to the answers that emerge. Imagine yourself acting on the answers and directions that you received . . . Imagine yourself calling upon the wisdom and love of this wise guide to help you in the days to come. Now in whatever way is best for you . . . bring closure to the visit with this inner guide. You can come back here any time you wish. All you have to do is take the time.

IMAGERY FINDING ONE'S SPECIAL PLACE[7]

Begin by placing your body in a comfortable position, arms and legs uncrossed, back well supported. Now take three deep breaths, and during each breath relax you even more. Let the exhalation be a letting go kind of breath, letting go of tension. With each breath take in what you need and with each out breath, release anything you don't need. Bring your attention to the top of your head. Feel your scalp relax and let your brow soften and smooth out. Allow the muscles around your eyes to relax. And let any tension flow out through your cheeks as you exhale. Suggest that your jaw relax. Imagine a wave of relaxation flowing down your shoulders, into your arms, elbows, and forearms, all the way into your hands and fingers. Now focus on your chest, releasing any tension around your heart or lungs, relax the muscles around your ribs. Wrap that relaxation around your back and let a wave of relaxation travel all down the spine. Allow the muscles along the spine to lengthen and release. Soften and relax the buttocks and pelvis. Let the belly be very soft so that the breath moves easily

---

[7]Source: Shames, K. (1996). *Creative imagery in nursing.* New York: Delmar Publications.

down into the abdomen. Invite the legs to join in the relaxation now, as it moves through the thighs, knees, calves, ankles, and feet. Let any last bit of tension or tightness drain out through your feet or toes. When you feel relaxed and comfortable, let me know with a nod of your head. As your body remains relaxed and comfortable, imagine yourself in a very special place, somewhere that is full of natural beauty, safety, and peace. It may be a place you have been to before or it may be a place you want to create in your imagination. Take some time and let yourself be drawn to one place that is just right for you today. Let me know when you are present there (wait for response). Describe what it is like there. What do you see? Are there any smells? Are there any sounds? What is the temperature like? Where are you in this special place? How do you feel here? Take some time to do whatever you would like to do here, to relax or do some activity. Feel free to do whatever you want. This is your place.

In a few moments, it will be time to come back into a waking state. Know that you can return to this place again any time you want. Now gently bring yourself back, letting the images fade but keeping with you this relaxed and peaceful feeling. Remember what has been important about this experience. Become aware of the current time and place. Begin to move your body, take a deep breath, open your eyes, and feel relaxed and awake.

At this point, the guide can take a few minutes to allow the person to share his experience.

IMAGERY IN ONCOLOGY[8]

Cancer might well be the most feared disease of our time. Many people live their lives in dread and fear of cancer. The traditional medical treatments are terrifying and excruciating. Many nurses find it beneficial to work with the client's negative images and beliefs.

Some nurses have reported making tapes (there are also some available commercially) in which the client is encouraged to imagine chemotherapy or radiation therapy as something positive. Some clients prefer to view it as beams of energy or light.

The practitioner might ask "How do you imagine the chemotherapy?" Despite the response, the nurse can be helpful in supporting the transformation of the images into something beneficial and positive. "Imagine the medicine going into exactly the cells that most need it. The side effects will be minimal." There are a great variety of techniques and applications that enhance the healing journey through the experience of cancer.

---

[8]Source: Shames, K. (1996). *Creative imagery in nursing.* New York: Delmar Publications.

QUICK USES OF IMAGERY IN THE CLINICAL SETTING[9]

IVs

When a patient is receiving intravenous fluids, he can envision fluid flowing to every part, removing toxins and flushing them out. The patient can see nutrients providing nourishment to every cell.

Pain Medications

Similarly, the patient can enhance the benefits of pain medication by envisioning its soothing effects as it travels through the bloodstream, sedating any irritated areas and bringing a deep sense of relief throughout. (It is suggested that relaxation be used at the first sign of discomfort; focus the patient on the breath. Imagine the body releasing its natural medicine to all areas that are tense or uncomfortable. If pain begins to interfere with activity or rest, ask for medication before becoming so uncomfortable that it would be difficult to work with relaxation and the following imagery.)

"Imagine the pain medication to be exactly the strength it needs to be. See, feel, or sense the muscles around the painful area softening and relaxing as you breathe into the discomfort. See or feel the pain medication moving to that area numbing it as if it deposited a layer of frost.

"Imagining a dial registering a number from 1 to 10 that represents your pain now. See the number come down to your tolerance level. Allow an image to form of a special, quiet, restful place and allow yourself to be there as you rest."

Antibiotics

Some patients like to imagine their antibiotic medication in the bloodstream as hunters stalking their prey. They can envision that the medication stays where the most protection is needed, particularly around burns or incisions, ready to pounce. If more medication is needed, there is an endless supply in the imagination.

Anticoagulants

Likewise, clients using anticoagulant agents can envision their blood becoming thinner, flowing to exactly the right places to prevent clotting. They can

---

[9]Source: Olson, M. (1997b). *Healing the dying.* New York: Delmar Publications.

see the medication as extraordinarily efficient and relish in watching as it does its magic.

Oxygen

As you take a deep breath, send nourishing healing oxygen into every cell of your lungs, expanding each cell like a balloon. As you exhale, imagine letting the balloons completely deflate and blow any tension or toxins that remain in the body out into the air. Continue doing this slowly for a few minutes, watching the balloons expand and contract.

Healing Image

Imagine little workers repairing the muscles and bones while they are resting, allowing the healing process to begin. See the bone rich in calcium, and see little bone cells growing like coral, increasing in number and density.

Ideal Images

Many clients continue to envision their healing process long after the crises have passed. One way to do this is to imagine themselves in 3 or 6 months. They can imagine themselves exactly as they would wish to be. They can observe how they look, how they walk, their facial expressions. They might imagine themselves running or swimming, looking healthy and happy.

It is also a good practice for nurses to see themselves as they want to be. Focus on the image; how does it feel to be whole? Many nurses find that using imagery supports their patients totally and empowers them in their work. According to one nurse, after incorporating imagery frequently, "I finally felt if I were making a difference, despite the disempowering aspect of the environment."

DIAPHRAGMATIC BREATHING

Diaphragmatic breathing is a useful technique to learn for relaxing and to begin the centering process. Consciously realizing the path each inhalation takes through the respiratory passages, and allowing each breath to move to the bottom of the respiratory tree by moving the diaphragm downward and outward moves the whole person toward feeling more relaxed. As the slow, long exhalation occurs, a person feels shoulders moving downward and tensions slowly leaving the body. To help with stress at work, a nurse should practice diaphragmatic breathing at home, in either a supine or sitting position. Putting one's hand on the abdomen is an easy way to know if the abdomen is involved in the breath, or if shallow, tense breaths are a pattern. Once a pattern of abdominal breathing is the norm, the nurse can think words like, "I can feel this way whenever I take a deep breath and cross my fingers." Connecting the relaxed feeling to the physical act of crossing fingers (on another physical cue) helps the body to remember how it feels to relax. A nurse who regularly practices this technique will have the ability to break the cycle of stress and muscle tension identified even at the bedside of a dying patient in just a few seconds. The pattern is:

- Recognize the feeling of tension
- Take an abdominal breath
- Use a physical cue that has been practiced
- Allow the shoulders to sag and relaxation to be experienced during the exhalation

This technique, or pattern, is useful by itself to help relax for a few minutes or to lead to more profound states of relaxation.

RESOURCES

Academy for Guided Imagery
P.O. Box 2070
Mill Valley, CA 94942
p. (800) 726-2070
f. (415) 389-9342

Acupuncture
National Acupuncture and Oriental Medicine Alliance
14637 Starr Road, SE
Olalla, WA 98359
(253) 851-6896

American Association for Music Therapy (AAMT)
P.O. Box 27177
Philadelphia, PA 19918
(215) 265-4006

American Psychological Association
750 First Street, NE
Washington, DC 20002-4242
(800) 374-2721

Aromatherapy
National Association for Holistic Aromatherapy
836 Hanley Industrial Court
St. Louis, MO 63144
(888) ASK-NAHA/
(888) 275-6242

Biofeedback
Association for Applied Psychophysiology & Biofeedback
10200 W. 44th Avenue, Suite 304
Wheat Ridge, CO 80003
(303) 422-8436

Compassionate Touch
20 Swan Court
Walnut Creek, CA 94596
(510) 935-3906

Herbal Medicine
American Holistic Medical Association
6728 Old McLean Village Drive
McLean, VA 22101
(703) 556-9245

Homeopathy
National Center for Homeopathy
801 N. Fairfax Street, Suite 306
Alexandria, VA 22314
(703) 548-7790

Maharishi Vedic University
1401 Ocean Avenue
Asbury Park, NJ 07712
(908) 774-9446

National Association of Music Therapy (NAMT)
8455 Colesville Road, Suite 930
Silver Springs, MD 20910
(301) 589-3300

Reiki
International Center for Reiki Training
29209 Northwestern Highway,
#592
Southfield, MI 48034
(800) 332-8112

Therapeutic Touch
Nurse Healers-Professional Associates, Inc.
1211 Locust Street
Philadelphia, PA 19107
(215) 545-8079

Transcendental Meditation
(888) 532-7686

Transcendental Meditation Program
(888) LEARN TM
www.tm.org

Education Plan 2.1 Plan for Achieving Competencies: Holistic Integrative Therapies in Palliative Care

Knowledge	Attitude	Skills	Undergraduate Behavioral Outcomes	Graduate Behavioral Outcomes	Teaching/Learning Strategies
Assumptions and philosophy of holistic care and healing within the context of dying.	*Accept the assumptions and philosophy of holistic therapies in end-of-life care. *Appreciate the ability to heal within the context of dying.		*Verbalize an appreciation for holistic, complementary care for patients and families.	*Evaluate the relationship between the use of holistic, complementary modalities and quality of life for patients and families.	*Document personal assumptions/philosophy regarding healing, holistic care, and the value of complementary therapies in a journal. *Develop a case study that reveals healing at the end of life.
Discussion of specific holistic therapies and application to palliative care.	*Affirm the benefits of holistic, complementary therapies at the end of life.	*Demonstrate the steps of simple holistic, complementary therapies.	*Inform patient and family about the value and availability of holistic healing therapies. *Administer simple holistic integrative therapies in the care of patients and families at the end of life.	*Administer more complex holistic healing therapies.	*Conduct a selected holistic, complementary therapy in class, seminar, or post-conference each week.

Education Plan 2.1 *(continued)*

Knowledge	Attitude	Skills	Undergraduate Behavioral Outcomes	Graduate Behavioral Outcomes	Teaching/Learning Strategies
Healing journey: tasks for dying consciously	*Personally consider the tasks for dying consciously.	*Engage in activities that promote emotional or spiritual tasks of dying consciously.		*Role model activities that promote emotional or spiritual tasks of dying consciously.	*Rehearse the dying process by creating a story of students'/nurses' own death and sharing this story and associated feelings with a fellow student, faculty, or colleague. *Document in a journal a written plan to complete unfinished business.
Self-care for the healer	*Value self-care.		*Perform healing therapies with colleagues to reduce caregiver stress. *Engage in self-care activities daily.	*Role model comprehensive self-care behaviors. *Identify alternative self-care strategies.	*Create an inventory of self-care activities within the last month and evaluate their adequacy. *Perform one self-care activity each day with journal documentation.

REFERENCES

Abrahms, E. (1999). Reiki. In N. Allison (Ed.), *The illustrated encyclopedia of body-mind disciplines* (pp. 133–136). New York: The Rosen Publishing Group, Inc.

Allison, N. (1999a). Guided imagery. In N. Allison (Ed.), *The illustrated encyclopedia of body-mind disciplines* (pp. 71–73). New York: The Rosen Publishing Group, Inc.

Barrett, E., & Kolkmeier, L. (1997). Relaxation. In B. Dossey (Ed.), *Core curriculum for holistic nursing* (pp. 182–187). Gaithersburg, MD: Aspen Publications.

Benson, H. (1995). *Beyond the relaxation process.* New York: Berkley Books.

Borysenko, J. (1990). *Guilt is the teacher, love is the lesson.* New York: Warner Books.

Bourne, E. (1995). *The anxiety & phobia workbook,* Second Edition. New Harbinger Publications, Inc.

Credit, L., Hartunian, S., & Nowak, M. (1998). *Your guide to complementary medicine.* New York: Avery Publishing Group.

Dossey, B. (1995a). Peaceful deathing and death. In B. Dossey, L. Keegan, C. Guzzetta, & L. Kolkmeier, *Holistic nursing a handbook for practice* (2nd ed.) (pp. 429–454). Gaithersburg, MD: Aspen Publications.

Dossey, B. (1995b). Imagery: Awakening the inner healer. In B. Dossey, L. Keegan, C. Guzzetta, & L. Kolkmeier, *Holistic nursing a handbook for practice* (2nd ed.) (pp. 609–666). Gaithersburg, MD: Aspen Publications.

Duke, J. (1997). *The green pharmacy.* New York: St. Martin's Press.

Frank-Schwebel, A. (1999). Music therapy. In N. Allison (Ed.), *The illustrated encyclopedia of body-mind disciplines* (pp. 366–369). New York: The Rosen Publishing Group, Inc.

Gatchel, R., & Maddrey, A. (1998). Clinical outcome research in complementary and alternative medicine: An overview of experimental design and analysis. *Alternative Therapies, 4*(5), 36–43.

Giasson, M., & Bouchard, L. (1998). Effect of therapeutic touch on the well-being of persons with terminal cancer. *Journal of Holistic Nursing, 16*(3), 393–398.

Guzzetta, C. (1995). Music therapy: Healing the melody of the soul. In B. Dossey, L. Keegan, C. Guzzetta, & L. Kolkmeier, *Holistic nursing a handbook for practice* (2nd ed.) (pp. 669–698). Gaithersburg, MD: Aspen Publications.

Hall, R. (1997). A comparison of three unconventional cancer therapies. *Alternative Health Practitioner The Journal of Complementary and Natural Care, 3*(3), 167–176.

Kolkmeier, L. (1995a). Self-reflection: Consulting the truth within. In B. Dossey, L. Keegan, C. Guzzetta, & L. Kolkmeier, *Holistic nursing a handbook for practice* (2nd ed.). Gaithersburg, MD: Aspen Publications.

Kolkmeier, L. (1995b). Relaxation: Opening the door to change. In B. Dossey, L. Keegan, C. Guzzetta, & L. Kolkmeier, *Holistic nursing a handbook for practice* (2nd ed.) (pp. 573–606). Gaithersburg, MD: Aspen Publications.

Krieger, D. (1997). *Therapeutic touch inner workbook.* Santa Fe, NM: Bear & Company Publications.

Laurant, R., & Shlien, J. (1984). *Client centered therapy and the person centered approach.* New York: Praeger.

Lusk, J. *30 scripts for relaxation, imagery, and inner healing.* Duluth, MN: Whole Persons Associates.

Macrae, J. (1987). *Therapeutic touch a practical guide.* New York: Alfred A. Knopf.

Mariano, C. (1998). Preparing nurses to deliver holistic care. *Spectrum, 10*(22), 14–15.

McBride, S., Graydon, J., Sidani, S., & Hall, L. (1999). Therapeutic use of music for dyspnea and anxiety in patients with COPD. *Journal of Holistic Nursing, 17*(3), 229–250.

McCraty, R., Barrios-Chaplin, B., Atkinson, M., & Tomasino, D. (1998). The effects of different types of music on mood, tension and mental clarity. *Alternative Therapies, 4*(1), 75–84.

Nelson, D. (1994). *Compassionate touch hands on caregiving for the elderly, the ill and the dying.* Barraytown, NY: Station Hill Press, Inc.

Olson, M. (1997a). Death and grief. In B. Dossey (Ed.), *Core curriculum for holistic nursing*. Gaithersburg, MD: Aspen Publications.

Olson, M. (1997b). *Healing the dying*. New York: Delmar Publications.

Payne, R. (1998). *Relaxation techniques a practical handbook for the health care professional*. New York: Churchill Livingston.

Quinn, J. (1985). In D. Kunz, *Spiritual aspects of the healing arts*. Wheaton, IL: Theosophical Publishing House.

Roach, S., & Nieto, B. (1997). *Healing and the grief process*. New York: Delmar Publications.

Robins, J. (1999). The science and art of aromatherapy. *Journal of Holistic Nursing, 12*(1), 5–17.

Rossman, M. (1999). Interactive guided imagery. In N. Allison (Ed.), *The illustrated encyclopedia of body-mind disciplines* (pp. 77–78). New York: The Rosen Publishing Group, Inc.

Schroeder-Sheker, T. (1994). Music for the dying. *Journal of Holistic Nursing, 12*(1), 83–99.

Shames, K. (1996). *Creative imagery in nursing*. New York: Delmar Publications.

Tinnerman, G. (1999). Using self care strategies to make lifestyle changes. *Journal of Holistic Nursing, 17*(2), 169–183.

Worden, J. (1982). *Grief counseling and grief therapy: A handbook for the mental health practitioner*. New York: Springer Publication Company.

PART 2

Social Aspects of Palliative Care

June 11, 2000

 I remembered Candy as soon as I saw her name on my patient list. When I walked in the house, I couldn't believe what a difference a year made! A hospital bed was now in the living room and Candy was sitting in a chair with oxygen on. She was short of breath with minimal activity. I was there to give her a Vancomycin infusion, so I had plenty of time to catch up on what had been going on with her. Apparently after her discharge from our agency a year ago, she had done well, although she was never able to return to her nursing position. Despite all of her holistic and medical therapies she continued to develop problems. She had a bowel obstruction, which resulted in a colostomy, and then the incision opened and was still not healed at the top or the bottom. Due to cardiac failure, she had significant peripheral edema. It was as though everything that could have gone wrong, did go wrong.

 She was not on our hospice service but rather receiving home care while she still pursued a cure for her disease. She told me she wasn't "ready to give up yet," and that no one had told her how long she had left. I asked her if she had ever asked her oncologist this question and she said she hadn't . . . she said she wasn't ready to think about death yet. I respected what she was telling me and didn't pursue it further. My intuition was that she had less than 6 months to live.

 In looking through her chart, there was no documentation of an advanced directive or appointment of a health care proxy. When I asked her about these documents, she said that she did not want to give control for her health care over to anyone. I explained that advance directives would allow her to maintain control over health care decisions at the end of life. We had a long talk about advanced directives, specifically her wishes and preferences regarding life-prolonging therapies when all efforts were viewed as medically futile. Laughing, she said she should have her friends over for an "advance directive" party and invite a notary to make them all official. She still maintained her sense of humor even in the face of death. She decided to appoint her husband as her health care proxy, believing that he would advocate in her best interest and communicate with members of the interdisciplinary team her end-of-life wishes. Candy showed tremendous strength and courage. By making such personal decisions, she hoped to maintain a sense of personal dignity as death approached.

3

Death and Society

Marilyn Bookbinder and Margaret Kiss

AACN Competencies

#1: Recognize dynamic changes in population demographics, health care economics, and service delivery that necessitate improved professional preparation for end-of-life care.

#13: Identify barriers and facilitators to patients' and caregivers' effective use of resources.

#15: Apply knowledge gained from palliative care research to end-of-life education and care.

> In the end, the question comes down to one of control over how a particular life ends and who has the power to make that decision and implement it.
>
> —Robinson, 1990

At the turn of the 20th century, Americans died from diseases such as yellow fever, small pox, diphtheria, and cholera. Death was often rapid with little time to say "good-bye" to loved ones. In 1900, life expectancy was less than 50 years of age for both men and women, while in the year 2000, the median age of death is 77 years old. Currently, Americans are struggling to develop a health care system that is both cost-effective and can ensure both a "good life" and "good death." This chapter addresses the changes and issues surrounding death in society in the 20th century, their impact on quality patient care, and the role of educators in preparing nurses to care for patients and families experiencing life-threatening illness. As we begin this new millennium, two landmark studies from the 1990s, specifically the Study to Understand Prognosis and Preferences for Outcomes and Risks of Treatments (SUPPORT, 1995) and the Institute of Medicine's Report (IOM, 1997) provide evidence of the need to improve the care of the dying in America. This is the challenge of nurses and all health professionals as we enter the 21st century.

CHANGES IN THE DEFINITION OF DEATH IN SOCIETY

Over the last few decades, the concept of "death" has raised many moral and ethical dilemmas for society. The New Encyclopedia Britannica (1999) defines death as "the total cessation of life processes that eventually occurs in all living organism." It goes on to say that "human death has always been obscured by mystery and superstition, and its precise definition remains controversial, differing according to culture and legal systems." Indeed, the experience of death has changed, as death in the first half of the century usually occurred from an acute or unexpected event, while today, many deaths occur following degenerative diseases that entail a long and declining course. In 1967, Kubler-Ross's seminal research and interviews with dying patients raised our awareness about the dual concept of death: death—the event, and dying—the process. Her psychological stages of dying, specifically denial, anger, bargaining, depression, and acceptance, though questioned today, have revolutionized our thinking about death. Although no consensus currently exists about when "dying" or "end of life" begins, the American Geriatrics Society (AGS) (1997) offers clinicians guidelines for making this determination with the statement, "people are considered to be dying when they have a progressive illness that is expected to end in death and for which there is no treatment that can substantially alter the outcome."

Although the "precise determination of death" is not a focus for this chapter, nurses may care for those patients whose families' fear being declared dead prematurely, for example, when the determination of death is extended to assure viability of organs for transplantation. The ability to prolong life and sustain life with artificial means necessitates the need for additional definitions of death. For legal purposes, "brain death" is considered to be the irreversible cessation of circulatory and respiratory function or the irreversible cessation of all functions of the entire brain, including the brain stem. Bioethicists and sociologists recommend the notion of "social death," referring to individuals who have lost their personhood by losing function of their cortex (Brody, 1988). Botkin and Post (1992) proposed that death be viewed as a "syndrome" requiring that a cluster of related attributes be present before a diagnosis of brain death can be made.

The different views of death reflect the multidimensional nature of the concept. Professionals need to be cognizant of varying definitions of death and the issues raised by each perspective. Some issues include:

- When should we remove life support and how should we support families?
- What are the risks/benefits of feeding versus not feeding patients at the end of life?
- When and from whom should we remove organs for transplantation?
- What skills and training do nurses need to serve as advocates to dying patients and families?
- What evidence is available to help nurses provide "best practices" in caring for patients and families experiencing life-threatening, and terminal illness?

In palliative care, death is also viewed as an outcome measure for improving end-of-life care. The Institute of Medicine's (IOM) report (1997) provides some conceptual benchmarks from which quality outcome indicators can be developed. A "good death" is defined as: one free from avoidable stress and suffering for patients and families and caregivers; in general accord with patients' and families' wishes; and reasonably consistent with clinical, cultural, and ethical standards. In contrast, a "bad death" is one in which there is needless suffering, disregard for patients' or family's wishes or values, and a sense among participants or observers that the norms of decency have been offended

The fear of experiencing a "bad death" seems warranted by the conclusions of a 5-year study of the end-of-life care received by 9,000 dying hospitalized patients. The *Study to Understand Prognosis and Preferences for Outcomes and Risks of Treatments* (SUPPORT, 1995) was designed both to increase understanding of hospitalized dying and to devise an intervention to promote more humane care of dying patients. The SUPPORT data confirmed the high reports of pain among dying patients (more than 50%), clinicians' lack of training in pain management, and institutional limitations on the delivery of pain control interventions. In addition, the SUPPORT data confirmed that patients' end-of-life treatment preferences, whether written or verbally communicated to nurses or family members, were often ignored by physicians or were otherwise ineffective in furthering the autonomous choices made by patients (SUPPORT, 1995).

TABOOS IN ACKNOWLEDGING DEATH

Death in the United States remains a taboo topic. Taboo, a Polynesian word, refers to something sacred or unclean. The object of a taboo in Polynesia is believed to have a power, or mana, so strong that only priests approach it. It is believed in some cultures that breaking the taboo requires ritual purification, or even death of the offender, to cleanse the community (The Concise Columbia Electronic Encyclopedia, 1994). Awareness of the objects, words, or acts associated with religious or cultural rituals are important in supporting and communicating with members of varying social/religious groups and planning end-of-life (EOL) care. For example, early American Indians shot arrows in the air to ward off evil spirits; military funerals often use this same ritual when guns are fired in the air as the last salute. Indeed, the traditional tombstone may have originated to keep the "bad spirits" down deep in the ground.

As death approaches, some individuals are inspired to search for meaning, peace, or transcendence that can replace fear and despair with hope and serenity (Byock, 1997). For others, grief, shame, guilt, and anger become overwhelming emotions, which prolong the period of grief or surface later in other areas of the mourner's life. In many households, it is taboo to speak of death, especially in the presence of children. Parents often consider death as morbid and "too much" for children to handle. Children may even be sent off to a relative and told a lie such as "Mommie has gone on a long trip" to avoid the topic. Unfortunately, when the child eventually learns the truth problems can arise such as unresolved guilt, distrust for grown-ups, and poor coping skills. Discussions about death make most people uncomfortable, including health care providers, and can trigger people's feelings about their own demise. Clearly, the SUPPORT study (1995) findings validate the need for improved physician-patient communication regarding goals of care and end-of-life decision making.

In addition to providing quality care to an ever-aging and diverse population, clinicians need to integrate patients' and families' racial, ethnic, cultural, and religious and nonreligious rituals and beliefs into care planning. Nurses should assess patients' perceptions, preferences, and behaviors and individualize communication and care strategies so as to respect these differences in the context of their organizational systems. Consumers are becoming more educated and vocal about their needs and options, especially those having Internet access, to sophisticated medical information. While information empowers some patients, it can create confusion for others and place them in a quandary regarding decision making (Desbiens, Mueller-Rizner, Hamel, & Connors, 1998). It is important that clinicians develop consensus about how they will evaluate patient and family education regarding end-of-life issues, and provide culturally relevant resources and other sources of support.

MORBIDITY AND MORTALITY STATISTICS FOR THE UNITED STATES: LEADING CAUSES OF DEATH

Statistics from 1995 show that black women can expect to live to 74 years compared to 79.6 years for white women; black men can expect to live 65.4 years compared to 73.4 years for white males (IOM, 1997). These data reflect an increase of nearly a quarter of a century in life expectancy in the United States that can be attributed in part to advances in sanitation, nutrition, and immunization, which have eradicated or greatly reduced diseases. The four leading causes of death in the United States continue to be heart disease (33%), cancer (23%), cerebrovascular disease (7%), and chronic obstructive pulmonary disease (4.6%). Accidents account for another 4.0% and pneumonia another 3.7%. In 1996, National Vital Statistics from the Centers for Disease Control and Prevention revealed that the U.S. death rate decreased and reached an all-time low of 491.6 deaths per 100,000. The largest decline in age-adjusted death rates among the leading causes of death was for Human Immunodeficiency Virus infection, which dropped 28.8% in 1996, compared with the previous year. While mortality rates differ by age and race, the general mortality rate of 1996 continued the downward trend.

WHERE ARE PEOPLE DYING?

Little is known about where dying patients spend their last few months of life, however, mortality statistics from 1992 indicate that 57% of deaths occurred in hospitals, 15% in nursing homes, 20% in residences, and 6% elsewhere, including those declared dead on arrival at the hospital (IOM, 1997). About 55 to 60% of persons older than age 65 die in the hospital (Kaufman, 1998). Recent findings from SUPPORT Investigators (Pritchard, 1998) support the national polls that while most people prefer to die at home the majority died in the hospital. The number of patients dying in-hospital varied between 29% and 66% in the five research sites across the United States, with 23 to 54% of these cases being Medicare beneficiaries. Investigators found that measures of hospital availability and use were the most powerful predictors of the place of death. The chance of dying in a hospital was increased for residents of regions with a greater availability of hospital beds. The risk was decreased in regions that had greater nursing home and hospice availability and use. Variations within groups were not explained by sociodemographic, clinical, or patient preferences.

In previous centuries the majority of people died at home. By the mid-seventies, more than 70% of deaths were occurring in hospitals and other institutional settings (National Hospice Organization, 1997b). The shift in the location of dying had a dramatic impact on the nature of dying. Patients dying at home were usually cared for by family members with little or no high technology equipment. The institutionalization of death raised a new set of challenges and problems for caregivers. Challenges include: increased decision making about the extent of aggressive treatments; how to support and provide proper care for the dying; how to deal with the isolation and depersonalization of institutions; and how to best meet the nonphysical but critically important sociological, spiritual, and emotional needs of patients and family members. Additional regulations placed on institutions from managed care organizations often resulted in earlier discharges, shortened lengths of stay and follow-up home care needs far greater than previously experienced. This is validated in data from 1988 through 1994, in which program payments for Medicare-covered home care services grew more than 500%, from $1.7 billion to $12.7 billion, and the number of certified home health agencies grew from approximately 5,700 to 7,800 (HCFA, 1996; IOM, 1997).

The literature describes an often fragmented approach to the care of the dying in institutions which led to undermining the patient's identity, wishes, and sense of self-worth. Institutionalization often served to isolate the family and to rob them of the opportunity to confront their own impending loss and adapt to the new roles and responsibilities ahead. Given proper support, most experts agree that families are able to resolve issues and become a strong source of support and caregiving for the patient. Ira Byock's (1997) book, entitled "Dying Well," illustrates through stories the prospect for growth and ability to achieve death-with-dignity at the end of life for patients and families. The hospice movement grew in response to this fragmentation of health care; the two strongest proponents for change came from the community and health care professionals who recognized inadequacies in end-of-life care.

DEATH TRAJECTORIES

Americans are living longer with chronic or terminal illnesses, resulting in the need for increases in assistance, symptom management, and hospice care services. There are many paths leading toward death. Patients who understand that they have a progressive disease from which they will likely die may not see themselves, or be seen by their families and friends, as dying. This group is differentiated from those thought to be imminently dying (i.e., likely to die within minutes to days), and those who are terminally ill but not thought to be actively dying (i.e., having a life expectancy of days to months and sometimes years). The latter group may have a period of prolonged "chronic living-dying" between the diagnosis of incurable illness and imminent death (McCormick & Conley, 1995). Patients in this group may be able to carry out their daily activities while coping with the prospect of death. Pediatric patients, for example, can live years to decades with illness such as cystic fibrosis. In the case of chronically ill older adults, premature death may suddenly occur from a superimposed viral illness, such as pneumonia.

The National Institute on Aging's agenda (NIA, 2000) for the years 2001 to 2005 has targeted three areas for research: 1) preventing or reducing age-related diseases, disorders, and disability; 2) maintaining physical health and function; and 3) enhancing older adults' societal roles and interpersonal support, and reducing social isolation. The aging population is at increased risk for developing multiple chronic or life-threatening diseases, including heart disease, cancer, stroke, respiratory diseases, and other terminal illnesses, such as Alzheimer's disease. Health care costs can increase and quality of life and independence may be compromised for older adults and the terminally ill by weakness, falls, delirium, urinary incontinence, sleep disturbances, and serious depression. Living months or years with disease presents patients, families, and clinicians with social, moral/ethical, and medical dilemmas.

Technologies that sustain life with artificial means have increased our ability to prolong life, yet they have raised many moral, ethical, and legal dilemmas for Americans. Some bioethicists contend that the real political struggles of the 20th century have not been over legal rights, but over control in the "way" individuals live their lives. Supreme Court rulings regarding the right to: abortion; to die; cause death; make family decisions; live; control one's own body; health care; refuse hydration; and to self-determination are examples of health care issues brought forth in the last few decades (Annas, 1993).

Nurses are an essential voice in these discussions in their roles as patient and family advocates, clinicians, leaders, health care policy makers, educators, and as researchers. Education in the legal, moral/ethical principles, and decision-making models are essential for nurses to have an impact in determining the quality of care offered to individuals at the end of life and empowering patients to take an active role in achieving this outcome.

PATIENT-REQUESTED EUTHANASIA AND ASSISTED SUICIDE

Assisted suicide is described as a practice by which health care providers supply, but do not directly administer, the means for a patient to voluntarily hasten his or her own death. This is usually done by prescribing lethal doses of medication that the patient then ingests (IOM, 1997). Patient-requested euthanasia refers to a practice in which the means of hastening death are administered directly by the health care provider (Matzo & Emmanuel, 1997), for example, injecting the patient with a lethal dose of medication. Brody (1992), a nationally known physician/ethicist, originated the term "assistance in dying" and claimed that patients capable of decision making could request assistance to achieve a "good death."

Since the 1970s there have been notable events that have shaped a new conceptualization and legal system related to the end of life and causing or assisting death (Table 3.1). The activities of Dr. Kevorkian, a nonlicensed pathologist who has admitted to assisting over 130 people to commit suicide, fueled the media and heightened public awareness about euthanasia and assisted suicide. One example of media coverage was the viewing of Dr. Kevorkian administering a lethal injection to a 52-year-old man with Lou Gehrig's disease on the "60 Minutes" television series (November, 1998). Although he was found guilty in 1999 of second degree murder and sen-

---

TABLE 3.1   Events Raising Public Awareness About Assisted Dying

- The first "right to die" case of Karen Ann Quinlan, NJ. Parents request permission to withdraw use of a respirator on their comatose young daughter.
- California "Natural Death Act" empowered patients to specify end-of-life wishes in a living will.
- Patient Self-Determination Act. Hospital patients are informed of their right to make treatment decisions.
- Opinion poll shows majority of Americans support assisted suicide.
- Study to Understand Prognosis and Preferences for Outcomes and Risks of Treatments (SUPPORT). Five-year study results include inadequate pain management at end of life.
- Dr. Kevorkian's activities criticized by physicians and ethicists for assisting more than 130 people to commit suicide.
- Americans continue to view assisted dying as a reasonable alternative to the fear of dying a lonely, undignified, prolonged, and painful, institutionalized death.
- Death with Dignity Act legalizes physician-assisted suicide in Oregon.
- Dr. Kevorkian found guilty of second-degree murder and sentenced to 10 to 25 years in prison.

---

tenced to 10–25 years of imprisonment, many Americans still view assisted dying as a "responsible alternative" to their fear of dying a lonely, undignified, prolonged, painful, or institutionalized death (Annas, 1995).

Although Oregon became the first state to legalize assisted suicide (but not euthanasia) in 1997 via the "Death with Dignity Act," physicians are cautious in granting their patient's requests for such assistance. A recent survey found that physicians granted approximately one in six requests for a prescription for a lethal dose of medication, and one in 10 requests actually resulted in suicide (Ganzini et al., 2000). The authors documented that effective palliative care interventions led some patients to change their minds about committing suicide. These data confirm other results that show patients who receive good symptom control at the end of life choose life over death (Coyle, 1992; Foley, 1995). The IOM (1997) cautions professionals in states considering legalizing assisted suicide that no one who chooses suicide does so because the health care system has failed to meet the needs of dying patients.

Although public debates about assisted dying have focused almost exclusively on physician practices (Bachman, Alcser, Doukis, Lichtenstein, Corning, et al., 1996), nurses' reports of their experiences with assisted dying are increasing. Schwarz's (1999) integrated review of bioethics and nursing literature (from 1990–1999) reveals the dilemmas faced by many nurses in discriminating between "hastening" and "assisting" death when caring for patients with severe symptom distress at the end of life. When 80 nurses were interviewed about the circumstances under which they felt justified in performing patient-requested euthanasia, 21% of the nurses were ethically able to justify active euthanasia and 16% indicated that they viewed patient autonomy and the presence of severe suffering as justifications (Davis et al., 1995). In Asch's 1996 study of 1,139 critical care nurses' self-reported clinical experiences with assisted dying, 16% (n = 129) reported participating in assisted suicide or patient-requested euthanasia. Recurring themes in their comments included concerns about overuse of life-sustaining technology, a profound sense of responsibility for the patient's welfare, a desire to relieve patient suffering to overcome the perceived unresponsiveness of physicians toward that suffering. Matzo and Emmanuel's (1997) survey of 441 oncology nurses (71% response rate) revealed that 131 (30%) nurses received up to 20 requests for lethal drugs in the previous year. Of this group, 1% (n = 6) acknowledged helping a patient to commit suicide and 4.5% (n = 20) reported performing patient-requested euthanasia.

Ferrell, Virani, Grant, Coyne, and Uman (2000) surveyed 2,333 nurses' perspectives on end-of-life care; their results support the need for closer examination of nurses' participation in assisted dying. Less than 1% of the nurses report participation but these findings are troubling and indicate the need to better understand nurses' conduct despite the ANA Code for Nurses prohibiting such practices. There is much support for the argument that if good symptom management were provided to dying patients, requests for assisted dying could be virtually eliminated (Coyle, 1992; Hall, 1996; Kazanowski, 1997; Kowalski, 1997; Murphy, 1992). This is especially important since skilled palliative care and hospice clinicians report being capable of making the dying process tolerable, if not completely comfortable, for almost 95% of their patients (Coyle, 1992; Foley, 1996; Quill, 1993).

Research regarding nurses' practices are needed. The questions to be answered involve the barriers that nurses encounter when trying to provide the best end-of-life care and access to palliative or hospice care for dying patients? Nurse educators, in particular, are challenged to help their students caring for highly symptomatic dying patients to distinguish between those acts presumed to be morally and professionally permissible and illegal acts of "assisted" dying (Schwarz, 1999).

EVIDENCE OF THE NEED TO IMPROVE END-OF-LIFE CARE

Two major studies within the last decade have identified priority areas for end-of-life care; the SUPPORT study (1995) and the Institute of Medicine Report (1997). Few clinical research projects have generated as much public interest or as many published articles as the SUPPORT study. This $29 million multiyear research project (funded by the Robert Wood Johnson Foundation), revealed the failure of the American Health Care System to provide effective and compassionate care to seriously ill and dying patients. The study began with a 2-year prospective observational study (phase I) of 4,301 patients followed by a 2-year controlled clinical trial (Phase II) in which 4,804 patients and their physicians were randomized by specialty group to an intervention group (n = 2652) or control group (n = 2152). The "intervention" took the form of a specially trained nurse who had multiple contacts with patient, family, physician, and hospital staff to: elicit preferences; encourage attention to pain control; facilitate advance care planning and physician/patient communication.

Results from Phase I documented the lack of communication between patients and physicians and provided characteristics about hospital deaths. Specifically, the results indicated that 46% of DNR orders were written within 2 days of death; 47% of physicians knew when their patient wanted to avoid CPR; 38% of patients who died spent at least 10 days in the ICU; 50% of patients who died in the hospital had moderate to severe pain (reported by families) at least half the time; and there was a high use of hospital resources. No improvements were found in the above outcomes following the Phase II nurse intervention. The findings from the SUPPORT study have provided the impetus for leaders in all health disciplines to develop and implement initiatives in research, education, and practice to improve end-of-life care for patients and their families.

The second major landmark report was produced by the Institute of Medicine (IOM), entitled "*Approaching Death: Improving Care at the End of Life*" (1997). This report is based on the collaborative efforts of a committee of 12 experts in medicine and nursing who cared for chronically ill and severely ill patients. The IOM report summarized issues that should be addressed regarding end-of-life care: 1) the state of the knowledge in EOL care; 2) evaluation methods for measuring outcomes; 3) factors impeding high-quality care; and 4) steps toward agreement on what constitutes "appropriate care" at end of life. The committee's four major findings, listed below, suggest starting points for quality improvement (QI) work in terms of patient care, organizations, education, and research:

- Too many people suffer endlessly at the end of life both from errors of omission (when caregivers fail to provide palliative and supportive care known to be effective) and from errors of commission (when caregivers do what is known to be ineffective and even harmful);
- Legal, organizational, and economic obstacles conspire to obstruct reliably excellent care at the end of life;
- The education and training of physicians and other health care professionals fail to provide them with knowledge, skills, and attitudes required to care for the dying patient; and
- Current knowledge and understanding are inadequate to guide and support consistent practice of evidence-based medicine at the end of life.

The IOM report concluded that the current knowledge is inadequate to guide the practice of clinicians in end of life care. Funding and resources targeted to improve care at the end of life are national in scope and include national, state, and local initiatives. There is also funding from private foundations such as the Open Society Institute's "Project on Death in America," the Commonwealth Fund, the United Hospital Fund as well as various professional organizations.

PALLIATIVE CARE AS AN AREA OF SPECIALTY PRACTICE

The hospice concept originated in the Middle Ages when pilgrims traveling to the Holy Land found their minds and bodies restored when they stopped at "way stations" attended by religious orders. Hospices, originally opened by the Irish Sisters of Charity in Dublin, Ireland (1879), moved to London by 1905. Dame Cicely Saunders, a nurse, who later became a social worker and physician, is credited with opening Saint Christopher's Hospice in London where she championed the need for a multidisciplinary approach and "around the clock" administration of opioids when caring for dying patients. Her approach to care focused on comfort, skilled nursing, family counseling, physical therapy, and addressing spiritual needs (Storey, 1996). These fundamental elements of care characterize quality palliative care.

Florence Wald, another nurse recognized for her pioneer work in the hospice movement in the United States, envisioned the need to maximize the quality of life for the terminally ill. Following a trip to St Christopher's, in the 1960s, she returned home to conduct a feasibility study of the need for a hospice in Connecticut. The United States subsequently opened their first hospice in Branford, Connecticut in 1974 (Friedrich, 1999). Wald, inducted into the Women's Hall of Fame in 1998, is known for her exemplary work in influencing hospices throughout the country, promoting holistic and humanistic care for the dying, and advocating for nurses' education regarding care at the end of life. The Hospice model serves as the "gold standard" for offering the best end-of-life care to patients and their families.

SIMILARITIES AND DIFFERENCES BETWEEN HOSPICE AND PALLIATIVE CARE

Palliative care found its roots in the hospice movement. The World Health Organization (WHO, 1990) defines palliative care as "the active total care of patients whose disease is not responsive to curative treatment when control of pain, of other symptoms and of psychological, social and spiritual problems is paramount. The goal of palliative care is the best possible quality of life for patients and their families" (p. 152). Palliative care affirms life and regards dying as a normal process that is neither hastened nor postponed. Palliative care provides: relief from pain and other distressing symptoms; integrates the psychological and spiritual aspects of patient care; and offers a support system to help the family cope during the patient's illness and in their own bereavement (Storey, 1996).

Portenoy (1998) describes the differences between palliative and hospice care; access to hospice has been traditionally limited to patients who have a life expectancy of less than 6 months and are no longer pursuing active treatment, palliative care is offered from the time a patient is diagnosed with a life-threatening illness. Due to a typically late referral to hospice, the length of stay for hospice patients is relatively short and averages only about

20 days (Avellanet, 2000). Physicians are less reluctant to refer patients to the palliative care team because it does not carry the absolute association with death that Hospice care does. Hospice programs usually require a Do Not Resuscitate order, insurers may not allow high-tech life-prolonging therapies or they may limit access to medical specialists. While palliative care programs also strive to relieve the pain and suffering associated with any life-threatening illness, they do not mandate foregoing of life-prolonging therapies. The goal of treatment remains achieving the optimal quality of life for patients and families.

The Medicare Hospice benefit is based on a probability prediction that an individual with a terminal or incurable illness will not survive for longer than 6 months. Palliative care experts, however, have long recognized the need to provide access to comprehensive services earlier in the disease trajectory. According to Portenoy (1998), the model of palliative care addresses both disease-specific therapies as well as supportive-comfort therapies that promote the optimal function and well-being of patients and their family caregivers. The Canadian Palliative Care Association's Model (1995) documents how palliative care needs intensify at the end of life. The core issues of palliation, comfort, and function are salient throughout the course of the disease. A palliative care model recognizes the need to address symptom distress, physical impairments, and psychosocial disturbance even during the period of aggressive primary therapy with goals of cure or the prolongation of life (Portenoy, 1998).

Factors that have contributed to the palliative care movement in the United States include the: growing aging population; assisted suicide debate; reduced patient autonomy; and inappropriate end-of-life care (i.e., overtreatment of medical care and undertreatment of pain and depression). Quality outcomes of good palliative care ensure that: patients' values and decisions are respected; comfort is a priority; psychosocial, spiritual, and practical needs will be addressed; and opportunities will be encouraged for growth and completion of unfinished business (Portenoy, 2000).

WHAT PALLIATIVE CARE SPECIALISTS PROVIDE

Palliative care specialists (advance practice nurses and physicians) address diverse quality of life concerns and promote interdisciplinary care emphasizing distinction of life and of dying, promotion of comfort and relief of suffering, and respect for autonomy and family involvement. As specialists they serve as role models and educators in clinical practice. They work to develop the theoretical and empirical body of knowledge in palliative care through research, develop and implement institution-based models of palliative care, and institute quality improvement programs. Palliative care special-ists focus on complex patients, such as those with multiple or difficult symptom control problems who require comprehensive care for multiple needs (e.g., needing family support or nursing home-based management for monitoring and titration of medication), and comprehensive care of the imminently dying. Although palliative care is now recognized as a specialty, Palliative Care, as a model of care, is a therapeutic approach ideally inte-grated into the care of all patients with life-threatening disease across the illness/dying trajectory (Portenoy, 1998).

CHANGES IN HEALTH CARE ECONOMICS

COST-CONTAINMENT IN PRACTICE SETTINGS

During the Clinton Administration (1992–2000), health care spending and allocation of resources resulted in the rapid expansion of managed care organizations in the United States. Managed care offers a broad menu of ways health services are accessed and paid for. This system is designed to save money by controlling patient access to expensive secondary and tertiary services and technology, and by setting limits on reimbursement.

The cost of end-of-life care in the United States is projected to escalate with the population's life expectancy. A recent analysis, from the National Medical Care Expenditure Survey (Cohen, Carlson, & Porter, 1995), found that for those persons 65 or older that died in 1987, spending during the last 6 months of their life accounted for an estimated 5.5% of total spending or 32.6 billion dollars. Other data sources (Scitovsky, 1996) suggest that expenditures may not increase so much by age alone, but rather by the cause of death. For example, cancer, chronic obstructive pulmonary disease (COPD), and renal disease cost more in Medicare payments than accidents and heart attacks.

End-of-life care is primarily funded through Medicare, Medicaid, the Veterans Administration and other public programs, with an estimated 60% of hospice patients being covered by Medicare (Vladeck, 1995). Although hospice coverage is now offered by nearly 80% of large and medium-sized employers (IOM, 1997), many patients and families miss the opportunity to access hospice services because of inadequate end-of-life discussions with their health care providers.

Managed care systems utilize management trends such as product-line management, total quality management (TQM) or continuous quality im-provement (CQI), and innovations that streamline delivery systems. Goals of managed care are aimed at reducing waste and cost, increasing customer satisfaction, and improving clinical outcomes (Johnsson, 1992). Health care providers are challenged with balancing the needs of their patients and the constraints of what insurers will provide. Reducing cost while providing quality care are the goals of hospital management; it is estimated that about 70% of nurse manager responsibilities will be allocated to quality improvement activities in the next decade.

TREATMENT DECISION MAKING: ESTIMATING PROGNOSIS

Physicians and nurses struggle with decisions about appropriate care for patients who are near death. Predicting how long someone will live with an incurable illness is a difficult and complex task. Lynn, Teno, and Harrell (1995) describe the construction of a model for more accurate prognostications of death. It includes a risk of death estimate plus 14 patient characteristics; diagnosis, serum sodium level, temperature, respirator rate, heart rate, oxygenation, creatinine level, mean blood pressure, bilirubin and albumin levels, Glasgow coma score, age, days in hospital, and having cancer as a co-morbidity. These authors assert that their statistical model coupled with the physician's estimates is better than either one alone.

Weeks, Cook, O'Day, Peterson, and Wenger (1998) examined data from 917 adults with Stage III or IV non-small cell lung and metastatic colon cancer in Phases I and II of the SUPPORT study across five U.S. teaching sites. Results indicated that patients were substantially more optimistic about their prognosis than their physicians were. In 82% of the physician-patient pairs, the patients' estimate of their chance of living 6 months was higher than the physicians; in 59%, the patient estimate exceeded the physician estimate by two prognostic categories. Patients who were more optimistic about their prognosis lived longer than patients who were less optimistic. Patients who believed that they would survive at least 6 months favored life-extending therapy over comfort care at more than double the rate of those who believed they had less than 6 months to live. Patients greatly overestimated their chances of surviving 6 months while physicians' prognostic estimates were more precise in that physicians (estimating 90% survival) accurately predicted 71% of the deaths.

These studies indicate two important findings. First is the need for better communication between physicians and their patients about prognosis. This discussion could help patients make more informed treatment decisions consistent with their values and could facilitate earlier access to palliative or Hospice care. The second relates to the need to better understand the source of patients' beliefs, preferences, and the ways in which they arrive at decisions about their care. This may be critical in designing interventions that are effective in changing end-of-life patterns of communication and care.

CHANGES IN SERVICE DELIVERY: IMPROVING END-OF-LIFE CARE

HOSPITALS IN NEED OF BETTER END-OF-LIFE CARE

The IOM (1997) study findings suggest a need for improved end-of-life care in four major areas: patient suffering, obstacles to obtaining excellent end-of-life care, education and training of professionals, and research to support "best practices" at the end of life. Because most deaths (70%) occur in hospitals, our comments will focus on areas identified as priorities for improvement in clinical settings.

ELIMINATING PATIENT SUFFERING

Research results indicate that there is an overwhelming need for improved symptom management at the end of life for both adults and children. Patients at the end-of-life experience many of the same symptoms and syndromes regardless of their underlying condition. To decrease patient and family suffering at the end of life and improve symptom control, in-hospital programs are adopting a palliative care model that offers comprehensive care for seriously ill patients and their families. Three Palliative Care Programs (Beth Israel Medical Center and Calvary Hospitals in New York, and The Cleveland Clinic in Ohio) are currently providing leadership in this area and making strides in developing the delivery of "palliative care" within acute care settings. More nurses with specialized palliative and hospice care expertise are needed to provide patient care, serve as role models for staff, assure that standards are evidence-based, and develop monitoring and evaluation programs to meet benchmarks set by professional organizations for quality care at the end of life. This work is especially important because nearly 30 years after the start of the Hospice movement in the United States, only half of adults who die of cancer receive Hospice care. Nurses have an important role in identifying and facilitating access to specialty services such as palliative and Hospice care for patients and families.

Palliative care services are lacking for children as well. In a Boston study of 165 children with cancer, 49% died in the hospital, and half of these were in the ICU. According to parents, 89% of the children suffered "a lot" or a "great deal" from at least one symptom in the last month of life; mostly pain, fatigue, and dyspnea (Wolfe et al., 2000). Currently only a handful of organized palliative care services for children exist in the United States. Palliative care programs designed for adults are inappropriate and ineffective for children (Stevens, Dalla Poza, Caelletto, Cooper, & Kilham, 1994; Whitman, 1993). One reason cited was the unwillingness of providers and parents to relinquish curative, invasive therapies even when there was little or no realistic hope for favorable outcomes. Often aggressive therapy is not abandoned until shortly before death so families and providers have little or no time to address their emotions or begin to grieve.

REMOVING BARRIERS TO PROVIDING EXCELLENT END-OF-LIFE CARE

Several structures are needed in organizations to identify and remove barriers to providing effective end-of-life care. A "top down and bottom up" approach is necessary, meaning that a mandate from top administration that includes support and resources coupled with a multidisciplinary team of experts, masterful in using a systematic process for creating change, is needed (Bookbinder et al., 1995). Structures geared toward reducing variation in practice and optimizing the achievement of "best practices" and outcomes can serve as a benchmark against which we can measure and constantly improve. In addition to hospital-required policies and procedures, structures include standards of care, guidelines, and tools that direct patient care management such as protocols, algorithms, care paths, flowsheets, and standardized orders.

Quality structures can be internally initiated or externally imposed. For example, by the Year 2001, hospitals seeking accreditation by the Joint Commission on Accreditation of Healthcare Organizations (JCAHO, 2000) are required to implement new pain management standards, including care at the end of life. This national initiative requiring relief of pain and suffering occurred within 15 years of the American Pain Society's quality assurance pain standards for acute and cancer pain (Max, Donovan, Miaskowski, Ward, Gordon, et al., 1995) and pain guidelines (WHO, 1990). This dramatic change in society's culture regarding the need for pain relief offers hope to palliative care initiatives aimed at good end-of-life care.

Protocols and algorithms have become popular clinical tools in a managed care era of "doing more with less time and resources." These tools aim to streamline processes of care and deliver consistent and timely interventions. Tools such as the *Palliative Care Clinical Practice Protocol for Dyspnea* (HNA, 1996) and *Symptom Management Algorithms for Palliative Care* (Wrede-Seaman, 1999) provide clinicians with a methodology for assessing symptoms, etiology, directions for treatment options, and guidelines for pharma-cological and nonpharmacological interventions.

Pathways (carepaths), flowsheets, and standardized orders are products of a managed care era that intend to "reduce variation" in services and practices, and thereby reduce costs (Association of Community Cancer Centers, 1998; Blancett & Flarey, 1998; Gordon, 1996; Haward, 1998; Janken, Grubbs, & Haldeman, 1999; Wakefield, Johnson, Kron-Chalupa, & Paulsen, 1998; Zander, 1991). Although the many needs of dying patients have been identified (SUPPORT, 1995), few end-of-life clinical pathways have been developed and tested (National Hospice Organization, 1997c; Bookbinder, 2000). Goals for these pathways include: 1) respecting patient autonomy, values, decisions; 2) continually clarifying goals of care; 3) minimizing symptom distress at the end of life; 4) optimizing appropriate supportive interventions and consultations; 5) reducing unnecessary interventions; 6) supporting families by coordinating services; 7) eliminating unnecessary regulations; 8) providing bereavement services for families and staff; and 9) facilitating the transition to alternate care settings, such as Hospice, when appropriate (Bookbinder, 2000).

Palliative and Hospice care experts are working to produce and implement the materials needed to build "safe and competent" infrastructures that will improve patients' and families' quality of living and dying. As members of multidisciplinary teams, nurses can lead efforts to implement structures that can improve the care of dying patients. This includes selecting and evaluating tools for practice and determining the strength of the evidence to reliably predict positive patient outcomes. Evaluation and testing of palliative care structures and their appropriateness, effectiveness, and cost of care are greatly needed (Higginson, 1993; Kristjanson, 1986).

Kirchhoff and Beckstrand's (2000) recent survey of 199 critical care nurses (69% response rate) documented perceptions of obstacles and helpful behaviors regarding the provision of end-of-life care. Six of the "top ten" obstacles related to issues involving the patient's families that made patient care at the end of life more difficult. Examples cited included the family not fully understanding the meaning of life support, not accepting the patient's poor prognosis, requesting more technical treatment than the patient wished, and being angry. Additional barriers related to problems with physicians. The "most helpful" behaviors were those that made dying easier for patients and their families, such as, agreement among physicians about care, dying with dignity, and the family's acceptance of the prognosis.

IMPROVING EDUCATION OF PROFESSIONALS

Nurse educators are beginning to identify appropriate and effective strategies for teaching care of the dying patient and their family. Results of recent nursing studies describe the impact of continuing education programs. Significant positive effects on attitudes toward care of dying patients were found when nurses in high-risk areas were randomly assigned to a 6-week experiential and didactic educational program (Miles, 1980). In a more recent study, Hainsworth (1996) randomly assigned a self-selected sample of nurses to a control (n = 14) and intervention (n = 14) group consisting of discussions, video, music, and role-playing over a 3-week period. Although significant differences were not quantified, the investigator suggested that future research include educational programs that are longer than 3 weeks, teach specific and extensive content in end-of-life care, and assess behavioral changes in patient care.

A survey of 90 (73% response rate) medical students, residents, interns, fellows, and attending physicians in a large Northeast tertiary care center revealed the need for systematic and standardized training in dealing with terminally ill patients (Borr Sand, Blackoff, Abrahm, & Healy, 1998). The most important topics identified by the sample were pain management, quality of life, and do-not-resuscitate status. Topics related to grieving, reaction to stress (bad news), and fostering the doctor-patient relationship were viewed as less important topics. When asked to describe an important personal or professional experience with death and how this affected their practice, physicians reported that the death of a loved one generated empathy toward others. The authors note that empathy is a key component missing in medical training programs.

The SUPPORT (1995) study documented nurses' opinions that improved communication, time, and repeated information about end-of-life issues were necessary for families to make decisions regarding interventions for life-threatening illnesses (Hiltunen et al., 1995). These findings highlight the role of the nurse as companion and confidant to patients and families and support a shared decision-making model in end-of-life treatment discussions. This is especially relevant given that only 15% of patients nationally have an advance directive. National efforts are underway to educate professionals in the United States. The American Medical Association's Education for Physician's on End-of-Life Care (EPEC) (Emanuel, von Gunten, & Ferris, 1999) curriculum, supported by a grant from the Robert Wood Johnson Foundation, is a 2-year initiative designed to educate physicians across the United States on essential clinical competencies in end-of-life care. A complementary program entitled the *End of Life Nursing Education Consortium* (ELNEC), also funded by the Robert Wood Johnson Foundation, is being developed and scheduled to begin in 2001 to educate nurses nationally regarding nursing care at the end of life. The American Association of Colleges of Nursing is developing this initiative in collaboration with the City of Hope researchers and educators, Dr. Betty Ferrell and Dr. Marsha Grant.

BUILDING EVIDENCE-BASED PRACTICE

Although few end-of-life care practices are currently based upon strong scientific evidence (IOM, 1997), research is available to help nurses shape their role in providing state-of-the art care to patients and their families at the end of life. Research results indicate the need for health care settings to: a) systematically identify and remove obstacles to excellent care at the end of life; b) identify end-of-life issues in vulnerable populations, such as children, older adults, and the chemically dependent; d) test models and tools (algorithms and carepaths) aimed to improve symptom control and end-of-life outcomes, such as comfort and distress; e) develop programs to educate professionals in end-of-life care and evaluate the various formats for education; and f) develop professional competencies which demonstrate "best practices" at the bedside. Also important is the need for professionals to: a) improve communication and understanding about treatment goals and outcomes among physicians, nurses, patients, and families; b) understand the contributing factors to nurses' reported behaviors in assisted suicide; and c) determine patient prognosis and earlier preparation for end-of-life care planning, especially in the "chronic-living-dying" population.

Views toward death and dying in American culture continue to change at a relatively consistent pace as evidence is compiled documenting the need to improve the care of the dying and their families. This challenge to nurses and nurse educators is a formidable one as we enter the 21st century.

Education Plan 3.1 Plan for Achieving Competencies: Death and Society

Knowledge Needed	Attitudes	Skills	Undergraduate Behavioral Outcomes	Graduate Behavioral Outcomes	Teaching/Learning Strategies
Changes related to death in American society and the taboo in acknowledging death.	*Consider changes related to death in society of the 21st century as compared to the previous century. *Appreciate death as a normal part of the life cycle. *Validate the need for improved health care provider-patient/family communication regarding dying and death.		*Discuss dying and death with patients and families as a normal part of the life cycle rather than something that should be feared.	*Raise public awareness of the negative consequences of avoiding the discussion of dying and death.	*Explore the students'/nurses' first experience with death and their related perceptions. *Discuss taboos about death from students'/nurses' own cultural/religious perspectives. *Have students report on societal perspectives of dying and death as presented by mass media, i.e., television, newspapers, Internet, etc.

Education Plan 3.1 *(continued)*

Knowledge Needed	Attitudes	Skills	Undergraduate Behavioral Outcomes	Graduate Behavioral Outcomes	Teaching/Learning Strategies
Changing Demographics Related to Death: —Morbidity and mortality statistics; —Leading causes of death; —Where people die; —Different dying trajectories.	*Value patients' and families' desires to die at home with necessary support. *Support patients and families who are experiencing varying dying trajectories.		*Describe the changes in morbidity and mortality rates, leading causes of death, patient/family preferences of where to die, and different dying trajectories as they relate to nursing practice and health care delivery.	*Collaborate in research studies that provide epidemiological data related to dying and death.	*In small groups, have students/nurses discuss feelings and attitudes regarding different dying situations. Elicit their perceptions regarding nursings' roles and responsibilities in caring for patients and families experiencing varying dying trajectories.

Education Plan 3.1 *(continued)*

Knowledge Needed	Attitudes	Skills	Undergraduate Behavioral Outcomes	Graduate Behavioral Outcomes	Teaching/Learning Strategies
Desire for Hastened Death: —Euthanasia; —Physician-assisted suicide.	*Appreciate the need for quality palliative care so that the need for hastened death will not be perceived as necessary by patients with terminal illness. *Affirm the ANA Code of Ethics which states that nurses' participation in assisted suicide or euthanasia is unethical.		*Communicate to patients that palliative care will be provided to alleviate end of life suffering.	*Collaborate with other health professionals for greater access to palliative care for all patient populations.	*Discuss the Oregon Death with Dignity Act, the reasons individuals requested physician-assisted suicide and implications for nursing practice.

Education Plan 3.1 *(continued)*

Knowledge Needed	Attitudes	Skills	Undergraduate Behavioral Outcomes	Graduate Behavioral Outcomes	Teaching/Learning Strategies
Changes in health care economics: —Cost containment in practice settings. —Treatment decisions based on estimate of prognoses.	*Appreciate the impact of managed care on quality care offered at the end of life. *Acknowledge the difficulties in determining prognoses and estimating life expectancy.		*Balance the needs of patients and families at the end of life within the constraints of managed care systems. *Discuss with patients and families their role and responsibilities as members of an HMO. *Encourage patients and families to advocate for their end of life needs to their insurance companies. *Assist patients/families in selecting an HMO through discussion of relevant criteria.	*Address economic barriers to palliative care for all populations across all health care settings by proactive strategies at the administrative, institutional, and community levels. *Advocate for the needs of patients and families enrolled in HMOs who are experiencing life-threatening illness. *Evaluate models that prognosticate death for varying disease states in diverse patient populations.	*Invite an administrator of an HMO to class or conduct a telephone interview to discuss the care available to patients and families experiencing life-threatening illnesses. *Analyze newspaper and media reports regarding access to palliative care across populations and health care settings.

Education Plan 3.1 *(continued)*

Knowledge Needed	Attitudes	Skills	Undergraduate Behavioral Outcomes	Graduate Behavioral Outcomes	Teaching/Learning Strategies
Changes in service delivery to improve end of life care: —Improving patient suffering; —Removing barriers to end of life care; —Improving education of health professionals; —Building evidence-based practice.	*Express commitment to changes in service delivery that will improve end of life care.		*Participate in nursing initiatives which will improve patient suffering, remove barriers to end of life care, improve nursing knowledge regarding palliative care, and build evidence-based practice.	*Provide expert palliative care. *Serve as role models for staff. *Insure that standards are evidence-based. *Set up monitoring and evaluation programs to meet benchmarks set by professional organizations for quality care at the end of life.	*Assist students/nurses to identify leadership opportunities related to palliative care. *Have students/nurses develop continuous quality improvement with their clinical setting to evaluate an aspect of palliative care.

REFERENCES

American Geriatrics Society (1997). Measuring quality of care at end-of-life: A statement of principles. NY:NY: Author. (online) Available: http://www.americangeriatrics.org (March 5, 2000).

Annas, G. J. (1993). *Standard of Care: The Law of American Bioethics*. New York: Oxford University Press.

Annas, G. J. (1995). How we die. *Hastings Center Report, 25*, 512–514.

Asch, D. A. (1996). The role of critical care nurses in euthanasia and assisted suicide. *New England Journal of Medicine, 334*, 1374–1401.

Association of Community Cancer Centers (1998). *Oncology Critical Pathways*. Rockville, MD: Author.

Avellanet, C. (2000). 1999 Annual report of Jacob Perlow Hospice. Beth Israel Medical Center, New York.

Bachman, J., Alcser, K., Doukis, D., Lichtenstein, R., Corning, A., & Brody, H. (1996). Attitudes of Michigan physicians and the public towards legalizing physician-assisted suicide and voluntary euthanasia. *New England Journal of Medicine, 334*, 303–309.

Blancett, S. S., & Flarey, D. L. (1998). *Health care outcomes: Collaborative, path-based approaches.* Gaithersburg: Aspen.

Bookbinder, M. (2000). Quality care at end-of-life. In B. R. Ferrell & N. Coyle (Eds.), *Palliative care nursing*. Oxford University Press.

Bookbinder, M., Kiss, M., Coyle, N., Brown, M., Gianella, A., & Thaler, H. (1995). Improving pain management practices. In D. McGuire, C. Yarbro, & B. Ferrell (Eds.), *Cancer pain management* (2nd ed.) (pp. 321–361). Boston: Jones and Bartlett.

Borr Sand, R., Blackoff, G., Abrahm, J. L., & Healy, K. (1998). A survey of physicians' education in caring for the dying. *Journal of Cancer Education, 13*(4), 242–247.

Botkin, J. R., & Post, S. G. (1992). Confusion in the determination of death. *Perspective in Biology & Medicine, 36*(1), 129–138.

Brody, H. (1988). Brain death and personal existence: A reply to Green and Wikler. *Journal of Medicine and Philosophy, 4*, 8.

Brody, H. (1992). Assisted dying—A compassionate response to a medical failure. *New England Journal of Medicine, 327*, 1384–1388.

Byock, I. R. (1997). *Dying well.* New York: Riverhead Books.

Canadian Palliative Care Association (1995). Palliative care: Towards a consensus in standardized principles of practice.

Cohen, S. B., Carlson, B. L., & Porter, D. E. B. (1995). Health care expenditures in the last six months of life. *Health Policy Review* (American Statistical Association *Section on Health Policy*), *1*(2), 1–13.

Coyle, N. (1992). The euthanasia and physician suicide debate: Issues for nursing. *Oncology Nursing Forum, 19*, (Supplement 7), 41–46.

Davis, A. J., Phillips, L., Drought, T. S., Sellin, S., Ronsman, K., & Hershberger, A. K. (1995). Nurses' attitudes toward active euthanasia. *Nursing Outlook, 43*(4), 174–179.

Desbeins, N. A., Mueller-Rizner, N., Hamel, M. B., & Connors, A. F. (1998). Preference for comfort care does not affect the pain experience of seriously ill patients. *Journal of Pain & Symptom Management, 16*(5), 281–289.

Emanuel, L. L., von Gunten, C. F., & Ferris, F. D. (1999). *The education for physicians on end-of-life care (EPEC) curriculum.* American Medical Association & The Robert Wood Johnson Foundation.

Ferrell, B., Virani, R., Grant, M., Coyne, P., & Uman, G. (2000). Beyond the Supreme Court decision: Nursing perspectives on end-of-life care. *Oncology Nursing Forum, 27*(3), 445–455.

Foley, K. M. (1995). Pain, physician-assisted suicide, and euthanasia. *Pain Forum, 4,* 163–178.

Foley, K. M. (1996). Controlling the pain of cancer. *Scientific American,* 164–165.

Friedrich, M. J. (1999). Hospice care in the U.S.: A conversation with Florence S. Wald. *Journal of the American Medical Association, 281*(18), 1683–1685.

Ganzini, L., Nelson, H. D., Schmidt, T. A., Kraemer, D. F., Delorit, M. A., & Lee, M. A. (2000). Physicians' experiences with the Oregon Death with Dignity Act. *New England Journal of Medicine, 342*(8), 557–563.

Gordon, D. B. (1996). Critical pathways: A road to institutionalizing pain management. *Journal of Pain and Symptom Management, 11*(4), 252–259.

Hainsworth, D. S. (1996). The effect of death education on attitudes of hospital nurses toward care of the dying. *Oncology Nursing Forum, 23*(6), 963–967.

Hall, J. (1996). Assisted suicide: Nurse practitioners as providers? *Nurse Practitioner, 21,* 63–71.

Haward, R. A. (1998). Review of evidence-based cancer medline. *Annals of Oncology, 9,* 1073–1078.

HCFA (1996). Trends in Medicare home health agency utilization and payment: CYs 1974–1994. *Health Care Financing Review 1996 (Statistical Suppl.),* 76–77, 1996b.

Higginson, I. (Ed.). (1993). *Clinical audit in palliative care.* Oxford: Radcliffe Medical Press.

Hiltunen, E. F., Puopolo, A. L., Marks, G. K., Marsden, C., Kennard, M. J., Follen, M. A., & Phillips, R. S. (1995). The nurse's role in end-of-life treatment discussions: Preliminary report from the SUPPORT project. *Journal of Cardiovascular Nursing, 9*(3), 68–77.

Hospice Nurses' Association (HNA) (1996). *Hospice and palliative care clinical practice protocol: Dyspnea.* Pittsburgh, PA: Author.

Institute of Medicine (IOM) (1997). In M. J. Field & C. K. Cassel (Eds.), Approaching death: Improving care at the end of life. Committee on Care at the end of life, Division of Health Care Services, Institute of Medicine. Washington, DC: National Academy Press.

Janken, J. K., Grubbs, J. H., & Haldeman, K. (1999). Toward a research-based critical pathway: A case study. *The Online Journal of Knowledge Synthesis.* Clinical Column. Document Number 1C.

Johnsson, J. (1992). TQM approach may help solve physician practice problems. *Trustee, 45*(4), 11.

Joint Commission on Accreditation of Hospitals Organization (2000). Available: http://www.jcaho.org

Kaufman, S. (1998). Intensive care, old age, and the problem in America. *Gerontologist, 38*(6), 715–725.

Kazanowski, M. (1997). A commitment to palliative care: Could it impact assisted suicide? *Journal of Gerontological Nursing,* 36–42.

Kirchhoff, K. T., & Beckstrand, R. L. (2000). Critical care nurses perceptions of obstacles and helpful behaviors in providing end-of-life care to dying patients. *American Journal of Critical Care, 9*(2), 96–105.

Kowalski, S. (1997). Assisted suicide: Where do nurses draw the line. *Nursing & Health Care, 14,* 70–76.

Kristjanson, L. J. (1986). Indicators of quality of palliative care from a family perspective. *Journal of Palliative Care, 2,* 7–19.

Kubler-Ross, E. (1967). *On death and dying.* New York: Touchstone.

Lynn, J., Teno, J. M., & Harrell, F. E. (1995). Accurate prognostications of death: Opportunities and challenges from clinicians. *Western Journal of Medicine, 163,* 250–257.

Matzo, LaPorte M., & Emanual, E. J. (1997). Oncology nurses practices of assisted suicide and patient-requested euthanasia. *Oncology Nursing Forum, 24,* 1725–1732.

Max, M. B., Donovan, M., Miaskowski, C. A., Ward, S. E., Gordon, D., Bookbinder, M., Cleeland, C., Coyle, N., Kiss, M., Thaler, H., Janjan, N., & Weinstein, S. (1995). American Pain Society quality improvement guidelines for the treatment of acute pain and chronic pain. *JAMA, 274*(23), 1974–1880.

McCormick, T. R., & Conley, B. J. (1995). Patients perspectives on dying and on the care of dying patients. *Western Journal of Medicine, 163*(3), 236–243.

Miles, M. S. (1980). The effects of a course on death and grief on nurses' attitudes toward dying patients and death. *Death Education, 4,* 245–260.

Murphy, P. A. (1992). Perspective: Nursing—the real issue: *Trends in Health Care, Law, and Ethics, 10,* 124–127.

National Hospice Organization, Working Party on Clinical Guidelines in End-of-Life Care. (1997b). Changing gears: Guidelines for managing care in the last days of life in adults. Arlington, VA: Author.

National Hospice Organization (1997c). A pathway for patients and families facing terminal illness. Arlington, VA: Author.

National Institute on Aging (2000). Research agenda for 2001–2005 (online). *Available: http:// www.nih.gov/nia/strat-plan.* (Feb. 3, 2000)

Portenoy, R. K. (1998). Defining palliative care. Newsletter: Department of Pain Medicine and Palliative Care, 1(2) 1–2. Beth Israel Medical Center, New York. Available: http:// www.stoppain.org (January 4, 2000)

Portenoy, R. K. (2000). Quality outcomes of good palliative care. Paper presented at Beth Israel Medical Center, New York.

Pritchard, R. S., Fisher, E. S., Teno, J. M., Sharp, S. M., Reding, D. J., Knaus, W. A., Wenneberg, J. E., & Lynn, J. (1998). Influence of patient preferences and local health system characteristics on place of death. *Journal of the American Geriatric Society, 46,* 1242–1250.

Quill, T. E. (1993). Doctor, I want to die. Will you help me? *Journal of the American Medical Association, 270,* 870–873.

Schroeder, S. A. (1999). The legacy of SUPPORT. *Annals of Internal Medicine, 131*(10), 780–781.

Schwarz, J. K. (1999). Assisted dying and nursing practice. *Image: Journal of Nursing Scholarship, 31*(4), 367–373.

Scitovsky, A. (1996). Age and the high cost of health care. Paper presented at the First International Conference on Priorities in Health Care, Stockholm, Sweden, October 13–16.

Stevens, M. M., Dalla Pozza, L., Caelletto, B., Cooper, M. G., & Kilham, H. A. (1994). Pain and symptom control in pediatric palliative care. *Cancer Survey, 21,* 211–231.

Storey, P. (1996). *Primer of palliative care* (2nd ed.). Iowa: Kendall/Hunt.

The New Encyclopedia Britannica. (1999). Chicago: Encyclopedia Britannica.

The Concise Columbia Electronic Encyclopedia (3rd ed.) (1994). Columbia University Press.

SUPPORT Principal Investigators (1995). A controlled trial to improve care for seriously ill hospitalized patients: The Study to Understand Prognoses and Preferences for Outcomes and Risks of Treatments (SUPPORT). *JAMA, 274,* 1591–1598.

Vladeck, B. (1995). Medicare and managed care: Working together for the future. *Medical Interface, 8*(1), 50–52.

Wakefield, B., Johnson, J. A., Kron-Chalupa, J., & Paulsen, L. (1998). A research-based guideline for appropriate use of transdermal fentanyl to treat chronic pain. *Oncology Nursing Forum, 25*(9), 1505–1512.

Weeks, J., Cook, F., O'Day, S. J., Peterson, L., Wenger, N., Reding, D., Harrell, F. E., Kussin, P., Dawson, N., Connors, A. F., Lynn, J., & Phillips, R. S. (1998). Relationship between cancer patients' predictions of prognosis and their treatment preferences. *Journal of the American Medical Association, 2789*(21), 1709–1714.

Whitman, E. H. (1993). Terminal care of the dying child: Psychosocial implications of care. *Cancer, 71,* 3450–3462.

Wolfe, J., Holcombe, G. E., Klar, N., Levin, S., Ellenbogen, J. M., Salen-Schatz, S., Emanuel, E. J., & Weeks, J. (2000). Symptoms and suffering at the end of life in children with cancer. *New England Journal of Medicine, 342*(5), 326–333.

World Health Organization (1990). Technical Support Series 804, Cancer Pain Relief and Palliative Care. Geneva: WHO.

Wrede-Seaman, L. (1999). *Symptom management algorithms: A handbook for palliative care.* Yakima: Intellicard.

Zander, K. (1991). CareMaps®. The core of cost/quality care. *New Definition, 6*(3), 1–3.

4

The Nurse's Role in Interdisciplinary and Palliative Care

Lisa M. Krammer, Aileen A. Ring, Jeanne Martinez, Mary Jo Jacobs, and Mary Beth Williams

AACN Competencies

#6: Collaborate with interdisciplinary team members while implementing the nursing role in end-of-life care.

#14: Demonstrate skill at implementing a plan for improved end-of-life care within a dynamic and complex health care delivery system.

> Why are you afraid? I am the one who is dying! . . . But please believe me, if you care, you can't go wrong. . . . Death may get to be routine to you, but it is new to me.
>
> —Anonymous

This chapter will describe the significance of the interdisciplinary team process and the fundamental elements of effective interdisciplinary team process. In conclusion, the complex dimensions within nursing roles involved in successful family care at the end of life are presented.

PALLIATIVE CARE FRAMEWORKS

CONCEPTUAL MODEL OF CARE

In order to relieve suffering, palliative care nursing utilizes a conceptual framework for end-of-life care practice. An effective model of care for the delivery of palliative nursing, adapted from hospice nursing, is Dame Cicely Saunder's conceptual model of "whole person" suffering. Saunders espouses that "whole person" suffering has four dimensions; physical, psychological, spiritual, and social (Krammer, Muir, Gooding-Kellar, Williams, & von Gunten, 1999). Under this concept, suffering effects each domain of the bio-psychosocial-spiritual aspects of care. This conceptual model forms the basis for the description of palliative care nursing practice in this chapter.

DELIVERY MODEL OF CARE

Within the traditional, medical model of care, lies a perceived dichotomy between curative/death defying care and palliative care. It is almost as though the goal of care is *first* and *only* cure, then only if unable to cure, to relieve suffering. Often, this perceived dichotomy prevents or delays the introduction of palliative care measures for patients and their families. In order to provide quality, comprehensive, "whole person" care, should not the goals of curative and palliative care be woven together concurrently? It would seem to be generally appropriate to relieve suffering *at the same time* as pursuing curative life-prolonging therapies (Von Gunten & Muir, 1999).

An effective framework for the delivery of palliative care throughout the disease continuum can be most readily visualized as an "umbrella of care." Debate exists as to the beginning and end of the umbrella's arch. For some health care clinicians, palliative care starts with the initial diagnosis of an illness, at which time the management of symptoms and the psychosocial stressors of the disease upon the patient and family are vigorously addressed with active, curative focused therapy. While this scope may be considered ideal, the majority of palliative care providers emphasize the maximization of function and quality of life in those with far-advanced disease. For all providers, palliative care culminates in the management of complex physical, psychological, social, and spiritual issues which patients and members of their families will experience during the final phase of life and will include bereavement care for the family (Krammer et al., 1999).

With the emergence of palliative care as a distinct medical specialty (Carducci, Blacker, Perrone, & Alexander, 1999; von Gunten & Muir, 1999), an ever-growing number of hospitals have begun to develop comprehensive, academic palliative care programs (Bircumshaw, 1993), consisting of one or all of the following program elements: acute palliative care inpatient units (Kellar, Martinez, Finis, Bolger, & von Gunten, 1996), palliative consultation teams (von Gunten, Camden, Neely, Franz, & Martinez, 1998; Weissman, 1997), outpatient palliative care clinics and home hospice programs. This programmatic approach allows for patients with advanced progressive disease and their families to have access to palliative care expertise in all settings; including the acute care hospital, outpatient clinic, home or nursing home. With a comprehensive palliative care program, the interdisciplinary team will utilize the same philosophy and model of care as they work throughout the continuum with the patient and family in a coordinated and collaborative manner in achieving mutually established goals.

PRINCIPLES OF PALLIATIVE CARE

A core principle of palliative care across the entire disease spectrum and in all settings is the concept that the family constitutes the unit of care. The family rather than the disease are the primary focus of care. The constructs of family-centered care form the foundation of the palliative care philosophy. Palliative care addresses the meaning of disease, suffering, life, and death within the context of each family unit (Lillard & Marietta, 1989). Palliative care recognizes that each family member will experience the disease process and all of its implications within the context of his or her particular worldview, and individual careplans are developed to reflect these worldviews.

Another core palliative care principle is the commitment to collaborate through an interdisciplinary team process (Carducci et al., 1999). In order to facilitate a family in crisis to establish and then achieve mutually agreed upon goals, the palliative care team integrates and coordinates the assessment and interventions of each team member and creates a whole plan out of many parts. Good palliative care is significant in the manner in which it embraces cultural, ethnic, and faith differences and preferences, while interweaving the principles of ethics, humanities, and human values into every patient/family care experience (Loscalzo & Zabora, 1998; Rosen, 1999).

Further, clinical ethics is an essential footprint for the provision of end of life care. Whereas clinicians often learn the *theoretical* principles behind ethics (Beauchamp & Childress, 1994), palliative care necessitates that these principles be incorporated into the practice or "put into motion" 24 hours a day, 7 days a week (Roy & MacDonald, 1998). Palliative care embodies this concept of "ethics in motion" (C. Muir, personal communication, August 10, 1999) as each interdisciplinary team member, including patient and families, contemplate the ethical questions in advanced disease and in end of life decision making.

Ethical challenges present themselves to the palliative care interdisciplinary team on an hourly basis. The following vignettes are a sampling of the ethical issues faced by the interdisciplinary team in routine daily practice.

- Decision-Making Capacity/Respect for Autonomy
  Mr. T., a 32-year-old gentleman, with advanced AIDS-Dementia admitted with confusion and recurrent aspiration pneumonia. Patient has a disengaged family system, and no advanced directives. The palliative care team is challenged with the assessment of the risks/benefits in treating this recurrent infection. Given the patient's advanced dementia and with no surrogate decision maker known, the ethical questions are: a) Should the palliative care team institute life-prolonging treatment for Mr.T.?; b) How does the palliative care team elucidate and/ or clarify goals of care when a patient is unable to articulate and engage in decision making?
- Patient Autonomy/Truth Telling
  Mr. B., a 74-year-old gentleman with a history of small cell lung cancer and a one day history of extensive metastatic disease. Mr. B's wife died 3 years ago from lung cancer, and he has an involved family consisting of three adult children who are "devoted to his well-being." The children are united in efforts to ensure that the oncologist does not disclose the news of progressive disease to Mr. B. The children believe that if their father is fully informed of the extent of his disease he will give up the hope to live. Some of the ethical questions in this case are: a) What is the obligation of the palliative care team to tell vulnerable patients' bad news?; b) What are the obligations of the palliative care team towards the family when they tend to block the sharing of information with a patient who possesses decision-making capacity?
- Physician-assisted suicide
  Mrs. M., a 41-year-old woman with progressive amyotropic lateral sclerosis is admitted for management of acute onset of dyspnea. She is married with two school-aged children. Her parents and in-laws are alive and in good health. From the onset of her diagnosis 1 year ago, she shared with her primary physician, a neurologist, that suffering in her eyes means "the inability to breathe" and "the inability to speak." When the palliative care nurse was performing an initial assessment, the patient asked her "Is there any way you can help put me out of my misery?" The ethical questions are: a) Are there limits to patient autonomy

when a patient requests treatments and/or interventions which are either illegal or in conflict with quality clinical practice?; b) What are the limits on attempts to relieve suffering?

Each member of the interdisciplinary team has a unique relationship/ view with the patient and family. These varied perspectives reveal vital information that is invaluable when identifying and clarifying potential conflicts and facilitating resolution. It is through the use of an interdisciplinary team process that each ethical issue in palliative care is collaboratively and interdependently addressed and evaluated.

THE INTERDISCIPLINARY TEAM

Palliative care's reliance upon the interdisciplinary team as a key factor for successful outcomes requires an understanding of the distinction between interdisciplinary and multidisciplinary practice. In the traditional multidisciplinary team, the physician primarily directs care of the patient and the family needs may or may not be considered. (See Figure 4.1) Multiple disciplines of the health care team may be involved in the individual assessments and in the delivery of care, although efforts by these team members are often uncoordinated and independent. The primary mode of communication between disciplines is the medical chart. The result is often incomplete communication between professions, lack of accountability, and a tendency for each discipline to develop its own patient care goals. Family needs are often unidentified and most often, not incorporated into the overall plan of care.

In contrast, in an interdisciplinary model, communication and decision making between team members is collaborative with leadership shared and based upon primary patient/family needs and goals. The identity of the interdisciplinary team supercedes personal identities and agendas (Cummings, 1998), and the concept of the "sum of the whole is greater than its parts" is valued and respected. The interdisciplinary model facilitates team members to: (a) directly interact with the patient and family, (b) to share information among team members, (c) to provide consultation to one another, and (d) to work interdependently together in order to achieve the goals identified by the patient and family.

Table 4.1 lists the most common members of the palliative care interdisciplinary team, explains their function within the team, and discusses their interrelationship with the palliative care nurse. The nurse, as a coordinator of care and a core member of the interdisciplinary team, has the responsibility to spearhead the development of therapeutic relationships not just be-

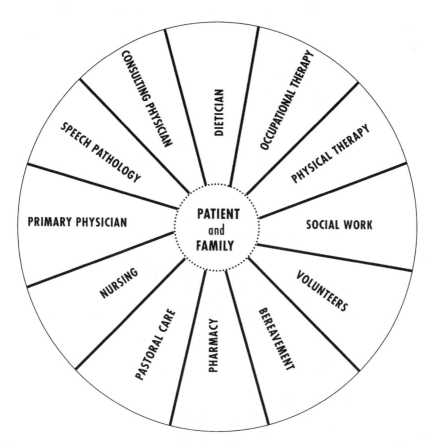

FIGURE 4.1   The multidisciplinary team.
Various members of the health care team contribute as individuals to the
care plan for each patient. However, the communication between each
discipline is often lacking and/or fragmented as represented by the individual pie pieces separated by heavy dark lines. Additionally, there is no mechanism to facilitate communication between the disciplines.

tween herself and the patient and family, but also with all pertinent members
of the team, which in turn ensures effective and goal-driven supportive
communication and patient outcomes. The goals of the patient and family,
their treatment preferences, and support needs are continually reassessed
by the palliative care nurse. A hallmark of quality palliative care is the
collaborative role that the nurse develops with the physician. Often, the

TABLE 4.1 The Interdisciplinary Team Member's Role, Function, and Interrelationship with the Palliative Care (PC) Nurse

Advanced Practice Nurse
Function: Incorporates the role of advanced clinician, educator, researcher, and consultant to families, staff, colleagues, and communities.
Interrelationship: Acts as a consultant, educator, role model, and mentor to the PC nurse to synergistically achieve quality outcomes for patients and families.

Bereavement Counselor
Function: Identifies through IDT assessment high risk family members for bereavement and provides anticipatory grief counseling. Coordinates bereavement services for families including counseling sessions, grief support groups, memorial services, and community outreach programs.
Interrelationship: Relies on the PC nurse assessment of the family upon a patient's death in order to begin bereavement care. Values the PC nurse's role in identifying high risk family members for grief and bereavement.

Patient/Family
Function: The focus of care of the interdisciplinary team. The goals identified by the patient/family direct the participation of other members of the team.
Interrelationship: The patient/family understands the PC nurse is the coordinator of interdisciplinary care and continuously confers with the PC nurse regarding patient/family needs.

Palliative Care Physician
Function: Consults with primary care physician and collaborates with IDT to provide expertise in pain management, communication, and treatment decisions at the end of life for patients and families.
Interrelationship: Understands the PC nurse has the greatest prolonged contact with the patient and family and relies upon the holistic assessment and interventions of the nurse in order to develop a comprehensive medical care plan in collaboration with the interdisciplinary team.

Pastoral Care Counselor
Function: Provides in-depth assessment of spiritual needs of patient/family including search for meaning and purpose of life. Acts as a liaison with community clergy and a resource for the interdisciplinary team regarding ethical questions, faith traditions, and world religions.
Interrelationship: Respects the spiritual assessment of the PC nurse and is consulted when family issues require advanced assessment and intervention. Acts as a resource for PC nurse when needing to debrief after a difficult death or experience.

TABLE 4.1   *(continued)*

Primary Care Physician
Function: Initiates a relationship with the palliative care team with referral of a new patient/family. Provides a medical history of the patient's illness and any other pertinent medical and psychosocial information; continues to be the primary physician or transfers the role to the PC physician.
Interrelationship: Assessments and interventions of the PC nurse and those of the interdisciplinary team are coordinated with the primary physician to establish a comprehensive plan of care for the patient and family.

Social Worker
Function: Provides history (via genogram) regarding the strengths, resources, and realities of patient/family system. Interventions include emotional support through individual, family, high risk, and bereavement counseling. Provides referrals for families to the community as needed for social services.
Interrelationship: Delivery of care involves ongoing collaboration with PC nurse who is continuously identifying psychosocial needs and outcomes of the patient and family.

Therapies (Pharmacy, Occupational, Physical, Dietary, Speech, Art, Music, Touch, Massage)
Function: Provide education and/or "hands-on" therapy of specialized discipline to maximize independence and quality of life of patient and family.
Interrelationship: Participates in plan of care when consulted by PC nurse and reports outcomes of interventions through collaboration with the PC nurse.

Volunteer
Function: Gives of time freely to contribute to patient and family needs by direct service, administrative support of the palliative care program, public relations, and community education.
Interrelationship: Reports observed family dynamics to PC nurse in order to revise plan of care if needed.

Volunteer Coordinator
Function: Recruits, screens, educates, supervises, and retains volunteer staff to provide supportive services to patients and families.
Interrelationship: Plans assignments of volunteers based upon identified needs of family by PC nurse; Involves PC nurse in volunteer training.

physician has had a long-term relationship with the patient and family, and as the needs for traditional medical model "curative" care lessen and palliative care measures increase, this may represent a "loss" for the physician. As the nurse develops a relationship with the patient and family; the collaborative relationship with the physician may also be a source of support for the physician personally along with professionally for decision making. The nurse is a primary conduit for information, critical assessments, and evaluation of the patient and family goals within the interdisciplinary team. A critical aspect of palliative care involves the identification and subsequent resolution of often divergent goals of the patient, family, or the health care team. The palliative care nurse is often in the ideal position to be instrumental in coordinating and affecting a comprehensive family-focused plan of care.

CHARACTERISTICS OF AN EFFECTIVE INTERDISCIPLINARY TEAM

A dynamic and outcomes-oriented interdisciplinary team requires collaboration, leadership, coordinated decision making, and conflict resolution. Collaboration is defined as the ability to work with others, especially on intellectual endeavors (Merriam-Webster, 1993). It is the process of collaboration that empowers team members to act as decision makers within the group. For example, if a question on nausea and vomiting arises, various members of the team may provide observations and opinions in an effort to maximize the relief of all components of nausea and vomiting. Using a true collaborative process, the ultimate decision maker regarding this aspect of care would not come to a conclusion solely benefiting oneself or one's own perspective, but rather the decision reflects the team's total input. Through collaboration, effective patient- and family-driven quality outcomes are achieved.

Palliative care differs from the traditional medical model in which the physician is the sole leader of the multidisciplinary team. In the palliative care model, leadership is filled by the member of the interdisciplinary team who is best educated and qualified to address and focus upon specific patient or family goals. In addition to achieving patient and family outcomes, leadership is essential to facilitate and optimize the professional potential of each team member's contribution (M. B. Williams, personal communication, Feb. 10, 1999).

Also, in the traditional multidisciplinary team, the physician, as team leader, is the primary decision maker for the care team. In contrast, in a true interdisciplinary team process coordinated decision making among team members are necessary to achieve quality patient and family outcomes. In order to sort out which member or members of the team that would be the most appropriate in contributing to the decision-making process, the following questions, developed by Ina Cummings (1998), should be considered: "Who has the information necessary to make the decision?", "Who needs to be consulted before the decision is made?", and "Who needs to be informed of a decision after it is made?" Certain levels of decision making may be made by individual members of the team (i.e., titrating a pain medication based on patient needs), whereas other levels will require the input from the entire team as a whole (i.e., developing a care plan). Poor, fragmented decision making results from failure to include appropriate team members in the decision-making process (Cummings, 1998).

Due to the interdependency among interdisciplinary team members, professional conflict will inevitably arise which may be beneficial and stimulating to an interdisciplinary team. Respect and trust in each team member's skills, knowledge, expertise, and motivation are imperative. Lack of respectful conflict will result in group uniformity which may stifle the creativity and the professional advancement and development of team members. Diverse ideas and opinions are often the impetus for innovative solutions for patient care problems and in the process, deepen the professional dialogue within the team. However, conflict becomes destructive when it is personalized or viewed as a threat to a member's role. Thus, the art in managing conflict is not to avoid it, but to manage it effectively so that team members, patients, and families can receive its full benefits. See Figure 4.2 for an algorithm for interdisciplinary team conflict management (Cummings, 1998).

THE DEVELOPING ROLE OF NURSING IN PRACTICING PALLIATIVE CARE

THE ESSENCE OF PALLIATIVE CARE NURSING

In the book *Intimate Death*, the author writes: "When death comes so close, and sadness and suffering rule, there is still room for life, and joy, and surges of feeling deeper and more intense than anything known before . . . to witness the preciousness of these last moments of life and to the extraordinary privilege of being able to share them has some value . . . to deepen our respect for the value of life itself . . . " (deHennezel, 1997).

In order to identify the essence of palliative care nursing, the values and beliefs of the role of the palliative care nurse and the qualities and themes

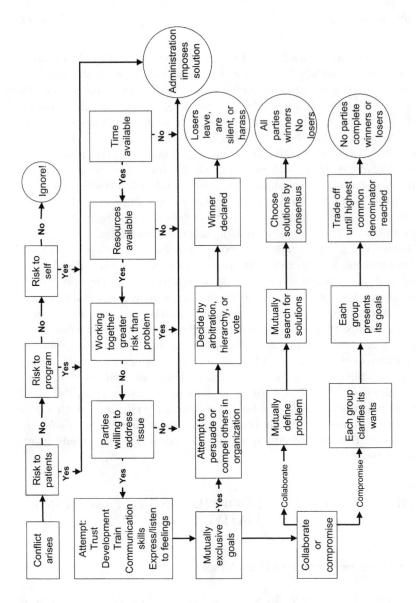

FIGURE 4.2 Interdisciplinary team conflict management flow chart.

128

inherent to the person that provides end-of-life care are to be delineated. As deHennezel describes, working with patients at the end of their life and with the families who are adjusting to illness and eventual loss, enables those who work with these families to learn not only about the value of life but also continuously transform themselves in the process.

The palliative care nurse combines the science of nursing with ethics, philosophy, the humanities, diverse world views, and individual and family life experiences in order to provide holistic care to families that are coping with a life-limiting illness.

THE NURSES' ROLE IN INTERDISCIPLINARY CARE

The following case example is that of an advanced practice nurse (APN) bringing a specific and well-defined set of qualities, knowledge, and judgments in caring for individuals and families at the end of life. This includes advanced scientific and biophysical knowledge, analytical skills, and a broad repertoire mastery of communication and interpersonal skills. Also, specialized knowledge and proficiency in the ability to incorporate ethics, humanities, cultural diversity, family, spiritual, and psychological issues into care is demanded (Weggel, 1997).

The J.D. Calkin Model of Advanced Nursing Practice (Spross & Baggerly, 1989) serves as an excellent model on which to base palliative care advanced practice nursing. Calkin defines the clinical judgment abilities of three nursing practice levels as novice, expert by experience, and the master's prepared nurse.

The following case study illustrates Saunder's four dimensions of human suffering within the context of Calkin's Advanced Nursing Practice Model. Also, the case study will demonstrate the APN subroles of expert clinician, educator, consultant, researcher, and collaborator (Spross & Baggerly, 1989).

Clinical Case Study . . . A 58 Year-Old Mother Suffering with Dyspnea Secondary to Head/Neck Cancer

Mrs. T. is a 58-year-old female who is married and has two children. She was diagnosed 5 months ago with advanced head and neck cancer. All curative interventions including surgical resection, chemotherapy, and radiotherapy have failed to halt the progression of her metastatic disease. Mrs. T's major distressing physical symptom is profound dyspnea that has limited her ability to bathe, cook, eat, get dressed, and walk. Essentially all independent activities of daily living have been stripped from her, and she is now confined to bed under the care of her husband. Currently, the treatment for her dyspnea consists of bronchodilators, oxygen, and steroids.

Mrs. T. is a retired school teacher and prior to her illness enjoyed reading and crafts. She is Lutheran and is a very active member in her church. Mrs. T's mother died 2 years ago from cancer, and since that time Mrs. T. has assumed the primary caregiver role for her elderly, ill father who lives in her home. Her daughter is to be married in 1 month.

BIO-PSYCHOSOCIAL-SPIRITUAL ASSESSMENT OF MRS. T AND HER FAMILY BY THE ADVANCED PRACTICE NURSE ON THE PALLIATIVE CARE UNIT

Through daily interactions with Mrs. T. and her family, the APN built a therapeutic, trusting relationship focused upon management of physical symptoms and their meaning for family and advanced care planning. Despite the multimodal therapy utilized to treat Mrs. T.'s dyspnea, she continued to feel like she was suffocating at all times which in turn increased her anxiety. The APN ordered intermittent oral morphine to relieve the sensation of breathlessness. Mrs. T and her family were hesitant to use morphine as they heard it was "addicting." The APN discussed the misconceptions associated with morphine use, and explained the distinctions between addiction, dependence, and tolerance. Mrs. T agreed to use it and immediately began to experience relief from her sensation of breathlessness and anxiety. Through providing education and support to Mrs. T and her family regarding this clinical issue, the APN was able to assist the patient and family in feeling prepared to make quality of life decisions, thereby strengthening their therapeutic relationship.

Respecting the value of nonpharmacological measures in relieving dyspnea, the APN recommended a fan to be directed at Mrs. T's face as she recalled recent research which demonstrated that cool air blowing on the trigeminal nerve diminishes the sensation of breathlessness.

The staff nurse reports to the interdisciplinary team that when Mrs. T. and her daughter discuss the upcoming wedding, Mrs.T requires more breakthrough opioid, which does not appear to relieve her dyspnea. After rounds, the APN gently explored with Mrs. T her feelings towards her daughter's future wedding. Mrs. T began crying and acknowledged the despair she is feeling regarding her inability to help with the wedding plans, and most importantly she feels she may not live to see the wedding day. The APN remained present with Mrs. T. allowing her to express all her fears. The APN reported back to the interdisciplinary team the interactions she had with Mrs. T., and based upon the APN's observations and recommendations, the interdisciplinary team developed an adjusted plan of care to increase psychosocial/spiritual support to Mrs. T to help process her feelings of loss and despair. This included increased visits from the chaplain and social worker, and the incorporation of Mrs. T's friends and fellow members of the church into the care plan. Through the interventions of the interdisciplinary team, Mrs. T was able to record a video for her daughter to play the day of her wedding in the event that she died prior to this momentous day.

With in-depth knowledge of family systems theory, the APN identified the need for the interdisciplinary team to address the already actualized loss of Mrs. T's role within the family including mother, wife, caregiver, and daughter. The bereavement counselor began meeting weekly with the daughter after being consulted by the APN to begin early interventions for "high risk grief status."

Having managed several patients with this type of cancer sequela, the APN knew of the potential high risk of tracheal occlusion due to the aggressive nature of this tumor histology. Mrs. T began to display specific clinical signs which heightened the APN's suspicions that Mrs. T's demise might be caused by complete tracheal occlusion. Anticipating the potential patient, family, and staff crisis in experiencing this event, the APN prepared the patient, family, and team with intense education and provided an algorithm of treatment strategies in case this should occur. Understanding that the treatment strategies would involve the use of sedative measures to avoid the patient dying with a feeling of suffocation, the APN prepared the patient and family, members of the interdisciplinary team, and the discipline of pharmacy by conducting in-services on issues surrounding sedative measures, including, treatment strategies, drug choices, therapeutic ranges of dosing, and ethical implications. Prior to these interventions, the APN consulted with the ethics team to collaboratively participate in education.

Progressively, Mrs. T showed signs and symptoms of tracheal occlusion. The interdisciplinary team enacted the well thought out and individualized careplan that aided in minimizing the fear of the family and staff, and patient suffering.

OUTCOME

Mrs. T's death occurred without the feared "suffocation" and she was able to spend her last minutes of life in private communication with her husband. Mrs. T. died 1 week before her daughter's wedding. Through the coordinated efforts of the interdisciplinary team, Mrs. T's family was able to discuss realistic expectations for this day and develop a plan to proceed with the wedding. All family members cherished viewing the message from their mother and wife on the wedding day.

DISCUSSION OF THE ROLE OF THE ADVANCED PRACTICE NURSE

- *Clinician*
  Utilized sophisticated and appropriate assessment tools and input of

all interdisciplinary team members to develop/lead development of comprehensive care plan. Developed new approaches and standards of care. Executed interventions. Advanced clinical knowledge of dyspnea and comfort measures to address physical symptoms and fears was demonstrated through utilization of innovative and ethically sound, scientifically based practice.

- *Educator*
  The APN facilitated complex philosophical, ethical, and clinical management discussions among physicians, family, and all interdisciplinary team members to achieve a positive outcome. The APN assessed the learning needs of Mrs. T, and her family and staff. The APN presented scientifically based education on the following issues: a) potential for role conflict, b) actualized loss/anticipatory grief, c) management of dyspnea, and d) the ethical considerations surrounding the use of sedative measures. The APN educated other disciplines (i.e., pharmacy) through in-services on the philosophy and treatment strategies of palliative care.

- *Researcher*
  The APN generated new knowledge through identifying research questions and by instituting novel approaches to address these questions. The APN investigated and integrated palliative care research strategies to formulate an individual plan of care for Mrs. T.(i.e., use of fan).

- *Collaborator*
  The APN mentored staff in bio-psychosocial-spiritual assessments and interventions. The APN built and preserved collaborative relationships, and identified resources and opportunities to work with community representatives. The APN facilitated the development/implementation of staff forums, in-services, physician/nurse collaboration, and ethics consultation. The APN demonstrated the value of collaboration with the patient and family, the interdisciplinary team, and other health care professionals in order to facilitate the best possible outcome.

- *Consultant*
  The APN consulted with the palliative care physician/ethics team to determine the appropriate treatment strategies for meeting the needs of the patient and family. Also, the bereavement counselor was consulted after the APN identified the actualized loss experienced by Mrs. T's family. As a consultant, the APN was consistently available to the patient and family, IDT, and other health care professionals to discuss and explain issues surrounding the palliative care philosophy.

By maintaining a consistent presence with the patient and family, and among interdisciplinary team members, the APN helped to minimize decision-making conflicts. With advanced knowledge in the humanities, the APN through language and image gave expression to the experience of illness, death, grief, and human suffering.

CONTINUING PROFESSIONAL EDUCATION

Knowledge, public opinion, and changes in health care are generating rapid changes and developments in the area of how we understand and treat patients and families who face life-ending illnesses. In order to fulfill the ever-expanding responsibilities of a palliative care nurse, the nurse is challenged to keep well-informed of new developments in bioethics, symptom management, family care, and public policy. Various forums and educational resources are available to support the palliative care nurse in keeping abreast of evolving issues in palliative care. Participation in professional societies (i.e., Hospice and Palliative Care Nurses Association) and continuing education strategies (i.e., journals, national conferences) along with attainment of specialty certification (i.e., National Board for Certification of Hospice and Palliative Nurses) collectively enhance the palliative care nurse's ability to deliver impeccable bio-psychosocial-spiritual care for patients and families.

CONCLUSION/FUTURE DIRECTION

Palliative care is an emerging specialty within health care, especially nursing. The philosophy and delivery of palliative care transcends to all areas of nursing where suffering accompanies illness. The palliative care nurse is a true leader with the interdisciplinary team and hence, is in an ideal position to establish standards for consistent practice, foster education, and promote research. It is a professional privilege to be in the field of palliative care nursing, as it brings hopefulness to areas of end of life care that have traditionally been avoided, for example ethics, pain, and human suffering. Equally applicable to the art of palliative care nursing practice is Henry David Thoreau's prose in which he states, "It is something to be able to paint a picture, or to carve a statue, and to make a few objects beautiful. But it is far more glorious to carve and paint the atmosphere in which we work, to effect the quality of the day—this is the highest of the arts" (Thoreau, H. D., 1943).

Education Plan 4.1 Plan for Achieving Competencies: Interdisciplinary Palliative Care

Knowledge Needed	Attitude	Skills	Undergraduate Behavioral Outcome	Graduate Behavioral Outcomes	Teaching/Learning Strategies
Palliative Care Movement	*Affirm the need for improved care of the dying and their family.	*Participate in activities supportive of palliative care nursing.	*Demonstrate commitment to offering quality care at the end of life.	*Assume leadership roles in organizing, implementing, and evaluating palliative care nursing initiatives.	*Report on information and resources available at three web sites related to palliative care. *Identify local initiatives targeting change in end of life care. *Participate in an advisory or board of directors meeting related to hospice/palliative care to identify the needs and planned initiatives/responses.

Education Plan 4.1 (*continued*)

Knowledge Needed	Attitude	Skills	Undergraduate Behavioral Outcome	Graduate Behavioral Outcomes	Teaching/Learning Strategies
Ethical issues related to palliative care.	*Consider nursing's position regarding ethical issues associated with palliative care.	*Act in accordance with published nursing position statements related to end of life care.	*Communicate nursing's position regarding ethical issues to the patient, families, and other health care providers.	*Analyze the implications of published nursing position statements related to end of life care. *Participate in the development of nursing position statements, policies, and standards related to ethical issues associated with palliative care.	*Debate ethical issues and nursing's position related to care at the end of life. *Write a personal position statement regarding an ethical issue related to end of life care.

Education Plan 4.1 *(continued)*

Knowledge Needed	Attitude	Skills	Undergraduate Behavioral Outcome	Graduate Behavioral Outcomes	Teaching/Learning Strategies
Role development as a palliative care nurse.	*Affirm students' or nurses' own personal and professional growth as a palliative care nurse.	*Demonstrate the integration of palliative care knowledge, attitudes, and skills in nursing practice.	*Provide competent, holistic, and compassionate end of life care for patients and families.	*Provide competent, holistic, and compassionate end of life care for patients and families in complex caregiving situations.	*Document through journaling an introspective narrative of students'/nurses' own personal and professional growth as a palliative care nurse. *Analyze a case study that documents the responses and practices of the nurse from novice to expert.

Education Plan 4.1 *(continued)*

Knowledge Needed	Attitude	Skills	Undergraduate Behavioral Outcome	Graduate Behavioral Outcomes	Teaching/Learning Strategies
Development, characteristics, and roles of an interdisciplinary palliative care team.	*Appreciate the unique contribution of each member of the interdisciplinary palliative care team. *Affirm the value of nursing's role on the interdisciplinary palliative care team.	*Effectively communicate with all members of the interdisciplinary team.	*Collaborate with members of the interdisciplinary palliative care team in determining goals and plans of care for patients and families experiencing life-threatening illness.	*Assume a leadership position as a member of the interdisciplinary palliative care team.	*Interview individual members of the palliative care team and discuss their unique contributions in post-conference or seminar. *Invite members of the interdisciplinary palliative care team to attend class to discuss their unique contributions, and barriers and facilitators to effective team functioning; *Attend an interdisciplinary team meeting and evaluate effective and ineffective methods of communication. Share findings in class or seminar.

REFERENCES

Beauchamp, T. L., & Childress, J. F. (1994). *The principles of biomedical ethics* (4th edition). Oxford, UK: Oxford University Press.

Benner, P. (1984). *From novice to expert: Excellence and power in clinical nursing practice.* Menlo Park, CA: Addison-Wesley Publishing Co.

Benner, P., Hooper-Kyriakidis, P., & Stannard, D. (1999). *Clinical wisdom and interventions in critical care. A thinking-in-action approach.* Philadelphia, PA: W. B. Saunders Company.

Bircumshaw, D. (1993). Palliative care in the acute hospital setting. *Journal of Advanced Nursing Practice, 18,* 1665–1666.

Byock, I. (1998). Hospice and palliative care: A parting of ways or a path to the future. *Journal of Palliative Medicine, 1,* 165–176.

Carducci, M. A., Blacker, S. E., Perrone, M. E., & Alexander, C. S. (1999). Palliative care in oncology practice. *Clinical Oncology, 2,* 1–12.

Children's Memorial Hospital. (1995). *Professional Performance Assessment.* Chicago, IL.

Cummings, I. (1998). The interdisciplinary team. In D. Doyle, G. Hanks, & N. MacDonald (Eds.), *Oxford textbook of palliative medicine* (2nd ed.) (pp. 20–30). Oxford, UK: Oxford University Press.

deHennezel, M. (1997). *Intimate death.* New York: Vintage Books.

Doyle, D., Hanks, G., & MacDonald, N. (1998). Introduction. In D. Doyle, G. Hanks, & N. MacDonald (Eds.), *Oxford textbook of palliative medicine* (2nd ed.) (pp. 3–8). Oxford, UK: Oxford University Press.

Ferris, F., & Cummings, T. (1995). *Palliative care: Towards a consensus in standardized principles of practice.* Ottawa: Canadian Palliative Care Association, p. 12.

Jonsen, A. R., Siegler, M., & Winsdale, W. J. (1992). *Clinical ethics: A practical approach to ethical decisions in clinical medicine* (3rd ed.). New York: McGraw-Hill.

Kellar, N., Martinez, J., Finis, N., Bolger, A., & von Gunten, C. F. (1996). Characterization of an acute inpatient hospice palliative care unit in a U.S. teaching hospital. *Journal of Nursing Administration, 26,* 16–20.

Krammer, L. M., Muir, J. C., Gooding-Kellar, N., Williams, M. B., & von Gunten, C. F. (1999). Palliative Care and Oncology: Opportunities for Oncology Nursing. *Oncology Nursing Updates, 6,* 1–12.

Lillard, J., & Marietta, L. (199x). Palliative care nursing: Promoting family integrity. In Gilliss C. L., Highley, B. L., Roberts, B. M., & Martinson, I. M. (Eds.), *Toward a science of family nursing* (pp. 437–461). Menlo Park, CA: Addison/Wesley Publishers.

Loscalzo, M. J., & Zabora, J. R. (1998). Care of the cancer patient: Response of family and staff. In Portenoy, R. K. & Bruera, E. (Eds.), *Topics in palliative care,* Vol. 2 (pp. 209–245) Oxford, UK: Oxford University Press.

Merriam-Webster. (1993). *Merriam-Webster's collegiate dictionary* (10th ed.). Springfield, MA: Merriam-Webster, Inc.

Rosen, E. J. (1998). *Families facing death: A guide for healthcare professionals and volunteers.* Revised edition. San Francisco, CA: Josses-Bass Publishers.

Roy, D. J., & MacDonald, N. (1998). Ethical issues in palliative care. In D. Doyle, G. Hanks, & N. MacDonald (Eds.), *Oxford textbook of palliative medicine* (2nd ed.) (pp. 97–138). Oxford, UK: Oxford University Press.

Saunders, S. (1998). Foreword. In Doyle, D., Hanks, G. & MacDonald, N. (Eds.), *Oxford textbook of palliative medicine* (2nd ed.) (pp. v–xiv). Oxford, UK: Oxford University Press.

Spross, J. A., & Baggerly, J. (1989) Models of advanced nursing practice. In Hamric, A. B. & Spross, J. A. (Eds), *The clinical nurse specialist in theory and practice* (2nd ed.) (pp. 19–40). Philadelphia: W. B. Saunders Company.

Thoreau, H. D., (1943). *Excerpts from writings on liberty*. Chicago, IL: Norman Press.

Weggel, J. M. (1997). Palliative care: New challenges for advanced practice nursing. *Hospice Journal, 12*, 43–56.

Weissman, D. (1997). Consultation in palliative medicine. *Archives of Internal Medicine, 157*, 733–737.

World Health Organization. (1990). *Cancer pain relief and palliative care*. Technical Report Series 804. Geneva: World Health Organization.

von Gunten, C. F., Camden, B., Neely, K. J., Franz, G., & Martinez, J. (1998). Prospective evaluation of referrals to a hospice/palliative medicine consultation service. *Journal of Palliative Medicine, 1*, 45–53.

von Gunten, C. F., & Muir, J. C. (1999). Palliative medicine—an emerging field of specialization. Cancer Investigation (Under review).

5

Ethical Aspects of Palliative Care

Judith Kennedy Schwarz

AACN Competencies

#12: Apply legal and ethical principles in the analysis of complex issues in end-of-life care, recognizing the influence of personal values, professional codes, and patient preferences.

#13: Identify barriers and facilitators to patients' and caregivers' effective use of resources.

> Should we inquire into the truth of the matter, or merely accept it on our own authority and that of others?
> —Socrates, in Plato's Euthypro (c.400BC)

Some decisions nurses make when providing end-of-life care seem particularly difficult; even experienced nurses may feel uncertain about whether they made the "right" decision. When the issue is what, all things considered, is the *right* thing to do—a moral or ethical question is asked. It is often exquisitely difficult to determine what the right response is when, for example, a terminally ill and suffering patient pleads with you to help speed her dying; you feel unable to help without causing her harm. An ethically hard case is one in which the good that you want to bring about can only be realized if the harm you seek to avoid is also brought about—when benefiting and harming cannot be disentangled (Cavanaugh, 1996).

Advances in scientific knowledge and developments in medical technology far exceed any social consensus about the circumstances for their appropriate use. The process of dying can now be prolonged almost indefinitely; this technological imperative (*can* do—implies *ought to*), has given rise to an unprecedented array of professional, moral, and legal questions within health care (Schwarz, 1992). The growing support for legalized assistance in dying reflects an increasingly fearful public. In particular, the fear centers on the possibility of dying a painful, protracted, or undignified death absent of personal control or meaning (Coleman & Fleischman, 1996). Research studies indicate that nurses also have fears about how to best provide care for dying patients. In one study, over half of the sample of 759 nurses reported acting against their consciences in providing end-of-life care and were also concerned that they were providing overly burdensome interventions to their dying patients (Solomon et al., 1993). Almost 80% of all American deaths occur in health care institutions, and most deaths are the result of degenerative diseases that are characterized by slow onset and an extended decline (Battin, 1991).

These facts raise such corresponding questions as: should end-stage Alzheimer patients receive technological interventions, including artificial nutrition and hydration, that prolong the inevitable process of dying? Or, how are we to respond to families of patients who are irreversibly comatose and insist that everything be done for their loved ones?

Decisions about death have increasingly become *conscious*, as the ability to sustain biological life increases. It is currently estimated that 70% of the deaths occurring in acute care or long-term care settings are arranged or negotiated by clinicians at the bedside (Orentlicher, 1990). Approximately 6,000 deaths are said to be arranged or planned each day in this country, some indirectly assisted or hastened through use of pain relieving analgesia or from decisions to discontinue or not initiate life-prolonging interventions (Quill, Cassel, & Meier, 1992).

Ethical and legal aspects of end-of-life decision making pose compelling challenges for nurses because they involve conflicts between values, principles, and priorities of care and require reasoned deliberation for their resolution. This chapter provides practicing nurses with the tools needed to identify and address the ethical issues in end-of-life care. In order to identify ethically relevant aspects of complex cases, nurses are encouraged to engage in values clarification and personal reflection. To effectively address the ethical issues in end-of-life care, nurses should use a decision-making framework that incorporates ethical theories, clearly defined moral concepts, and an understanding of the Code for Nurses (ANA, 1985).

Ethical and legal issues often seem intertwined in many end-of-life decisions. For example, the *identity* of who is *permitted* to speak for those incapable of decision making is a legal question. While applying a legal principle may clarify some aspects of cases, it may not satisfy the *moral* question of who *ought* to speak for that now silent person. Often the most difficult clinical conflicts occur at the junction of law and ethics—where an act that is illegal may seem morally required, or one that is legally required may seem morally inappropriate. Many of these cases resist satisfactory solutions. Although ethics and law function similarly in society in that they both sanction and guide behavior, they also differ in important ways. This chapter will focus on ethical issues in nursing care for those at the end of their life.

ETHICS AND ETHICAL THEORY

Ethics is a branch of philosophy that considers and examines the moral life. The word ethics comes from the Greek *ethos*, and originally meant character or conduct; the word moral comes from the Latin, *mores*, which means customs or habit (Davis, Aroskar, Liaschenko, & Drought, 1997). These two terms are frequently used interchangeably in nursing ethics to refer to conduct, character, and motivations involved in moral acts. They incorporate notions of approval or disapproval of both motivation and conduct, and sometimes are also applied to the character or virtues of the actor. Although these terms are commonly used interchangeably, there are some distinctions to be made between them.

The concept of morality is often used to refer to concepts of duty, obligation, and personal principles of conduct. Some authors maintain that morality exists at more of a social conventions level, and includes community expectations and standards of evaluation (Fowler, 1987). The term morals is frequently used interchangeably with values, and refers in particular to values or principles of conduct to which one is personally and actually committed (Jameton, 1984). The term ethics is distinguished by use of reflective thinking and practical reasoning and includes more overarching publicly stated and formal sets of rules or principles such as those found in professional ethics codes.

Normative ethics seeks ways to answer questions about right and wrong or good or bad in situations that call for a moral decision. Nursing ethics is both normative and practical, in that it makes use of ethical theory and analysis to examine and resolve what *ought to be done* in situations involving moral conflict in nursing practice. The term bioethics refers to the application of ethics and ethical analysis to moral and practical problems in biological sciences, medicine, and health care.

VALUES AND VALUES CLARIFICATION

Values have been called the cornerstone of nursing's moral art (Uustal, 1987). Few aspects of our personal or professional lives are value free. Values are ubiquitous; although often unspoken and frequently unexamined, they determine the nature of our moral choices. Values are foundational to our notions of good and bad, and inform our understanding of what constitutes benefit and harm, thus they are instrumental to the ethical decisions we make. Because our values influence the choices we make, they may also bias our judgments about the worth of our own view and negatively influence our judgments about the merits of others' choices, hence the need for values clarification. In the absence of reflection we may simply assume that others believe and would (should) do as we do. Uustal (1987) states that the price paid for unexamined values often included "confusion, indecision, and inconsistency" (p. 149).

Values clarification is a process of self-reflection that helps individuals identify, consider, and articulate the belief, purposes, and attitudes they prize and that drive their actions. Beliefs about death and what makes life worth living, our conclusions about the nature and significance of truth, or the meaning of paths not chosen, are all moral values. Fowler (1987) states that the purpose of values clarification is to assist individuals to identify those personal and professional values that influence behavior and their moral decision making. It is recognized that the essence of ethical conflict is the clash of values, principles, legal rules, and personal perspectives (Dubler, 1994). The need for values clarification is an essential first step in moral decision making.

Every nursing act that intervenes in the life of a patient has at least the possibility of enhancing or transgressing some value cherished by that patient. In situations of moral uncertainty or ethical dilemmas, questions of value will always be foundational. *Moral uncertainty* occurs when nurses are uncertain *if* a moral problem exists, are unsure about its nature, and unclear which values conflict and which principles might facilitate clarification. These situations often occur in nursing practice. Moral uncertainty may occur when a patient seems to be suffering unnecessarily, is refusing pain medication, but is unwilling or unable to explain their reason for refusing your efforts to help.

Moral dilemmas occur less frequently, and are understood as a situation in which two or more clear moral or ethical principles apply but they support mutually inconsistent courses of action. Each alternative course of action can be justified by a moral rule or principle, but one can only choose or satisfy one course of action at the expense of NOT satisfying the other. The nurse who believes s/he is duty-bound both to preserve life and reduce suffering may experience a dilemma when preserving life causes intense suffering or when suffering can only be reduced by interventions that may shorten life. There is no satisfying right answer to an ethical dilemma, but one should utilize reasoned [principled] thinking in order to be able to provide an rationale for the decision reached.

The third type of moral problem is the experience of *moral distress*, an emotion that occurs when nurses have identified and know what the right response that is called for, but institutional or other constraints make it almost impossible to pursue the right course of action (Jameton, 1984). The repeated experience of moral distress can lead nurses to experience moral passivity, burnout, or to leave the profession (Wilkinson, 1988). Nurses who experience moral distress from institutional constraints on their ability to practice as morally autonomous clinicians must seek support from colleagues and from other institutional and professional resources such as institutional and nursing ethics committees and state nursing associations. The experience of organization constraints on professional autonomy causes some nurse's scholars to rhetorically ask whether nurses who face ethical dilemmas are able to be ethical (Davis, 1994).

Resources to assist the nurse to effectively manage moral problems will be included in subsequent sections of this chapter. However, whatever the conflict, knowing one's own values and being sensitive to the values of others is an essential first step in ethical nursing practice.

ETHICAL THEORIES

Moral theories are methods of determining what counts when a decision must be made, and offer a method for weighing or ranking considerations identified as morally relevant to that decision. More succinctly, an ethical theory provides a framework of principles within which an agent can determine morally appropriate actions (Beauchamp & Childress, 1994).

It should be noted that nurses regularly explore and resolve ethical questions in their practice without recourse to ethical theories, and without a formal consideration of the nature of their foundational moral values. But sometimes the fact that people hold different foundational views can heighten moral conflict and diminish the options for resolution. The following scenario by Benjamin and Curtis (1992) illustrates the role that ethical theories can play in facilitating or hampering decision making. The case involves the question of whether everything should be done to prolong the life of a decisionally incapable elder gentleman in a nursing home. The staff must make the decision because there are no friends or family, and no prior indication of his wishes. Person A argues that he should be treated because not to do so would violate the duty to protect and preserve life. Person B agrees that the gentleman should be treated, but for a different reason. B argues that he should be treated because he is not in any pain, and although he is significantly cognitively impaired, he seems fairly content. In B's view, what one ought to do above all, is to maximize happiness, thus the man's life should be prolonged. As presented, the moral question can be answered in this case without agreement about the nature of basic ethical values and without similar systems for justification of those values.

Suppose the facts are changed a little, so that the gentleman is experiencing unmitigable pain and distress. In this case, B, with her foundational commitment to maximizing happiness, would revise her judgment and conclude that they should no longer strenuously attempt to extend the man's life. But the change in facts would be irrelevant to A, and her judgment that the patient's life should be prolonged would remain the same. This conflict is not likely to be resolved without further questions about the nature and justification of ethical principles that are the foundation to approaches of making ethical decisions.

Within bioethics, there are two major approaches to theoretical considerations—deontological and teleological systems of ethics. The deontological (from *deon,* Greek for duty) or Kantian approach to ethics, focuses on duties and obligations. Teleological theories (from *telos,* Greek for end) base the determination of whether an action is right or wrong on the action's consequences. These two ethical theories are increasingly subject to criticism for their overreliance on unrelated and often conflicting principles in dealing with moral problems in health care (Clouser & Gert, 1990), and by feminist moral theorists for their oppressiveness and indifference to the particularity of relationships (Gadow, 1996). These theories continue to dominate the ethical arguments used to resolve moral problems in health care, nurses must recognize them and be familiar with their use in decision making. These two theories will be described and contrasted to a decisional theory based on caring.

DEONTOLOGICAL MORAL THEORY

A deontological or Kantian approach to decision making focuses on duty and obligations. Kantian deontology is attributed to the 18th century moral philosopher Immanuel Kant. Deontologists maintain that whether an act is right or wrong depends upon the nature of the act itself when considered in terms of its inherent moral worth. Duty-based theories hold particular duties to be fundamental and make use of principles or their derivative rules in order to guide decision making. An example of duty-based theories include Natural Law, which identifies a duty to obey God's will and requires that one not kill, and the rules of traditional medical morality derived from the Hippocratic tradition that maintain that we should above all do no harm.

A deontological position requires commitment to the principle of universalizability—which means that once a moral decision is made, that same decision must be made in all similar situations regardless of the circumstances, time, or the identity of those involved. Such rules as, it is always wrong to directly take innocent human life, are considered valid when they meet certain conditions, identified by Kant as categorical imperatives. Proposed by Kant as a means to resolve conflicts between rules and principles, this imperative means that for a rule to be valid it must be applicable to everyone universally. This principle can be illustrated as follows: If it is morally acceptable for me to act as I do for my patient (e.g., not charging for services, stealing medications for her use, skipping home visits, etc.), so must it also be acceptable for every other nurse to act similarly for their patients.

Another form of this categorical imperative requires that persons should always be treated (and valued) as ends in themselves, and never solely as means. Thus nurses are required to respect individuals and their beliefs regardless of consequences and they are similarly obliged to respect persons' autonomous choices. Kant identified these categorical imperatives as unconditional commands that are morally required and obligatory in any circumstance (Davis et al., 1997). Within this theoretical perspective, it is simply one's duty to obey categorical imperatives without any exceptions, without reference to the consequences of the act, and in the absence of external or guiding authority. The moral standard includes keeping promises, avoiding or preventing harm, and respecting persons; these are principles that are morally required and are consistent with the rules provided in our professional code of ethics.

TELEOLOGICAL MORAL THEORIES

Teleological theories determine an action to be right or wrong based on the consequences of the action. The most important teleological theory for contemporary health care is utilitarian ethics (Fowler, 1987). Utilitarianism is best understood as a moral theory that asserts there is only one basic principle in ethics, the principle of utility, and this principle declares that we ought always to produce the greatest possible balance of value over disvalue for the greatest number of persons (Beauchamp & Childress, 1994). This position assumes that one can weigh and measure harms and benefits and arrive at the greatest possible balance of good over evil for the most people (Davis et al., 1997).

Utilitarians are disinterested in considerations of the agent's intentions, feelings, or convictions; all are viewed as irrelevant to the question of, What is the right thing to do? In the same fashion, utilitarians regard the question of whether a proposed action conforms to established social norms or ethical codes as relevant only to the extent that conforming (or not) has a bearing on the production of happiness or value over unhappiness (Aaras & Steinbock, 1995). In principle, at least, utilitarians are able to provide definite answers to specific questions about how one ought to act. The question of whether it is ever morally permissible to be untruthful depends upon context and circumstances; in those situations where telling a lie would, overall, produce more happiness or value than unhappiness, than telling a lie would be morally justified.

As with deontological theories, there are two versions of this theory—an act-utilitarian is primarily concerned with the consequences of particular acts, while a rule-utilitarian is more concerned about the consequences of general policies. To illustrate the difference between these versions— imagine that a nurse is trying to decide if it would be morally right to help a terminally ill patient die. An act-utilitarian would try to determine which alternative in this particular situation would maximize happiness and/or minimize suffering. The considerations included in making that determination would be the nature of the disease and the certainty of prognosis, the presence of a treatable depression, whether s/he really wanted to die or needed better palliative care, the impact in the patient's family, and the professional repercussions for the nurse.

By contrast, a rule-utilitarian uses the principle of utility to formulate and justify moral rules—and the correct moral rules are those that promote the greatest happiness for the greatest number (Aaras & Steinbock, 1995). In this particular case, the nurse would ask whether a general rule permitting assisted suicide would maximize happiness. Important considerations of this approach include questions about whether such a practice would put us on a slippery slope and threaten lives of other terminally ill patients who do not really want to die but might feel obliged or are susceptible to being coerced. Thus a rule-utilitarian might agree that while helping this particular patient to die might maximize happiness (or minimize suffering), it would still be wrong because of the larger negative consequences of a general policy permitting assisted suicide (Aaras & Steinbock, 1995).

How would a Kantian resolve this nurse's problem? Aaras and Steinbock (1995) suggest that the categorical imperative gives less guidance—it functions only to tell us what *cannot* be done, and not what *should* be done. The principle of universalizability is just one value in Kantian ethics; the other mandate is respect for persons. The question would then be reframed as, Does a policy of assisted suicide promote respect for persons or would such a policy lead to the devaluing of human life and to nonvoluntary killing of the weak, the vulnerable, and the poor?

Each of these theories has strengths and limitations, but neither ethical theories nor principles alone will provide a formula for resolving ethical questions. What they do provide is a framework for trying to reach workable solutions to complex and difficult questions (Aaras & Steinbock, 1995).

FOCUS ON CARING

An ethic of caring that focuses on relationships and responsibility is one aspect of the broader field of feminist ethics. This ethic stems in part from a critique of traditional ethical theories as biased in their representation of the experiences of men rather than women. Another dimension of feminist ethics is the analysis of oppression and dominance within relationships and social institutions. It is certain that power differentials between nurses (who are primarily female), physicians, patients, administrators, and payers illustrate just some of the relational inequalities that exist in most health care organizations (Davis et al., 1997).

The idea of an ethic of caring is particularly appealing to nurses because caring is considered to be the very foundation of their practice. Sara Fry, a contemporary nurse philosopher proposes caring as a fundamental value for the development of a theory of nursing ethics (Fry, 1989). Care for others is a core notion in an ethic of care, and is evident in the ANA Code for Nurses (1985), which mandates respectful care of the individual as its core tenet.

In an ethic of care, the decision maker focuses on identifying actions that promote and maintain relationships and views the patient as a unique individual within networks of relationships (Davis et al., 1997). Fry, Killen, and Robinson (1996) maintain that, "the actions and judgments made using care-based reasoning must be measured against what it means to be 'caring' within the context of the responsibilities the decision maker has to others . . . care-based reasoning does not involve the application of abstract ethical principles to the situation or impartiality on the part of the decision maker" (p. 42). Other scholars criticize the rejection of ethical principles as "an invitation to capriciousness" (Held, 1994, p. 75). An ethic of care is not yet adequately developed to function as a conceptual theory for identifying "right" actions in morally troubling situations (Davis et al., 1997; Fry, Killen, & Robinson, 1996).

ETHICAL PRINCIPLES AND CONCEPTS

The major ethical principles of significance to nurses are: respect for persons and autonomy; beneficence; nonmaleficence; and justice. The duties of veracity, fidelity, and confidentiality are moral rules derived from these principles that further guide and direct nursing actions. These moral rules are embedded in the provisions of the Code for Nurses (ANA, 1985). One particular rule that resonates for nurses who care for patients at the end of life is the proscription that, "the nurse does not act deliberately to terminate the life of any person" (p. 3). There may be occasions when moral agents feel obliged to question these rules and their appropriateness; under those circumstances they may wish to "appeal" to a higher level of moral authority (Veatch & Fry, 1995). Perhaps a nurse may question whether it is *always* wrong to "act deliberately to terminate the life of any person" and to ask whether other duties like mercy and compassion might sometimes prevail. This higher level of authority within a moral framework consists of ethical principles.

RESPECT FOR PERSONS AND THE PRINCIPLE OF AUTONOMY

The most fundamental ethical principle within nursing practice is the principle of respect for persons. The first provision in the Code for Nurses (ANA, 1985) calls for nurses to "provide services with respect for human dignity and the uniqueness of clients" (p. 1) unrestricted by any other considerations. Nurses are expected to, "take all *reasonable means* to protect and preserve life when there is *hope* of recovery or *reasonable hope of benefit* from life-prolonging treatment" (ANA, 1985, p. 2). In order to discern the meaning of such values as "hope" and "benefit," nurses must turn to the patient or to those who know them best.

The principle of respect for persons is broader and more abstract than the principle that addresses individual autonomy and self-determination. Respect for persons requires that each individual be treated as unique and entitled to treatment that is respectful of their human dignity. It is this principle of respect for persons that requires particular justification before we are permitted to interfere with the plans, privacy, or behavior of autonomous adult persons, and specifically constrains *paternalistic* decisions made by health professionals for patients with decision-making capacity.

The concept of autonomy is multidimensional and in its broadest sense incorporates the following: having a minimum of relevant information; self-determined choice; freedom to act on the basis of one's choices; and self-governance (Yeo, Moorhouse, & Dalziel, 1996). An autonomous (or decisionally capable) person determines their own course of action in accordance with a plan chosen by themselves. An autonomous action is understood as one done intentionally; made with understanding and without controlling influences that determine the action (Beauchamp & Childress, 1994).

How are nurses to understand this principle? This principle guides nursing actions in that nurses are *duty-bound* to respect patients' autonomous choices in all situations unless this principle is overridden by another moral principle of greater weight or standing (Fry, 1987). Such would be the case when questions are raised about whether the choice is truly autonomous, whether the choice is perceived as harmful to the individual or others, and in other situations where autonomous choice is not possible. In these situations the nurse's obligation to prevent harm to others or to benefit the patient may be determined to have greater moral weight.

It is the principle of respect for persons and autonomy that is the foundation of informed consent. According to this rule, persons must be given sufficient, accurate, and complete information necessary to make informed decisions about treatment choices. This includes decisions to accept, refuse, or to terminate treatments; whether or not these treatments are necessary for sustaining or prolonging life.

LIMITING AUTONOMY

Nurses who care for patients at the end of life may sometime wonder whether they ought to intervene to prevent harm that they fear may result from a patient's decision. Put another way, are clinicians ever justified in limiting or interfering with a person's autonomy? The two most frequently occurring ways that health care professionals infringe upon patient autonomy are through control of information (e.g., withholding, deceiving, or equivocating), or through preventing a patient from acting upon his or her choice (e.g., refusing to comply or assist, constraining, or forcing treatment) (Yeo, Moorhouse, & Daziel, 1996). This type of interference known as paternalism or *parentalism*, occurs often in health care and is done with the best of intentions, indeed, by definition is understood as an intervention that is imposed, for the patient's good or benefit.

In fact, such paternalistic actions as deception, breaking promises, or interfering with adult choices, are violations of moral rules that are never morally permitted unless a morally adequate reason is provided. To justify such violations, philosophers Culver and Gert (1982) argue that we must determine whether we would *publicly advocate* this kind of violation in all similar situations. "If all rational persons would agree that the evil prevented by universally allowing this violation would be greater than the evil caused by universally allowing it, the violation is strongly justified" (p. 149). This would be a difficult standard to meet for those who *presume* justification exists for telling lies we think benefit the other.

In considering circumstances when limitations on autonomy may be justified, "weak" paternalism is sometimes accepted to prevent persons from causing themselves *serious* harm. In this view, one would only be justified in interfering to prevent a *significant* harm from occurring, but only when the person's conduct is *substantially non-voluntary* or *non-autonomous* (Yeo, Moorhouse, & Daziel, 1996). To justify this type of interference, one would have to demonstrate that the presumption of autonomy or self-determination is no longer held, and that the person's choices were in fact no longer autonomous or freely chosen. Under this rule, we would be clearly justified in intervening if we discovered a patient attempting to jump out of a hospital window.

"Strong" paternalism, by contrast, involves limiting or interfering with the self-determination of someone whose autonomy is not in question (i.e., an adult capable of rational decision making), and is very rarely justified. For example, a decisionally capable person who, at the end of her life, makes a thoughtful and considered decision to stop eating and drinking, would be seriously wronged/harmed if a clinician were to override her decision and insert a feeding tube or intravenous line to prolong her life. Paternalistic behavior, regardless of how good the motives or the size of the benefit gained or the harm avoided, overrides the right of an adult to be treated as a person. To disregard a person's life plans and values in such a fashion is to show contempt for them as persons, or in Kant's terms, it is to treat them as mere means to an end, rather than ends in themselves.

Before an act of paternalism can be considered justified, each of the following conditions must be present:

1. The patient's capacity for rational reflection must be significantly impaired. This (*autonomy* condition) must be clinically determined and substantiated.
2. The patient is likely to be significantly harmed unless interfered with (the *harm* condition), and
3. It is reasonable to assume that the patient will, at a later time, with recovery of capacity for rational reflection, ratify or agree to the decision made to interfere (the *ratification* condition) (Benjamin & Curtis, 1992).

QUESTIONS ABOUT CAPACITY FOR AUTONOMOUS CHOICE

Patients should be assumed to have the capacity to make decisions for themselves unless there is clear evidence to the contrary (Beauchamp &

Childress, 1994). Patient capacity is often neither completely present nor totally absent, as is particularly the case in some elderly persons who may evidence a level of capacity that waxes and wanes. When capacity waxes and wanes, caregivers should take advantage of opportunities to engage the patient in decision making and advance-care planning when their capacities are at their best (Lynn et al., 1999). Capacity is best understood as task specific, in that a higher level of capacity is required for decisions associated with serious consequences (i.e., agreeing to a proposed surgical intervention) compared to decisions about choosing meals or where to eat them (Mezey, Mitty, & Ramsey, 1997). A capacity determination is a clinical judgment made by caregivers that know the patient best. When the consequences of the capacity determinations are particularly grave or the determination is contentious, clinicians may wish to seek a psychiatric consultation.

There are occasions when nurses may question whether a decision reflects what the patient *really wants* or whether the choice was *really made* autonomously. They want to know whether the patient is capable of making an autonomous choice and whether they should comply with a decision that seems inconsistent with previously stated values or is detached from contextual reality.

ASSESSING DECISION-MAKING CAPACITY

A decisionally capable person is able to understand a proposed intervention [or its termination], deliberate regarding major risks and benefits, make a decision in light of that deliberation, and communicate the choice to others. (Mezey, Mitty & Ramsey, 1997). The following is information that decisionally capable patients should understand:

- His or her condition for which the intervention is recommended.
- The nature of the recommended intervention.
- The risks and benefits of the recommended intervention, of alternative interventions, including no intervention or treatment.

Caregivers should determine the following:

- The patient acknowledges that treatment is recommended.
- The patient understands how the proposed treatment or lack of treatment can affect their quality of life.
- The patient's decision is not substantially based on a delusional belief (Yeo, Moorhouse, & Daziel, 1996, pp. 99–100).

These criteria are intended to establish *whether* the patient is *capable* of making a rational choice, and not whether the choice being made is rational.

DECIDING FOR OTHERS

If a patient lacks the capacity to make informed choices, other means must be identified for surrogate decision making. There are three standards for surrogate decision making—written advance directives, substituted judgment, or best interest. These three standards are ordered so that advance directives have priority over the other two, and substituted judgment has priority over the best interest standard (Lynn et al., 1999). The best of all situations is a thoughtfully drafted advance directive applied by a surrogate decision maker who knows the patient's values and wishes well.

The substituted judgment is a subjective standard that is ideally based on knowledge of the patient's wishes, values, views about particular interventions, and quality of life determinations. This standard allows the surrogate to decide as though the patient were speaking. Realistically, a surrogate's knowledge about the patient's goals and values is typically not entirely clear and decisive regarding a particular choice of treatment (Lynn et al., 1999). These authors state that, "in practice, surrogate decision making for incompetent patients often has to draw on all three standards for decisions about an incompetent patient's care" (p. 273). The "best interests" standard is used when the patient's treatment wishes, or values, are unknown. Under these circumstances, the decision maker must objectively weigh the expected benefits and/or burdens associated with the treatment recommended by the health care team and determine what would be best for this patient.

Nurses have an important role to play in surrogate decision making; the surrogate must be encouraged to focus on what the now incompetent patients would want if he or she was able to speak. It is often very difficult for grieving family members to put aside their own distress about the implications of honoring patient preference, especially when the decision involves withholding or withdrawing life sustaining treatments. While the patient retains capacity, he or she should be encouraged and guided by nurses to discuss their end-of-life choices with family members of other potential surrogate decision makers. Nurses are well positioned to describe to patients and their loved ones the actual effect of such often traumatic, life-prolonging interventions as CPR, tube feedings, and mechanical ventilation. As Perrin (1997) notes, "advance directives are unlikely to have an effect on care if a health care provider, proxy or family member does not support and advocate for following the person's wishes" (p. 25). In the absence of a thoughtful discussion that includes general end-of-life values and wishes about the use of such specific interventions as artificial nutrition and hydration, the legally appointed surrogate is ill-prepared to identify or implement the right decision for the patient.

BENEFICENCE AND NONMALEFICENCE

Beneficence, known generically as doing good, is often hard to separate from nonmaleficence, or the duty to not inflict harm. Some philosophers argue that the principle of beneficence includes four parts:

1. One ought not to inflict evil or harm (what is bad).
2. One ought to prevent evil or harm.
3. One ought to remove evil.
4. One ought to do good or promote good (Frankena, 1973).

These four rules are prioritized in that the first takes precedence over the second, which is in turn more compelling than the third, which takes moral precedence over the fourth, all things being equal (Frankena, 1973). Although it can seem difficult in clinical practice to distinguish preventing harm from providing benefit, Benjamin and Curtis (1992) believe that it is easier to get agreement on what constitutes a harm than on what constitutes a benefit. When the duty not to inflict harm conflicts with the duty to provide benefit, there is agreement that, all things being equal, there is a greater obligation not to injure others than to benefit them (Beauchamp & Childress, 1994).

NONMALEFICENCE

In health care, the principle of maleficence is understood as requiring clinicians to avoid intentionally causing patients *unnecessary* harm or pain, whether psychological or physical. Neither the principle of nonmaleficence nor any of its derived moral rules are absolute. We often do harm to patients in order to benefit them or to prevent a greater harm from occurring. What is morally relevant is whether causing the harm is morally justified. Under most circumstances, death is considered a major harm; the question of whether causing death is ever justified is an issue of significance to nurses who provide care at the end of life.

Patients at the end of their lives may be particularly vulnerable to harm. They are harmed when they receive unwanted or unnecessary interventions, overtreated with burdensome technological interventions that serve only to prolong dying, and they are also harmed when treatments are withdrawn without their consent or agreement. They are most certainly harmed when their pain is not adequately managed due to the nurse's fear that the patient's death might be hastened as a result of pain management with high dose opiates. The Code for Nurses (ANA, 1985), in addition to telling nurses that they may not "act deliberately to terminate life," also identifies an additional nursing duty; "the nurse may provide interventions to relieve symptoms in the dying client even when the interventions entail substantial risks of hastening death" (p. 4).

BALANCING GOOD AND EVIL—THE PRINCIPLE OF DOUBLE EFFECT

Any discussion that includes attempts to distinguish between harming and benefiting patients must consider the principle of double effect. This principle, developed by Roman Catholic moral theologians in the Middle Ages, is applied to situations in which it is impossible to avoid all harmful action, and a decision must be made about whether one potentially harmful action is preferable to another (Quill, Dresser, & Brock, 1997). This principle is used to justify claims that results of an act that would be morally wrong if caused intentionally are permissible if foreseen but unintended. The principle is often cited to explain why certain forms of care at the end of life that result in death are morally permissible and others are not (Cavanaugh, 1996; Coyle, 1992; Latimer, 1991; Quill, Lo, & Brock, 1997).

The following four conditions must be present for the principle of double effect to justify claims that an act that causes evil consequences is not always morally prohibited (Davis, 1987):

1. the action itself must be good or at least morally indifferent;
2. the individual must *sincerely* intend only the good effect and not the evil;
3. the evil effect cannot be the means to the good effect, and
4. there must be a proportionately grave reason for permitting the evil effect—that is, there must be a favorable balance between the good and the evil effects of the action.

Nurses may appeal to this principle in morally difficult situations where it is not possible to benefit a patient by an action without at the same time causing harm. The classic example is that of the terminally ill pulmonary patient who is experiencing both great pain and a low respiratory rate. The treatment of choice, injecting morphine sulfate, will quell the pain but might also quell the respiratory rate. The nurse has a moral duty to prevent and/or remove evil (pain) that appears to conflict with the duty to benefit patients (protect and preserve life), a dilemma indeed. The answer to the question of whether the nurse may administer the morphine is clearly yes. Applying the criteria of double effect illustrates why this is so:

1. The action of giving an injection of morphine is itself morally indifferent.
2. The *intended* effect is to relieve the pain *not* to depress the respirations.
3. Respiratory depression is not the means by which the pain relief is obtained.
4. The relief of pain and the related reduction of suffering combine to provide a sufficiently important reason—or proportionately greater good than the harm that is incurred—respiratory depression and likely death (Davis, 1987). This moral analysis is consistent with the position found within the Code for Nurses (ANA, 1985).

JUSTICE

The last principle that may facilitate nurses' decisions about end-of-life care is justice, which is understood broadly as fairness. Justice involves the determination of what someone or some group is owed, merits, deserves, or otherwise it entitled to (Yeo, Moorhouse & Donner, 1996). At the societal (macro) level of resource allocation, the concept of justice includes questions of how scarce resources ought to be distributed and what should "count" as morally relevant differences between individuals in order to justify differences in treatment. Micro-allocation issues involve determining which particular person will receive a specific and limited resource. A number of criteria for making such selections include: likelihood of medical benefit, random selection criteria, and present and future quality of life criteria (Yeo, Moorhouse, & Donner, 1996). It is generally agreed that, if a treatment will not medically benefit a patient, it is considered *futile,* and as such, its use is morally and professionally unwarranted. Medically futile interventions should not be proposed or offered to patients or families.

At the individual level of end-of-life care, clinicians cite justice in support of claims for dying patients to receive access to a level of palliative care equal to that of curative care (Coyle, 1992). In the current era of cost containment and social injustice, some fear that those who are already marginalized and disadvantaged by poverty, chronic or terminal illness, old age, or by cultural and racial status may feel a duty to die in order to spare families financial or emotional strain (Robinson, 1990). Individual nurses at the bedside will not resolve these complex issues. They require for their solution, interdisciplinary understanding and cooperative effort among all affected parties within society (Aroskar, 1987). Meanwhile, the Code for Nurses (ANA, 1985) stresses that nurses' commitment is to particular patients regardless of their "social or economic status, personal attributes, or the nature of their health problem" (p. 2), and regardless of the cost of their care to society. The challenge for caregivers is to reach ethically supportable decisions that are fair to individual patients while using available resources responsibly.

ELEMENTS OF A DECISION-MAKING FRAMEWORK

When nurses must choose between alternative courses of action that seem equally unattractive, they experience an ethical dilemma. The decision made will have significant implications for the well-being of the patient, involved family members, and for others effected by the choice. The nurse's ability to provide an ethically defensible rationale for decisions is recognized as a foundation to professional practice and the integrity of individual nurses (Davis et al., 1997). Rushton and Reigle (1993) argue in support of a shared decision-making model that promotes patient well-being and self-determination. According to this model the health care team offers expert knowledge, treatment recommendations, and advice about medically available and appropriate options to the patient [patient/family unit]. The patient decides which option will best promote their life goals and values. The nurse is particularly well positioned to understand the values that inform patients' choices and to appreciate the context of the patient's whole life, including the patient/family unit, their cultural, religious, and spiritual affiliations, and other unique preferences. The nurse is a vitally important member of this decision-making team.

When a clinical problem is identified as ethical and conflicts in moral values or ethical principles are present, the following steps will assist the nurse to successfully discuss, analyze, and develop an ethically supportable decision.

1. Review the overall situation—identify what is going on in this case?
2. Gather all relevant facts about the patient and her/his contextual situation including:

   • significant medical and social history
   • decision-making capacity
   • existence of any advance treatment directives—written, appointed or verbal, and any pertinent institutional policies.

3. Identify the parties or stakeholders involved in the situation, including those who will be affected by the decision(s) made.
4. Identify relevant legal data, including both state and/or federal laws.
5. Identify specific conflicts of ethical principles or values. Identify and consider nursing guidelines and the profession's code and position statements.
6. Identify possible choices, their purpose, and their probable consequences to the welfare of the patient—the focus of primary concern. Identify and make use of such interdisciplinary and institutional resources as institutional and nursing ethics committees, ethicists, chaplains, social workers, and other experienced colleagues.
7. Identify practical constraints to decision making, for example, institutional, legal, organizational, political, and economic.
8. Take action if you are the decision maker and implementer of the decision(s) made.
9. Review and evaluate the situation after action is taken in order to determine what was learned that will help in the resolution of similar situations in patient care and/or policy development (Cassells & Gaul, 1998; Davis et al., 1997).

CONCEPTUAL CONFUSION AND DIFFICULT DECISIONS IN END-OF-LIFE CARE

The final segment of this chapter will explore issues of patient autonomy and decisions about end-of-life interventions that range from instances of allowing or permitting death, to hastening or intentionally causing death and how these decisions are understood by nurses.

AUTONOMY AND THE REFUSAL OF LIFE-SUSTAINING TREATMENT

If the concept of autonomy means anything at all, it means the right to accept or refuse medical treatments. Decisions about the use or withdrawal of life sustaining treatments (LST) are complex and value-laden; decisions about their use may also forestall or hasten the time of death. Decisions regarding use of LST may also shape the patient's experience of the final stage of life; where it occurs, by whom it is attended, and the degree of comfort or suffering. Nurses generally find it easier to accept and comply with patient wishes when they agree with the decision. A decision by a young woman with anorexia-nervosa to refuse food is considerably more troubling than that of an older adult recovering from a serious stroke who indicates a wish not to be resuscitated in the event of a cardiac arrest (Yeo, Moorhouse, & Dalziel, 1996).

The concept of life-sustaining treatments includes any medical or nursing intervention, procedure, or medication, no matter how simple or complex, that is necessary for continued life. In the past, some treatments were considered ordinary and morally required, while others were called extraordinary and considered optional. This distinction between ordinary and extraordinary treatments has a prominent history within the Roman Catholic tradition and was used to determine whether a patient's refusal of treatment should be classified as suicide. Within that faith tradition, refusal of ordinary means was considered suicide (Beauchamp & Childress, 1994).

The terms *optional* (or *nonburdensome*) include (from the patient's perspective) all medications, treatments, and operations that offer a reasonable hope of benefit and can be obtained and used without excessive expense, pain, or other inconvenience. *Extraordinary* (or *burdensome*) treatments are those that are very costly, unusual, difficult or dangerous, or do not offer a reasonable hope of benefit to the patient (Davis et al., 1997). What should be of moral concern for nurses is not *what* the intervention is, but *whether* the benefits of its continued use outweigh its associated burdens, as determined by the patient or surrogate decision maker.

WITHHOLDING AND WITHDRAWING LIFE-PROLONGING TREATMENTS

Many health care professionals and family members are more comfortable not initiating life-sustaining treatments, than stopping them once begun. However, the question to be answered is whether this psychological fact has any moral significance (Beauchamp & Childress, 1994). Some clinicians regard withdrawing LST as "letting die," an act sometimes referred to as *passive euthanasia*, while others view withdrawing LST as an *act* that feels more like causing death, or killing. Withdrawing LST may be experienced as morally problematic for some nurses, particularly those who emphasize the "sanctity of life" and believe that continued life is an intrinsic good, regardless of burdens imposed by illness. However, nurses should be familiar with the existing legal and moral consensus that recognizes *no* moral distinction between withholding or withdrawing LST.

This consensus began to emerge in the early 1980s when a presidential commission was created to explore significant ethical issues in health care (President's Commission, 1983). One of their reports, entitled *Deciding to Forego Life-Sustaining Treatment* maintains that, "neither criminal nor civil law—if properly interpreted and applied . . . forces patients to undergo procedures that will increase their suffering when they wish to avoid this by foregoing life-sustaining treatments." The commission further held that, "the distinction between failing to initiate and stopping therapy—that is, withholding versus withdrawing treatment—is not in itself of moral [or legal] importance. A justification that is adequate for not commencing a treatment is also sufficient for ceasing it."

There is a clear ethical consensus that LST may be withheld or withdrawn under certain circumstances; in particular, when its use is against the patient's wishes (providing the patient is fully informed and freely consenting); when it will or has begun to harm the patient; or when it does not or will not benefit the patient in the future (Beauchamp & Childress, 1994; Davis et al., 1997). The ANA (1994b) in its position statement on assisted suicide, very clearly identifies the following treatment decisions as morally acceptable for nurses: honoring the refusal of unwanted treatments that are either disproportionately burdensome or nonbeneficial to the patient and withholding or withdrawing life-sustaining treatments under the previously specified patient circumstances. These interventions are also distinguished from assisted suicide.

WITHDRAWING ARTIFICIAL NUTRITION AND HYDRATION

Often the most difficult decisions about withholding treatments are those that involve simple noninvasive therapies like the use of antibiotics as well as those that are symbolically linked to caring and nurturing interventions, like providing food and fluids. The artificial provision of nutrition and hydration must be distinguished from the provision of food and water; they are morally and professionally dissimilar. Although dying patients typically experience a decline in appetite as death nears, nurses would continue to offer fluids and food so long as any interest or pleasure in eating remained. The administration of artificial nutrition and hydration is viewed differently. An emerging moral and legal consensus concludes that artificial nutrition and hydration is a medical treatment that may be refused or withdrawn on the same grounds as any other medical intervention, the estimation of its associated benefit or burden to the patient (Beauchamp & Childress, 1994; Veatch & Fry, 1995).

This conclusion is also supported by the nursing profession in the form of a Position Statement on foregoing nutrition and hydration (ANA, 1992). In those cases where a patient is unable to make her or his wishes known, or is unable to evaluate the benefits or harms of refusing artificial nutrition and hydration, a surrogate decision maker should be relied upon to determine what is in the patient's best interests. Nurses should also know whether their state's legislative policy restricts or limits surrogates' rights to decide about the administrations of artificial nutrition and hydration, as some states, like New York, require surrogates to have prior knowledge about the patient's wishes about their use before they are permitted to decide.

FROM LETTING DIE TO ASSISTED DYING: BACKGROUND ISSUES

Nurses who regularly care for dying patients may experience requests for assistance in dying from patients or family members. Every public opinion poll taken over the past 40 years has shown support by a majority of Americans for the idea of physician-assisted dying for those who are terminally ill and suffering (Quill, Cassel, & Meier, 1992). Many Americans have come to view assisted dying as a "reasonable alternative" to their fear of dying a lonely, undignified, prolonged, painful, or institutionalized death (Annas, 1995; Coleman & Fleischman, 1996).

Physician-assisted suicide (PAS) was legalized in Oregon in October 1997; over 60% of that state's citizens voted their support for the Death With Dignity Act. In the first year that PAS was legally available to terminally ill, decisionally capable citizens of Oregon, 16 after ingesting lethal amounts of drugs, compared with 27 people in the second (Sullivan, Hedberg, & Fleming, 2000). According to preliminary information, the reasons these individuals gave for wanting to die included: loss of personal autonomy and control of bodily functions; an inability to participate in activities that made life enjoyable; and desire to control the manner of dying (Sullivan et al., 2000). The experience of unmanaged pain was not cited as a factor. While only physicians are authorized to write the prescription for lethal medication, some warn that nurse practitioners with prescriptive authority will increasingly be asked by their patients as well as by physician colleagues to participate in assisted suicide (Hall, 1996). Oregon nurses must now decide whether and how they will participate in caring for dying patients who choose to ingest a lethal dose of medication, and how to respond in the event that the suicide attempt fails.

DEFINITIONS AND THE NEED FOR CONCEPTUAL CLARITY

Nurses experience uncertainty about the location of the moral, legal, and professional boundaries in end-of-life nursing care (Solomon et al., 1993). They may also find it difficult to distinguish professionally sanctioned end-of-life nursing interventions from those that are not (Schwarz, 1999). This difficulty may in part be caused by imprecisely defined or understood terminology used in end-of-life interventions, thus for purposes of clarification, use of the following definitions is recommended.

Assistance in Dying is an act that directly and intentionally brings about the death of a decisionally capable adult who voluntarily requests such assistance as a means to end suffering that cannot be otherwise relieved in a manner acceptable to that person. This concept includes both assisted suicide and voluntary active euthanasia (Brody, 1992).

Suicide is traditionally understood as the act of taking one's own life, and the act of doing so was decriminalized in 1961. Although the concept of "rational suicide" is increasingly acknowledged, most of those who commit suicide are irrational and suffer from clinically recognized psychiatric disorders and clinicians are obliged to prevent them from harming themselves (Davis et al., 1997).

Assisted suicide is the provision of the means to end life (e.g., a prescription for a lethal amount of drug, the lethal drug itself, or other measures) to an adult who is capable of ending life, with knowledge of that person's intentions (ANA, 1994b; Brody, 1992; Quill, Lo, & Brock, 1997).

Voluntary active euthanasia is a deliberate and intentional act that causes the death (often by the administration of a lethal injection) at the voluntary request of an adult who is incapable of causing his or her own death (Brock, 1992; Brody, 1992; Quill, Lo, & Brock, 1997).

Nonvoluntary euthanasia is a deliberate and intentional act that causes the death of a person who is incapable of expressing his or her wishes about dying, and *involuntary euthanasia* would be direct and intentional killing of a competent person who explicitly refuses receiving euthanasia (Brock, 1992).

Each of these interventions is morally distinct from honoring a patient/surrogate refusal of treatment, withholding or withdrawing of overly burdensome LST, and risking a hastening death through treatments aimed at relieving suffering or controlling pain.

Nurse Participation in Assisted Dying—What Do We Know?

Little is currently known about how often nurses are asked by patients for help in dying, and even less is known about the nature, circumstances, or frequency of their response to those requests (Schwarz, 1999). Only two descriptive studies have asked American nurses about their own clinical experiences regarding requests for assistance in dying (AID) and their response to such requests (Asch, 1996; Matzo & Emanual, 1997). Asch surveyed 1,600 critical care nurses (73% return rate) about their experiences with AID. Although 16% (n = 129) of the respondents stated they had participated in assisted suicide or euthanasia at least once, methodological and design problems associated with this study make these findings difficult to evaluate (Scanlon, 1996).

In the most recent study by Matzo and Emanual (1997), 441 of 600 (74% return) New England Oncology Nursing Society members indicated their response to patient requests for AID. This study replicated a previously completed study of the practices and attitudes of New England oncology physicians toward patient requests for AID. More physicians than nurses assisted patients' suicides (11% to 1%), but nurses were more likely than physicians to have performed patient-requested euthanasia (4% to 1%). Of the 441 responding nurses, 131 (30%) reported receiving up to 20 requests for lethal drugs in the previous year, and 111 nurses (25%) reported up to 20 requests for lethal injections. One percent (n = 6) of the nurses acknowledged helping a patient commit suicide, and 4.5% (n = 20) reported performing patient-requested euthanasia. Eleven nurses (2%) acknowledged injecting a lethal drug into a patient more than once in the previous year (Matzo & Emanual, 1997). Nurses reported that they did not discuss these experiences with their nurse colleagues.

In a national survey of physician practices regarding AID, Meier et al. (1998) report that more than half (57%) of the 38 physicians who described a recent experience with active euthanasia, asked a nurse to inject the lethal drug. As this research was designed and implemented by physicians to explore physicians' experiences, the question of how these nurses responded to the physician's requests was neither asked nor answered (Schwarz, 1999).

THE PROFESSIONAL VIEWS ABOUT ASSISTED DYING

Nurses should know that it is not uncommon for incurably ill or dying patients to look forward to death, have occasional thoughts about suicide (Foley, 1995; Quill, 1995), or to long for an end to the dying process (Coyle, 1992). Nurses and physicians are encouraged to recognize requests for assistance in dying. Assisted suicide or active euthanasia can be viewed as pleas for help (Coyle, 1992; Foley, 1995), and the nurse should explore what the patients are actually telling them. Often there is a need for better pain management (Ersek, Scanlon, Glass, Ferrell, & Steeves, 1995), emotional support (Quill, 1993; Scanlon & Rushton, 1996), or for someone to actively listen (Dixon, 1997).

Expert palliative care clinicians know that the experience of uncontrolled and persistent pain often results in patients with advanced disease feeling hopeless, becoming depressed, and likely to have thoughts about suicide (Coyle, 1992; Foley, 1995). When symptoms of pain and suffering are adequately managed most patients do not request AID. The dying process can be made tolerable, if not ideally comfortable, with good palliative or hospice care for 90% to 95% of dying patients (Coyle, 1992; Foley, 1996; Quill, 1993). Coyle (1992) cautions that, "wanting to die is not the same as wanting to be killed" (p. 45), and maintains that nurses should not participate in assisted dying. She argues for greater access to comprehensive palliative care for symptom management in dying patients and acknowledges that a "small minority" of patients probably will continue to request AID despite adequate symptom control. "Intensive and ongoing supportive care is required for these patients and their families" (Coyle, 1992, p. 45).

Nurses hold varied views about nurse participation in assisted dying and often justify their position by referring to their own clinical experience (Schwarz, 1999). Crucial to most who argue in support of assisting in dying are duties of beneficence, compassion for irremediable suffering, and the obligation to respect the autonomy of competent persons (Daly, Berry, Fitzpatrick, Drew, & Montgomery, 1997). Some experienced hospice nurses argue for those "very occasional" patients who, despite receiving skilled palliative care, prefer death to the life they are left with (Stephany, 1994).

ANA POSITION STATEMENTS ON NURSE PARTICIPATION IN ASSISTED DYING

The professional nursing organization opposes nurse involvement in both active euthanasia and assisted suicide; participation in either action is considered a breach of the Code for Nurses (ANA, 1985) and the ethical traditions of the profession. The justification for opposing nurse participation in active euthanasia is based on the principle of respect for persons, and nursing's historical commitment "to promote, preserve, and protect human life" (ANA, 1994a, p. 2).

Opposition to assisted suicide is based on the nurse's "obligation to provide comprehensive and compassionate end-of-life care which includes the promotion of comfort and the relief of pain, and at times, foregoing life-sustaining treatments" (ANA, 1994b, p. 1). The rationale for opposing nurse participation in assisted dying refers to the profession's central moral axiom, respect for persons, as well as the duty to "do no harm." The ethic of care and the profession's covenant with society that historically has been to promote, preserve, and protect human life (ANA, 1994b) are also factors.

ASSISTED DYING DISTINGUISHED FROM HASTENING DEATH

Experienced palliative care nurses recognize that death sometimes occurs secondarily as an *unintended though foreseen* side effect of high dose opiates used to manage refractory symptoms in dying patients. Despite the clear legal and moral consensus supporting the appropriateness of such interventions, when a patient dies immediately after a nurse provides additional analgesia, it can be a very disquieting experience. The fear of hastening death is well documented as one of the primary reasons nurses may be reluctant to provide adequate pain relief to suffering patients (Solomon et al., 1993).

In addition to reviewing the earlier discussion of the application of the principle of double effect to this issue, nurses are encouraged to also consult the ANA (1991) position statement on the promotion of comfort and relief of pain in dying patients. Nurses are supported in their obligation to provide "increasing titration of medication to achieve adequate symptom control, *even at the expense of life, thus hastening death secondarily*" (p. 1).

BARRIERS IN THE PRACTICE ENVIRONMENT TO SOUND ETHICAL PRACTICE

Nurses need to find ways to talk to each other and validate their experiences, tell their stories of despair or triumph, and share their experiences of moral uncertainty. Nurses may experience conflict between their own moral values and the values of the profession and they have the right to remain true to their conscientious moral and religious beliefs. Although prohibited from compromising legitimate patient choices or imposing their values on others, nurses who are ethically opposed to certain patient interventions will find support for their position in the Code for Nurses (ANA, 1985). They have the right to withdraw from providing care, assuming arrangements can be made for the patient's safe transfer to the care of another.

It is undoubtedly true that some of the barriers that constrain nurses from participating in ethical decision making are situations over which the nurse has no control. For example, most nurses practice as employees in health care organizations whose goals are business-oriented and whose focus is utilitarian (institutional values providing the greatest "good" for the greatest number). Nurses, by virtue of their education, experience, and moral commitment to caring are focused on doing good for individual patients. Conflict inevitably arises between the nurses' role as caregivers/patient advocates, institutional employees, and as clinicians expected to implement physicians' orders. The experience of being the nurse in the middle combined with the moral distress of being unable to do the right thing may result in the nurse perceiving that they are unable to act as morally autonomous agents.

PREVENTING BURNOUT

Nurses who care for dying patients may often find themselves in situations of ethical conflict; burnout is one potential consequence. To avoid the experience of burnout, nurses should: seek support from peers; share experiences of uncertainty; and seek ethics advice and support for the development of skills in identifying and resolving ethical problems in clinical practice. It is most important for nurses to acknowledge their own suffering and sense of frustration in caring for patients at the end of life. For example, when we identify a treatment approach that appears to be in a patient's best interest but we are unable to implement it (perhaps due to disagreements among team members and/or family members about what's in the patient's best interests) can be very upsetting and discouraging. Sometimes, with reflection, a morally acceptable compromise can be identified, one that preserves the underlying values of the concerned parties. Agreement to try a trial of therapy and to reassess within a specified time can help resolve some of the uncertainty.

Hospitals and health care organizations that provide support systems for nurses that encourage and facilitate moral growth and understanding will employ nurses who are less likely to succumb to moral passivity. Nurses should be encouraged to create their own opportunities for support regarding end-of-life issues and may consider the following interventions:

- Use of an ethics consultant can be a source of guidance and help nurses acquire the necessary skills for future application.
- Ethics committees, multidisciplinary and nursing, should be available to nurses for case consultation regarding ethical conflicts. Nurses should be members and work in concert with professional colleagues. Multidisciplinary institutional ethics committees also develop institutional policies and guidelines and plan programs for the ethics education of staff members.
- Interdisciplinary ethics rounds present an ideal opportunity for individuals working in different patient-care disciplines to regularly discuss troubling cases that may not require an immediate decision. Such meetings provide an opportunity for analysis, exploration, and sharing of different points of view. Thus, when ethical problems do occur, a foundation exists to provide guidance about the most effective way to respond.

CONCLUSION

In conclusion, nurses should be encouraged to continue to care as they struggle together with patients and their loved ones, professional colleagues, and concerned others in their attempt to identify what, all things considered, ought to be done in situations of moral conflict. And this, "to the extent that care of the dying draws us into their lives, we experience the gifts and deprivations of their own deaths and painfully anticipate the death of our loved ones and even ourselves" (Dixon, 1997, p. 297).

Education Plan 5.1 Plan for Achieving Competencies: Ethical Aspects of Palliative Care

Knowledge Needed	Attitudes	Skills	Undergraduate Behavioral Outcomes	Graduate Behavioral Outcomes	Teaching/Learning Strategies
Ethical decisions at the end-of-life: —Difficulties of right and wrong; —Influence of medical technology; —Conflicts between values, principles and priorities of care.	*Appreciate the difficulties regarding end-of-life decision making. *Recognize the utility and limitations of nurses' code of ethics. *Acknowledge how personal values influence behaviors and moral decision making.		*Address the ethical issues in end-of-life care. *Use a decision-making framework that incorporates ethical theories and moral concepts in end-of-life decision making.	*Assist nursing and other colleagues when faced with moral dilemmas or moral distress.	*Present cases that pose moral dilemmas and create moral distress related to end-of-life care. Discuss the conflicts, values, principles, and priorities inherent to the case.

Education Plan 5.1 *(continued)*

Knowledge Needed	Attitudes	Skills	Undergraduate Behavioral Outcomes	Graduate Behavioral Outcomes	Teaching/Learning Strategies
Ethics and Ethical Theory: —Terms and definitions; —Normative ethics; —Values and values clarification; —Deontological and teleological theories; —Ethic of caring	*Be sensitive to the values of others.	*Engage in value clarification and personal reflection related to end-of-life care and decision making.	*Articulate the relationship of ethics and ethical theory to nursing practice and palliative care.	*Apply ethics and ethical theory and analysis to moral and practical problems in health care.	*Explore and debate ethical questions related to end-of-life care, i.e., physician-assisted suicide, euthanasia, withholding or withdrawing treatments, DNR. Ask students/nurses to defend a position other than their own. *Debate an ethical issue from a deontological, telelogical, and feminist perspective.

Education Plan 5.1 *(continued)*

Knowledge Needed	Attitudes	Skills	Undergraduate Behavioral Outcomes	Graduate Behavioral Outcomes	Teaching/Learning Strategies
					*View films such as "Dax's Case: Who Should Decide," or "Is This Life Worth Living." *Discuss the values presented, the ethical issues, and possible resolution of the ethical/moral problem using ethical theory to assist with decision making. *Encourage students/nurses to relate an ethical issue from their personal history and explore how it has determined their present stand.

Education Plan 5.1 *(continued)*

Knowledge Needed	Attitudes	Skills	Undergraduate Behavioral Outcomes	Graduate Behavioral Outcomes	Teaching/Learning Strategies
Ethical Principles and Concepts: —Respect for persons and the Principle of Autonomy; —Limiting autonomy as a result of paternalism.	*Respect human dignity and the uniqueness of all people. *Affirm patients' right to determine their course of actions in accordance with their values, beliefs, and preferences.		*Apply ethical principles and the nursing code of ethics in nursing practice. *Provide the patient/family with accurate and complete information necessary to make informed decisions about treatment choices.	*Participate on ethics committee to determine ethical decisions for patients in palliative care.	*Present cases in which patient autonomy has been undermined or not respected. Discuss appropriate nursing responses and actions to support autonomy.

171

Education Plan 5.1 *(continued)*

Knowledge Needed	Attitudes	Skills	Undergraduate Behavioral Outcomes	Graduate Behavioral Outcomes	Teaching/Learning Strategies
Assessing decision-making capacity	*Acknowledge that decision making capacity is often neither completely present nor completely absent.		*Collaborate with advanced practice nurses and other health professionals in determining the decision-making capacity of a patient. *Encourage patients who are competent to discuss their end of life wishes with family or other surrogate decision makers. *Discuss with patients and family the benefits and burdens of life-prolonging interventions.	*Assess decision-making capacity of the patient in conjunction with other members of the interdisciplinary team.	*Round with the interdisciplinary team to determine the decisional making capacity of selected patients. Discuss the process in class or post-conference.

Education Plan 5.1 (*continued*)

Knowledge Needed	Attitudes	Skills	Undergraduate Behavioral Outcomes	Graduate Behavioral Outcomes	Teaching/Learning Strategies
Beneficence and Nonmaleficence and the Principle of Double Effect	*Affirm the principles of doing good and avoiding harm to the patient. *Acknowledge the Principle of Double Effect and its relationship to pain management. *Affirm nurses' moral duty to prevent/and or remove evil, such as pain.		*Avoid causing unnecessary harm or pain to the patient. *Refer the Principle of Double Effect in morally difficult situations regarding the provision of quality end-of-life care.	*Explain the Principle of Double Effect to health care providers, particularly in relationship to providing adequate pain management.	*Discuss cases of pain management with regard to the Principle of Double Effect.
The Principle of Justice	*Adhere to the principle of justice in the allocation of resources for all populations.		*Support access to resources for all patients.	*Collaborate with other health professionals to insure that access to health care and available resources are fairly distributed across all patient populations.	*Discuss an issue related to the allocation of health care resources, such as organs availability or access to opioids. Determine as a group the barriers to fair allocation, and strategies to overcome barriers.

Education Plan 5.1 *(continued)*

Knowledge Needed	Attitudes	Skills	Undergraduate Behavioral Outcomes	Graduate Behavioral Outcomes	Teaching/Learning Strategies
Elements of a Decision-Making Framework	*Appreciate the values that inform patient's choices.		*Utilize the steps of the decision-making process to discuss, analyze, and develop an ethically supportable decision regarding end-of-life conflicts.	*Educate other health professionals regarding the elements of the decision-making process regarding end-of-life conflicts.	*Identify an ethical conflict or problem. As a group utilize the steps of the decision-making process to arrive at a decision.

Education Plan 5.1 *(continued)*

Knowledge Needed	Attitudes	Skills	Undergraduate Behavioral Outcomes	Graduate Behavioral Outcomes	Teaching/Learning Strategies
Controversies, complexities, and difficult decisions in end-of-life care: —Autonomy and life sustaining treatments; —Withholding and withdrawing life prolonging treatments; —From "Letting Die" to "Assisted Dying."	*Judge the benefits to burdens of life-sustaining treatments. *Consider life withholding and withdrawing of life-prolonging therapies as non-distinct and morally and legally appropriate options in end-of-life care. *Appreciate that nutrition and hydration are medical interventions that may be refused or withdrawn, whereas the provision of food and water is appropriate to offer so long as there is interest expressed by the patient.		*Refer difficult ethical situations to the institutional ethics committee.	*Participate on ethics committee to determine ethical decisions for patients in palliative care.	*Based on a case study, debate the issues of withholding or withdrawing life-sustaining therapies. Have students role play the family, physician, nurse, ethicist, and clergy presenting each perspective and determining a solution to the dilemma. *Have students/nurses attend an ethics committee meeting. Based on this meeting, have them present a case in question, the varying viewpoints, and the decision to the class.

Education Plan 5.1 *(continued)*

Knowledge Needed	Attitudes	Skills	Undergraduate Behavioral Outcomes	Graduate Behavioral Outcomes	Teaching/Learning Strategies
Nurse Participation in Assisted Dying: —The Profession's Position; —ANA Position Statements	*Affirm the ANA position regarding physician-assisted suicide and euthanasia.		*Respond to requests for physician-assisted suicide as patient's pleas for help for better pain management, emotional support, or the need for active listening or presence.	*Explore with patients their requests for assisted suicide. *Coordinate interdisciplinary team efforts to provide effective palliative care to decrease the requests for assisted suicide.	*Discuss professional experiences of students/nurses in which they were asked to participate in assisted suicide. Discuss the students'/nurses' feelings and responses. *Review the ANA Position Statements related to End of Life Care. Identify the ethical/legal principles that support the position statements, and discuss the implication for palliative care.

REFERENCES

Aaras, J. D., & Steinbock, B. (1995). *Ethical issues in modern medicine* (4th ed.). Mountain View, CA: Mayfield.

American Nurses Association (1985). The code for nurses with interpretive statements. Kansas City: Missouri: ANA.

American Nurses Association (1991). *Position statement on the promotion of comfort and relief of pain in dying patients.* Washington, DC: American Nurses Association.

American Nurses Association (1992). Position statement: Foregoing nutrition and hydration. Kansas City: Missouri: ANA.

American Nurses Association (1994a). *Position statement on active euthanasia.* Washington, DC: American Nurses Association.

American Nurses Association (1994b). *Position statement on assisted suicide.* Washington, DC: American Nurses Association.

Annas, G. J. (1995). How we lie. *Hastings Center Report* (Special Supplement), 25, S12–S14.

Aroskar, M. A. (1987). The interface of ethics and politics in nursing. *Nursing Outlook, 35,* 269.

Asch, D. A. (1996). The role of critical care nurses in euthanasia and assisted suicide. *New England Journal of Medicine, 334,* 1374–1401.

Battin, M. P. (1991). Euthanasia: The way we do it, the way they do it. *Journal of Pain and Symptom Management, 6,* 298–305.

Beauchamp, T., & Childress, J. (1994). *Principles of biomedical ethics* (4th ed.). New York: Oxford University Press.

Benjamin, M., & Curtis, J. (1992). *Ethics in nursing* (3rd ed.). New York: Oxford University Press.

Brody, H. (1992). Assisted dying—A compassionate response to a medical failure. *New England Journal of Medicine, 327,* 1384–1388.

Cassells, J., & Gaul, A. (1998, Jan.). An ethical assessment framework for nursing practice. *Maryland Nurse,* 9–12.

Cavanaugh, T. A. (1996). The ethics of death-hastening or death-causing palliative analgesic administration to the terminally ill. *Journal of Pain and Symptom Management, 12,* 248–254.

Clouser, K. D., & Gert, B. (1990). A critique of principlism. *Journal of Medical Philosophy, 15,* 219–236.

Coleman, C. H., & Fleischman, A. R. (1996). Guidelines for physician-assisted suicide: Can the challenge be met? *Journal of Law, Medicine & Ethics, 24,* 217–224.

Coyle, N. (1992). The euthanasia and physician-assisted suicide debate: Issues for nursing. *Oncology Nursing Forum, 19,* 41–46.

Culver, C., & Gert, B. (1982). *Philosophy in medicine: Conceptual and ethical issues in medicine and psychiatry.* New York: Oxford University Press.

Daly, B. J., Berry, D., Fitzpatrick, J. L., Drew, B., & Montgomery, K. (1997). Assisted suicide: Implications for nurses and nursing. *Nursing Outlook, 45,* 209–214.

Davis, A. J. (1987). The boundaries of intervention: Issues in the noninfliction of harm. In M. D. Fowler, & J. Levine-Ariff (Eds.), *Ethics at the bedside: A source book for the critical care nurse.* Philadelphia: J. B. Lippincott.

Davis, A. J. (1994). Selected issues in nursing ethics: Clinical, philosophical, political. *Bioethics Forum, 10,* 10–14.

Davis, A. J., Aroskar. M. A., Liaschenko, J., & Drought, T. S. (1997). *Ethical dilemmas & nursing practice* (4th ed.). Stamford, CT: Appleton & Lange.

Dixon, M. D. (1997). The quality of mercy: Reflections on provider-assisted suicide. *Journal of Clinical Ethics, 8,* 290–302.

Dubler, N. (1994, April). Introduction: Bioethics and alternative dispute resolution. In N. Dubler & L. Marcus (Eds.), *Mediating Bioethical Disputes* (A practice guide). New York: United Hospital Fund of NY.

Ersek, M., Scanlon, C., Glass, E., Ferrell, B., & Steeves, R. (1995). Priority ethical issues in oncology nursing: Current and future directions. *Oncology Nursing Forum, 22,* 803–807.

Foley, K. M. (1995). The relationship of pain and symptom management to patient requests for physician-assisted suicide. *Journal of Pain and Symptom Management, 6,* 289–287.

Foley, K. M. (1996, Sept.). Controlling the pain of cancer. *Scientific American,* 164–165.

Fowler, M. D. (1987). Introduction to ethics and ethical theory. In M. D. Fowler & J. Levine-Ariff (Eds.), *Ethics at the bedside: A source book for the critical care nurse.* Philadelphia: J. B. Lippincott.

Frankena, W. K. (1973) *Ethics* (2nd ed.). Englewood Cliffs, NJ: Prentice-Hall.

Fry, S. T. (1987). Autonomy, advocacy, and accountability: Ethics at the bedside. In M. D. Fowler & J. Levine-Ariff (Eds.), *Ethics at the bedside: A source book for the critical care nurse.* Philadelphia: J. B. Lippincott.

Fry, S. T. (1989). Towards a theory of nursing ethics. *Advances in Nursing Science, 11,* 9–22.

Fry, S. T., Killen, A. R., & Robinson, E. M. (1996). Care-based reasoning, caring and the ethic of care: A need for clarity. *Journal of Clinical Ethics, 7,* 41–47.

Gadow, S. (1996). Aging as death rehearsal: The oppressiveness of reason. *Journal of Clinical Ethics, 7,* 35–40.

Hall, J. (1996). Assisted suicide: Nurse practitioners as providers? *Nurse Practitioner, 21,* 63–71.

Held, V. (1994). Feminism and moral theory. In J. E. White (Ed.), *Contemporary moral problems* (4th ed.). St. Paul, MN: West.

Jameton, A. (1984). *Nursing practice: The ethical issues.* Englewood Cliffs, NJ: Prentice-Hall.

Latimer, E. J. (1991). Ethical decision-making in the care of the dying and its application to clinical practice. *Journal of Pain and Symptom Management, 6,* 329–336.

Lynn, J., Teno, J., Dresser, R., Brock, D., Lindemann Nelson, H., Kielstein, R., Fukuchi, D. L., & Itakura, H. (1999). Dementia and advance-care planning: Perspective from three countries on ethics and epidemiology. *Journal of Clinical Ethics, 10,* 271–285.

Matzo, M. L., & Emanual, E. J. (1997). Oncology nurses' practices of assisted suicide and patient-requested euthanasia. *Oncology Nursing Forum, 24,* 1725–1732.

Meier, D. E., Emmons, C., Wallenstein, S., Quill, T., Morrison, R. S., & Cassel, C. K. (1998). A national survey of physician-assisted suicide and euthanasia in the United States. *New England Journal of Medicine, 338,* 1193–1201.

Mezey, M., Mitty, E., & Ramsey, G. (1997). Assessment of decision-making capacity: Nursing's role. *Journal of Gerontological Nursing, 23,* 28–35.

Orentlicher, R. (1990). The right to die after Cruzan. *Journal of the American Medical Association, 264,* 18.

Perrin, K. O. (1997). Giving voice to the wishes of elders for end-of-life care. *Journal of Gerontological Nursing, 23,* 18–27.

President's Commission for the Study of Ethical Problems in Medicine and Biomedical and Behavioral Research (1983). Deciding to forego life-sustaining treatment. Washington, DC: United States Government Printing Office.

Quill, T. E. (1993). Doctor, I want to die. Will you help me? *JAMA, 270,* 870–873.

Quill, T. E. (1995). When all else fails. *Pain Forum, 4,* 189–191.

Quill, T. E., Cassel, C. K., & Meier, D. E. (1992). Care of the hopelessly ill: Proposed clinical criteria for physician-assisted suicide. *New England Journal of Medicine, 327,* 1380–1384.

Quill, T. E., Dresser, R., & Brock, D. W. (1997). The rule of double effect: A critique of its role in end-of-life decision making. *New England Journal of Medicine, 337,* 1763–1771.

Quill, T. E., Lo, B., & Brock, D. W. (1997). Palliative options of last resort: A comparison of voluntarily stopping eating and drinking, terminal sedation, physician-assisted suicide, and voluntary active euthanasia. *Journal of American Medical Association, 278,* 2099–2104.

Robinson, B. (1990, Winter). Question of life and death: No easy answers. *Ageing International,* 27–35.

Rushton, C., & Reigle, J. (1993). Ethical issues in critical nursing. In M. Kinney, D. Packa, & S. Dunbar (Eds.), *AACN's clinical reference for critical care* (pp. 8–27). St. Louis: CV Mosby.

Scanlon, C. (1996). Euthanasia and Nursing Practice—Right Question, Wrong Answer. *The New England Journal of Medicine, 334*(21), 1401.

Scanlon, C., & Rushton, C. H. (1996). Assisted suicide: Clinical realities and ethical challenges. *American Journal of Critical Care, 5*, 397–405.

Schwarz, J. K. (1992). Living wills and health care proxies: Nurse practice implications. *Nursing & Health Care, 13*, 92–96.

Schwarz, J. K. (1999). Assisted dying and nursing practice. *Image, 31*, 367–373.

Solomon, M., O'Donnell, L., Jennings, B., Guilfoy, J., Wolf, S., Nolan, K., Jackson, R., Koch-Weser, D., & Strachan, D. (1993). Decisions near the end of life: Professional views on life-sustaining treatments. *American Journal of Public Health, 83*, 14–22.

Stephany, T. M. (1994). Assisted suicide: How hospice fails. *American Journal of Hospice & Palliative Care, 10*, 1–5.

Sullivan, A. D., Hedberg, K., & Fleming, D. W. (2000). Legalized physician-assisted suicide in Oregon—the second year. *New England Journal of Medicine, 342*, 598–604.

Uustal, D. B. (1987). Values: The cornerstone of nursing's moral act. In M. D. Fowler & J. Levine-Ariff (Eds.), *Ethics at the bedside: A source book for the critical care nurse*. Philadelphia: J. B. Lippincott.

Veatch, R. M., & Fry, S. T. (1995). *Case studies in nursing ethics*. Boston: Jones and Bartlett.

Wilkinson, J. M. (1988). Moral distress in nursing practice: Experience and effect. *Nursing Forum, 23*, 16–28.

Yeo, M., Moorhouse, A., & Dalzeil, J. (1996). Autonomy. In M. Yeo & A. Moorhouse (Eds.), *Concepts and cases in nursing ethics* (2nd ed.). Peterbourough Ontario: Broadview Press.

Yeo, M., Moorhouse, A., & Donner, G. (1996). Justice. In M. Yeo & A. Moorhouse (Eds.), *Concepts and cases in nursing ethics* (2nd ed.). Peterbourough Ontario: Broadview Press.

6

Legal Aspects of Palliative Care

Gloria C. Ramsey

AACN Competencies

#12: Apply legal and ethical principles in the analysis of complex issues in end-of-life care, recognizing the influence of personal values, professional codes, and patient preferences.

#13: Identify barriers and facilitators to patients' and caregivers' effective use of resources.

> Every human being of adult years and of sound mind has a right to determine what shall be done with his own body. . . .
> —Justice Benjamin Cardozo
> *Schloendorff v. Society of New York Hospital* (1914)

Lay and professional communities throughout the world are struggling with bioethical and legal dilemmas brought about by the diffusion of medical technology. A heightened sense of self-determination and decision making associated with: termination of life-sustaining treatment; care of the dying; patient-requested euthanasia and assisted suicide; organ transplantation; genetic testing and engineering; resource allocation; and confidentiality engender bioethical and legal dilemmas in health care. These dilemmas have different practice ramifications for different health care professionals. Patient's well-being, not only in hospitals, nursing homes, and home care but also in rapidly diversifying health care locations, will best be served only if health care professionals are able to collaborate with each other and the patient and family in examining and resolving bioethical issues.

For nurses, in particular, advance care planning is a moral, as well as a legal issue. The moral question of what is right and/or best for the patient, what ought to be done and who is the best person suited to do the right or best thing evokes strong personal sentiments when discussing end of life care. These questions have the potential to provoke conflict among those involved in patient care—physicians, nurses, social workers, and others—and the questions for each are clouded by the individual's personal and professional ethics.

Moral questions pose a different dilemma for the family. Many times, families are faced with discussions regarding whether to stop treatment and let the patient die. A long drawn out death can have a debilitating and at times devastating effect on family members. Whether expected or sudden, few people are truly prepared for death. Dealing with one's mortality evokes a level of discomfort that most people would rather avoid. However, if the family has accepted the patient's diagnosis, prognosis, and impending death, then the confusion, misunderstanding, and guilt they can experience may be mitigated.

Decisions about advance care planning, and especially about foregoing treatment, call for careful thinking and communication. Decisions about care at the end of life ought to be made in accordance with an individual's wishes, preferences, beliefs, and values. No one should be subject to medical care against his or her wishes. Autonomy and self-determination are the foundation for such decisions.

Nursing faculty, nursing students, and practicing nurses address ethical and legal issues including advance care planning with patients and family members daily in clinical practice. With increased medical technology and competing interests of dying patients, their families, and significant others, the wish of many to die with dignity is a concern for health care professionals. Nurses are in a key position to address the escalation of bioethical dilemmas that result in wrenching situations for patients, families, providers, and the courts. Since the landmark cases of Karen Ann Quinlan in 1976 (*In re Quinlan*, (N.J. 1976) cert.denied, *Garger v. New Jersey*, (1976), and Nancy Beth Cruzan in 1990 (*Cruzan v. Director, Missouri Department of Health*, (1990), nurses, physicians, other health care professionals have shaped public policy regarding patient and surrogate participation in end of life decision making even when the patient is incapacitated and unable to make decisions.

LAW AND ETHICS: SAME OR DIFFERENT?

Law and ethics are similar in that they have developed in the same historical, social, cultural, and philosophical soil (Davis, Aroskar, Liaschenko, & Drought, 1997). Black's Law Dictionary defines law as "that which is laid down, ordained, or established; a body of rules of action or conduct prescribed by controlling authority and having binding legal forces; and that which must be obeyed and followed by citizens subject to sanctions or legal consequences" (1990, p. 884–885). The law may be better defined as the sum total of rules and regulations by which a society is governed. Ethics, on the other hand, are informal or formal rules of behavior that guide individuals or groups of people.

Law and ethics are different actions: Actions can be 1) ethical and legal; 2) unethical and illegal; 3) ethical and illegal; and 4) unethical and legal (Smith & Davis, 1980). For the nurse, the latter two possibilities present the most difficult situations and are the most challenging. Legal rights are grounded in the law and ethical rights are grounded in ethical principles and values. The law establishes rules that define a person's rights and obligations and the appropriate penalty for those who violate it. Moreover, the law describes how government will enforce the rules and penalties. There are many laws that affect the practice of nursing and nurses must be able to differentiate ethical issues from those that are strictly legal or clinical.

NURSING AND THE LAW

Legal and moral obligations are not new to nurses. The Nurse Practice Act, a legal statute regulating nursing, and the professional code of ethics are the foundations of nursing practice. Similarly, nurses are confronted with complex moral and legal questions on a regular basis when caring for dying patients. Questions such as: when does death occur?; does an individual have a right to choose death?; is there a difference between letting a person die and taking measures to hasten death?; and do you disclose a terminal diagnosis to a patient?; are a few of the ethical and legal issues in contemporary nursing.

Decision making at the end of life has been at the heart of many ethical dilemma discussions and legal cases in bioethics in the past 20 years. Since nurses are legally responsible and accountable for the health care patients and their families receive, nurses can no longer afford to view the questions of ethics and law as solely an academic exercise. Nor should ethical and legal considerations of today's health care issues remain solely in the purview of the organization's ethics committee or risk management departments. Nurses must understand the basis concepts of ethical decision making and know the relevant laws that address the current controversies to ensure that individual and societal rights and values are protected.

THE LAW AND END OF LIFE CARE: THE RIGHT TO DIE

The term *right to die* is used in the legal context to mean that an individual has a right to refuse medical treatment and the refusal of such treatment will cause death. Alan Meisel (1995) reminds us that the term *right to die* has some unfortunate connotations. To the lawyer, the word *right* is almost sacred. However, to the health care professional, the word is often seen as antithetical to the interests (rights) of health care professionals. The language he suggests denotes an adversarial relationship between patients and health care professionals. Moreover, he argues that many health care providers and laypersons confuse the word *right* with *duty*. When right is used with die, the phrase connotes to some that death is preferable to life or that patients have a right to die, and health care professionals have a duty to let them die, to abandon them, or even to kill them (Miesel, 1995). Taking the lead from the Cruzan decision where the court used the term "right to refuse life-sustaining treatment" in preference to "right to die," the focus here is primarily on how laws may affect the right to refuse life-sustaining treatment and quality of care at the end of life.

Nonetheless, the term *right to die* is increasingly used both popularly and in the legal contexts (Meisel, 1995, 2000). Although not used in all legal cases, and at times rejected by some lawyers and ethicists, the term is being used by the courts and sometimes in combination with phrases such as "death with dignity" (Meisel, 1995). However, during the recent United States Supreme Court decisions (*Washington v. Glucksberg*, 1997; *Vacco v. Quill*, 1997), which addressed whether there is a constitutional right to physician-assisted suicide, the Supreme Court unanimously ruled that there is no such right. The plaintiffs in these cases demanded a "right to die" with physician assistance, not a right to adequate end-of-life care (Burt, 1997).

The United States Supreme Court appeared to preserve the distinction between the withdrawl of life-sustaining treatment (Vacco, 1997) and assisted suicide or euthanasia (Glucksberg, 1997; Orentlicher, 1997). The right to refuse treatment (Cruzan, 1990) is a long established right that physicians are legally and ethically required to honor. Patients have a right to insist that their bodies not be touched without their consent. In light of the Supreme Court's rulings, physicians who provide palliative care, with the patient's consent and with the specific intent to relieve pain and suffering, are encouraged to continue this practice (Annas, 1997). Members of the Court seem to accept that there is a "right not to suffer," at least when death is imminent (Annas, 1997). Accordingly, there remains a *right to die*.

THE LAW AND END OF LIFE CARE: PURPOSE AND TYPES OF ADVANCE DIRECTIVES

Before exploring the purpose and types of advance directives, nurses must know that each state has it own law regarding the use of advance directives. Nurses should know the formalities for executing an advance directive, which type is recognized in their state, and what the limitations are, if any, for honoring an advance directive.

PURPOSE

Advance directives have three major purposes (Meisel, 1995). The first and perhaps most important is that they are a mechanism by which individuals can exercise control over their bodies. This document will allow them to direct the kind of medical care they want or do not want in the event that they lack decision-making capacity at the time a medical decision needs to be made. They are directions to others about the kind of medical care one would like to receive in advance of the need for that care. Advance directives generally are discussed in the context of the right to forego life-sustaining treatments. However, they also may be used to direct the administration of treatment. Advance directives pertain to decision making about any kind of health care, and they may be executed by an adult who is in good or poor health as long as they possess the requisite decision-making capacity to exercise their right to self-determination. Advance directives are intended to effectuate a person's own choice and self-determination even when the individual no longer possesses this capacity (Meisel, 1995).

The second purpose of advance directives is to provide guidance, especially to health care professionals, regarding how to proceed with decision making about life-sustaining treatment in the face of diminished capacity. When patients lack decision-making capacity, a great deal of confusion can arise in the clinical setting as to how health care decisions are to be made, who has the authority to make them, and what the treatment decisions should be. Advance directives contribute significantly to the willingness of health care professionals to proceed with a clinical approach to decision making rather than requesting judicial intervention when patients lack decision-making capacity.

The third purpose of advance directives, and the one which might be identified as most important by health care professionals, is that they provide immunity from civil and criminal liability when certain stated conditions are met. All advance directive statutes contain provisions that grant immunity to health care professionals when they act in good faith and in accordance with state statutes respecting advance directives (Meisel, 1995). Most litigated "right to die" cases end up in court because of the fear of liability, statutory immunity provisions provide an impetus for decision making by protecting health care professionals in the clinical setting.

TYPES OF ADVANCE DIRECTIVES

There are two types of advance directives, the living will and the durable power of attorney for health care. Advance directives generally give instructions and guidance regarding end-of-life wishes and preferences and/or appoint a proxy to serve as a surrogate in decision making. This section will discuss each of these, as well as other relevant issues pertaining to advance directives.

THE SUPPORT STUDY

In light of the increased attention to end-of-life issues in lay and medical publications, physicians are often unaware of their patients' preferences concerning end of life care. The Study to Understand Prognoses and Preferences for Outcomes and Risks of Treatment (SUPPORT) and its companion study, the Hospitalized Elderly Longitudinal Project (HELP), both studies of seriously ill hospitalized patients, documented the lack of communication between physicians and their very ill patients about end of life issues (Knaus, Harrell, Lynn, et al., 1995; Haidet, Hamel, Davis, et al., 1998). This landmark study which produced significant data, 67 manuscripts published in the literature as of December 31, 1999 (Phillips, Hamel, Covinsky, & Lynn, 2000), further documented the ineffectiveness of advance directives (Teno, Licks, Lynn, et al., 1997; Teno, Lynn, Phillips, et al., 1994; Teno, Lynn, Wenger, et al., 1997), the effect of serious illness on patients and their families (Covinsky, Goldman, Cook, et al., 1994; Covinsky, Landefeld, Teno, et al., 1996), the cost-effectiveness of life-extending interventions at the end of life (Hamel, Phillips, Davis, et al., 1997), and the influence of patient age and race on decision making (Phillips, Hamel, Teno, et al., 1996; Hamel, Phillips, Teno, et al., 1996; Hamel, Teno, Goldman, et al., 1999).

While the SUPPORT study's intervention on five specific outcomes: physician understanding of patient preferences, incidence and time of documentation of do-not-resuscitate (DNR) orders; pain; time spent in an intensive care unit (ICU), comatose, or receiving mechanical ventilation before death; and hospital resource use failed to make a difference, some of the SUPPORT/HELP findings did not influence clinical practice. For example, ineffectiveness of advance directives in SUPPORT has not dampened the importance for them in policy and clinical practice (Phillips, Hamel, Covinsky, & Lynn, 2000; Fins et al., 1999). In fact, subsequent studies indicate that a Durable Power of Attorney for Healthcare was significantly associated with both DNR orders and comfort care plans (Fins et al., 1999). These findings support patients, nurses, and physicians to engage in conversation addressing end-of-life care. Advance directives are no substitute for careful and sensitive communication and thinking between patients, surrogates, and healthcare professionals. However, when physicians understand patient preferences and there is clear communication about patient preferences, patients' choices are respected (Wenger, Phillips, & Teno, 2000). Nurses play a seminal role in facilitating this important and much needed communication (Murphy et al., 2000).

LIVING WILLS

A living will is a document that documents specific instructions to health care providers about particular kinds of health care treatment an individual would or would not want to prolong life. Living wills generally are used to declare wishes to refuse, limit, or withhold life-sustaining treatment under certain circumstances should the individual become incapacitated and is unable to communicate. An individual may execute a living will to instruct health care professionals not to administer any "extraordinary treatment," "heroic treatment," "artificial treatment," or "life support" in the event of terminal illness. Furthermore, living wills also can be used to give instructions about what kind of treatment an individual wants to have administered, although there are no reported cases in which an individual has requested the administration of a particular treatment through a living will (Meisel, 1995). However, in light of the health care debate about futile treatment, such use may become more prevalent.

While most states have detailed living will statutes, living wills are not recognized by statute in New York, Massachusetts, and Michigan (Meisel, 2000). In New York, however, the Court approved the use of living wills by stating that the "ideal situation is . . . [where] patient's wishes [are] expressed in some form of writing . . . " (*In re Westchester County Medical Center (O'Connor)*, 72 N.Y.2nd 517, 531 N.E.2d 607, 534 N.Y.S.2d 886, rev'g 139 A.D.2d 344, 532 N.Y.S.2d 133 (1988)). The "writing" provides a "clear and convincing" standard of proof (a very high standard of proof) to allow an individual's stated wishes to be respected.

DURABLE POWER OF ATTORNEY FOR HEALTH CARE

A Durable Power of Attorney for Health Care (DPAHC) is a document that permits an individual to designate another person to make health care decisions for them should they lose decision-making capacity. The person who is appointed by the patient to make decisions is called a health care proxy, health care agent, attorney-in-fact, or surrogate. The term "durable power of attorney" should be used to refer to the document used to appoint this person. The language used varies from state to state and nurses should become familiar with their own state's language. Moreover, an agent's authority may also vary from state to state.

One major distinction between a DPAHC and a living will is that the DPAHC may be used for all health care decisions, and not limited to withholding or withdrawing life-sustaining treatment. Further, a DPAHC does not require that an individual know in advance all the decisions that may arise. In fact, a health care proxy can interpret the patient's wishes as medical circumstances change and can make treatment decisions as the need arises.

A DPAHC vests broad decision-making authority to one person. In states with family consent laws, it is not clear how health care providers are expected to resolve conflict between family members who bear the same relationship to the patient in the absence of an advance directive. Generally, in states with family consent statutes, the laws provide some mechanism whereby one may resort to the courts to resolve disputes among family members. There are times when health care professionals receive conflicting instructions from various members of the same family. Appointing a health care proxy is extremely important when an individual chooses not to appoint a family member. For example, it is quite common for an HIV-positive patient or patient with AIDS to appoint a friend rather than a family member as a health care proxy under the DPAHC statute.

Advance directives should become effective only when it is determined that the individual is incompetent or lacks decision making. As long as the patient retains decision-making capacity, his or her decisions govern. When the patient is deemed to lack decision-making capacity, the health care proxy is authorized to make all treatment decisions on behalf of the patient and in accordance with the patients stated wishes, whether reduced to writing or verbally. The proxy is bound to make the kinds of decisions the patient would have made him or herself, had they the capacity to do so. Such decision making employs the standard of "substituted judgment." In situations where the patient has never been competent, and/or there is no clear and convincing evidence of what the person would have wanted, the proxy will be called on to make decisions on the basis of what he or she believes to be in the "best interest" of the patient. Under this approach, it is impossible to truly analyze the proxy's decision on the basis of the patient's right to self-determination. Rather, the effort is made to protect the interest of the patient and to carry out society's interest in providing appropriate health care for all.

COMBINATION DIRECTIVES

A number of states have a single advance directive statute that combines elements of a living will and a DPAHC into a single document. A combination document arguably avoids many of the pitfalls of each document alone. If the instructions are too general, the health care proxy has the authority to determine whether instructions should be applied under the specific circumstances. If the instructions are too specific and do not address the particular situation at hand, the health care proxy has the discretion to apply them or not. Nevertheless, a discussion between the patient and the health care proxy should occur regardless of whether there is a DPAHC or a combination directive. Communication is the most effective way to ensure that the patient's wishes are known and that the health care proxy is aware of their appointment.

ORAL ADVANCE DIRECTIVES

Although a written advance directive is preferable, especially in light of an emergency situation, courts view oral advance directives favorably, especially living wills. The courts have either enforced them per se or have heavily relied upon them in deciding whether to forgo life-sustaining treatment. Even when state statutes recognize written advance directives, oral directives have been found to be legally operative in a number of jurisdictions. The more specific the oral advance directive, the more likely it is to be enforced and have clinical and legal significance.

When made by individuals with full decision-making capacity, courts have considered the weight of the patients' statements when making a decision to terminate life-prolonging treatments. These statements include (Furrow, Greaney, Johnson, Soltzfus, & Schwartz, 1995):

- If the statements were made on serious occasions or were solemn pronouncements (were brought up when the parties were together).
- If they were consistently repeated.

- If they were made by a mature person who understood the underlying issues.
- If they were consistent with values demonstrated in other aspects of the patient's life (including the patient's religion).
- If they were made shortly before the need for the treatment decision.
- If they addressed with some specificity the actual condition of the patient.

Accordingly, such statements should be considered and documented by the health care providers when discussing advance directives with patients.

FAMILY CONSENT LAWS

Many people are under the impression that their family members will be allowed to make the proper decisions for them should the need arise and therefore, see no need to formally execute an advance directive (Furrow et al., 1995). Traditionally, health care professionals and the courts have also relied on families to make health care decisions for family members throughout the years, without any legal authority. In 1982, the President's Commission concluded that given this practice, family decision making had gained and should be accorded legal acceptance. The Commission pointed out five reasons why deference to family members is appropriate when done in consultation with the physician and other health care professionals:

1. The family is generally most concerned about the good of the patient.
2. The family usually is the most knowledgeable about the patient's goals, preferences, and values.
3. The family deserves recognition as an important social unit that within limits, ought to be treated as a responsible decision maker in matters that intimately affect its members.
4. Especially in a society in which many other traditional forms of community have eroded, participation in a family often is an important dimension of personal fulfillment.
5. Since a protected sphere of privacy and autonomy is required for the flourishing of this interpersonal union, institutions and the state should be reluctant to intrude, particularly regarding matters that are personal and on which there is a wide range of opinion in society.

Motivated by concern over the formal legal status of family decision making in the 1980s, state legislatures recognized and began to regulate it by statute. In 1995, with the exception of two (2) states, New York and

Missouri, the courts authorized family members and others close to the patient to make decisions (New York State Task Force on Life and the Law, 1995). In fact, the District of Columbia and 30 other states have statutes that explicitly grant family members and others close to the patient the right to make decisions for patients who lack capacity. Family consent statutes vary from state to state. Some have been added to state living will statutes to provide an alternative mechanism for making life-sustaining treatment decisions for individuals who do not have an advance directive, while others are freestanding statutes that either apply to life-sustaining treatment or health care decisions generally.

WHO SHOULD COMPLETE AN ADVANCE DIRECTIVE?

An advance directive can be likened to flood or fire insurance; one hopes never to have to use it but should the need arise, it is important to have the coverage. Therefore, all persons should be encouraged to complete an advance directive, a DPAHC if someone is available to serve as a health care proxy, and, in the event that no such person exists or based on personal preference, a living will. A DPAHC is preferable to a living will in that no one can accurately foretell the future, and interpretations of a living will may be difficult because of the lack of specificity and ambiguity in the terms used.

Even in states with family consent laws, people should be encouraged to complete an advance directive. This is especially important when a person is concerned that their family is unable or unwilling to comply with their wishes, or if the preferred health care proxy is at variance with the hierarchy of family members stipulated in the state's family consent statute.

THE PATIENT SELF-DETERMINATION ACT

The Patient Self-Determination Act (PSDA), (Pub.L.No. 101-508, '4206, 4751 [hereinafter OBRA], 104 Stat. 1388-115 to 117, 1388-204 to 206 (codified at 42 U.S.C.A. '1395cc(f) (1) & id. '1396a(a) (West Supp. 1994)) which became effective December 1, 1991, is the first federal law to focus on advance directives and the right of adults to refuse life-sustaining treatment. The Act was motivated by concerns that in the absence of clear directives regarding their views on life-sustaining treatment, patients do not have their view respected when they become incapacitated. The PSDA requires that facilities (i.e., hospitals, nursing homes, home health agencies, HMOs) participating in the Medicare and Medicaid program must provide written information to individuals about their right to participate in medical decision making and formulate advance directives. The key provisions of the legislation are as follows:

THE PATIENT SELF-DETERMINATION ACT—FACILITIES MUST PROVIDE

1. *Written information* to each ADULT individual concerning "an individual's rights under State law (whether statutory or as recognized by the courts of the State) to make decisions concerning such medical care, including the right to accept or refuse medical or surgical treatment and the right to formulate advance directives."
2. *Written policies* of the provider or organization respecting the implementation of such advance directives.
3. *Inquiry* as to whether a person has an advance directive.
4. *Documentation* in the patient's medical records whether the individual has executed an advance directive.
5. *Nondiscrimination,* that is, not to condition the provision of care or otherwise discriminate against an individual based on whether the individual has executed an advance directive.
6. *Compliance* with requirements of state laws respecting advance directives at facilities of the provider or organization.
7. *Education* for staff on issues concerning advance directives and provision for community education regarding advance directives.

Procedural guidelines for implementation are provided within the PSDA. However, the legislation does not delineate roles for health care professionals in meeting the legislative mandate. This allows for flexibility and innovation in the law's implementation and the creation of appropriate mechanisms to facilitate its purpose (ANA, 1991). Who assumes responsibility for dissemination of the information, assists in executing advance directives, and places documentation in the health care record varies according to state and health care setting.

Similarly, the PSDA does not provide guidance to resolve conflicts among family members and the patient nor does it address the difficult clinical and ethical questions related to decisionally incapacitated patients who have never executed an advanced directive. The PSDA neither creates nor affects requirements with respect to informed consent to medical care or determination of mental capacity. In sum, the PSDA has a narrow focus, that is, the handling of written directives for medical care made by persons who later become incapacitated.

DO NOT RESUSCITATE DIRECTIVES

Cardiopulmonary resuscitation (CPR) is an area in which nurses assume an active role in initiating or withholding treatment. Whether or not to initiate CPR calls for careful attention to ethical, legal, professional, and institutional policies. The ethical principles used to justify decisions regarding resuscitation are rooted in principles of autonomy, self-determination, respect for others, beneficence, nonmaleficence, and best interests.

Cardiopulmonary resuscitation was established to be used with witnessed arrests, sudden death in the young, drowning, and predictable arrests, such as in anesthesia and cardioversion (Hall, 1996). Hall reminds us that all patients who have cardiopulmonary arrest—for any reason, of any age, or with any condition, will have CPR performed in almost all hospitals or nursing homes in the United States unless there is a specific order written to the contrary (the DNR decision). "Slow codes" or "partial codes" or any actions that lead the patient's family to believe a full intensive code is being done when it is not are unethical and could give rise to legal implications (Meisel, 1995). Such practices are also not advisable from a risk management perspective. This kind of behavior unnecessarily exposes professionals and their institutions to potential liability. Moreover, if such actions deceive or injure the family they might be deemed illegal under a civil or criminal action for fraud (Hall, 1996).

Since CPR is automatic for every patient, physicians and nurses fear that if they do not start CPR on all patients that they are at risk of being sued; this is not true. Health care professionals are never required legally to do procedures that are clearly futile. In fact, nurses and other health care professionals might be sued for performing CPR without consent when the current medical literature indicates that such procedures are futile or the treatment will not be effective (Gazelle, 1998). Nurses and other health care professionals are not at great risk of being found liable for refraining from attempted CPR on some patients.

Similarly, with a policy of automatic resuscitation, obtaining a DNR (do not resuscitate) order is critical if the patient wishes to avoid this type of treatment. In 1988, New York became the first state to enact DNR legislation and it required that consent for CPR be presumed and if physicians do not want to resuscitate patients, they must obtain patient's consent before writing such an order (Swidler, 1989). Many other states have enacted DNR legislation since New York. The American Medical Association (1991) mandates that patients and families be consulted before a DNR order is written.

What nurses need to know about DNR directives is that patients have a right to refuse CPR and may request DNR orders after they have been informed of the risks and benefits involved. Open communication is important to ensure that the decision is acceptable to all parties involved. If the physician is unable to write a DNR directive or comply with the patient's request, the physician has a duty to notify the patient or family and assist the patient to obtain another physician. Not all statutes address the duty of the physician to transfer the patient if the physician is unwilling to implement the directive. Thus, nurses ought to be aware when such dilemmas are present and act to advocate on behalf of the patient. Moreover, nurses need to know which patients have a DNR directive, the institutional policy and law governing the use of directives, the patient's wishes regarding interventions to be withheld, and their own values toward the decision to withhold treatment (ANA, 1992). The medical record should clearly indicate the terms of the directive and whether the terms accurately reflect the patients' current stated preferences.

Surveys demonstrate strong support for advance directives among the general public (Gordon & Dunn, 1992). However, the low numbers of patients who complete advance directives is alarming. The literature suggests that more patients would complete advance directives if they had more information and assistance in completing them (Mezey, Ramsey, Mitty, & Rappaport, 1997; Emanuel, Barry, & Stoeckle, 1991). To that end, a number of educational interventions have been implemented to address these issues. Notwithstanding, few interventions increased advance directive completion by more than 18% (Hare & Nelson, 1991; Rubin, Strull, Fialkow, Weiss, & Lo, 1994; Sachs, Stocking, & Miles, 1992) and many did not increase completion at all (Robinson, DeHaven, & Koch, 1993). Even patients at higher risk of becoming decisionally incapable and who are more likely to understand the need for advance directives were not more likely to complete advance directives. Completion is however more concentrated among white patients with higher education and income levels (Hopp & Duffy, 2000).

There is evidence to suggest that despite the seemingly low effectiveness rates of educational interventions, heath care providers can make a tremendous difference in whether patients discuss end of life care with their family or friends or complete advance directives. One outpatient home care program elicited a 71% increase in advance directive completions among its 34 participants (Luptak & Bould, 1994). This intervention differed significantly from others by including multiple conversations with a regular health care provider during outpatient visits over a concentrated (2–4 month) period. Such conversations can have a positive effect on advance care planning discussions and advance directive completion.

Patients and providers may fail to discuss advance directives because patients expect providers to initiate a discussion, while providers wait for patients to raise the issue. For that reason, nurses have a very important role in end-of-life care and their relationship with patients and families bear on the decision-making process. As advocates and educators, nurses must educate patients and families to communicate their treatment preferences to their physicians whether they choose to reduce it to a written statement or not. Nurses should facilitate dialogue to empower patients and families to communicate their values, goals, and treatment preferences. Patients want their physicians with whom they have a relationship to initiate and discuss end of life care and living wills (Emanuel et al., 1991).

While many patients discuss advance care planning with their families, other patients find it difficult to initiate such discussions (Elpern, Yellen, & Burton, 1993). Health care professionals can open up discussion between families and patients by providing a format for such discussions or using advance directives to minimize conflicts between patients and their families. Patients indicate that they complete advance directives to ease the financial and emotional burden on their families and to support decision making (Elder, Schneider, Zweig, Peters, & Ely, 1992; Mezey, Kluger, Maislin, & Mittelman, 1996). Patients may decide that an advance directive is unnecessary because they believe that family members would know what to do when the time came. Studies show that patients who feel that others will make appropriate decisions were more likely to have adult children than those who did not (Elder et al., 1992). Health care providers should be aware of these sentiments and, where appropriate, involve family members in these discussions.

Patients who lack critical information about health care interventions or who hold erroneous beliefs about treatments may be unwilling to execute a directive (Kayser-Jones, 1990). In such cases, education may change people's treatment preferences. For example, patients who received written information about CPR both appreciated the information and changed their treatment preferences regarding it (Schonwetter, Walker, Kramer, & Robinson, 1993).

The extent to which a patient's age influences his or her willingness to execute an advance directive is unclear (Luptak & Bould, 1994); there is some evidence that older people are more likely to execute advance directives (DHHS, 1993). Providers need to consider that older people's values about the importance of health may be different than younger individuals. Not uncommonly, an older person might refuse to formulate an advance directive out of concern for the family and the conflicts that such a document might generate (Stetler, Elliott, & Bruno, 1992); they would rather defer decisions to the family (High, 1993; Danis, Garrett, Harris, & Patrick, 1994).

Another issue that influences patients' or families' comfort or discomfort in discussing advance directives concerns how one defines autonomy. Most people who complete an advance directive do so to assure that their individual wishes are followed; however, the western notion of autonomy is not applicable to cultures where the family rather than the individual is the locus of decision making. For such individuals, an advance directive may conflict directly with accepted norms of behavior and the decision-making process identified by that culture. Health care providers need to approach advanced directives with cultural sensitivity and cultural competence (Hopp & Duffy, 2000).

Fears that an advance directive permits providers to withhold care or will lead to substandard care may be at the root of the rejection of advance directives for some patients. People may be concerned that once an advance directive is completed and it contains a statement to withhold treatment, providers will devote less attention to their care and may withhold more treatment than was desired (Caralis, Davis, Wright, & Marcial, 1993). In a study by Elder et al. (1992), some individuals feared that an advance directive might allow care to be withheld too soon and could result in a shirking of societal duties. One person commented that he would not want to hear, "Sorry, we don't have the time or money to treat you." This fear is not only present among patients alone; nurses and other health care providers hold similar beliefs (Anderson, Walker, Pierce, & Mills, 1986; Davidson, Hackler, Caradine, & McCord, 1989).

Socioeconomic and cultural factors substantially influence decisions to complete an advance directive. Studies are confirming that people with less education, lower income, or who are African American or Hispanic are less likely to formulate advance directives (High, 1993; Robinson et al., 1993, Mezey, Leitman, Mitty, Bottrell, & Ramsey, 2000). Several explanations are plausible. Individuals with these sociodemographic characteristics are less likely to have regular access to care. For them, limiting any medical care would seem unnecessary because they already have too little, not too much. They are also less likely to have exposure to the concept of advance directives (Murphy, 1990; Mezey, Kluger, Maislin, & Mittelman, 1996). Furthermore, most physicians are white; people who have experienced discrimination throughout their lives may particularly distrust the intent of health care providers with respect to advance directives. Non-white patients are less likely than white patients to discuss end of life decisions with a white physician. Moreover, certain cultural factors in non-white communities may prohibit discussions of death and dying. For example, there are fears among the African American community that AIDS was developed to wipe out the community (Haas et al., 1993).

The location and timing of when a patient receives information about advance directives is also important. It is well recognized that an acute episode or emergency admission is an inappropriate time to receive this information, yet this is the point at which most hospitals are fulfilling their responsibilities under the PSDA. Information may be better utilized during the pre-admission period where patients can discuss advance directives in the comfort of their own home. Alternatively, information can be presented as part of the discharge process when the impact of hospitalization is still new, but without the distraction of acute symptoms.

In long-term care, discussing advance directives poses particular issues. In some cases, nursing home residents may not have any family or friends with whom to discuss such issues; or a relative may live at some distance and rarely visit. Health care providers can sensitize residents to the need for advance directives under such circumstances. Should the resident decide to execute a DPAHC, providers need to be vigilant that the health care proxy will be available, willing, and able to act in the resident's best interest. Residents with fluctuating decision-making capacity may vary in their ability to fully or even partially participate in decisions about their care. If that is the case, providers need to carefully and critically work at not abrogating resident's rights while shielding those who are decisionally incapable from inappropriately making decisions (Mezey, Mitty, Bottrell, Ramsey, & Fisher, 2000).

While end of life decisions are made by some with little difficulty or conflict, the vast majority of people are reluctant to confront their own mortality and are unwilling to execute an advance directive. A similar phenomenon exists with organ donation, where, even though most people support donation, few actually fill out organ donor cards (Overcast, Evans, Bowen, Hoe, & Livak, 1984). Some may feel that an advance directive will not be necessary in their individual case; tragedy will fall elsewhere. In the Hare and Nelson study (1991), physicians reported that 38% of patients were "interested and eager" to discuss a living will, 32% were "interested and willing, but not eager," 23% were "uninterested and somewhat resistant" to discussion, and 7% had been "openly resistant" to the discussion. Elpern et al. (1993) found that 44% of patients thought it "depressing to think about dying." Some may argue that no amount of education will be able to counteract the discomfort associated with discussing death and dying. However, nurses need to learn techniques to discuss death realistically and sensitively with patients and their families.

Health care providers, both professional and nonprofessional, raise a number of issues when they express their negative feelings about advance directives. Some may mistrust the validity of the information contained in the advance directive because they feel or fear that the patient did not fully understand the advance directives' content or purpose (Jacobsen, White, Battin, Francis, Green, & Kasworm, 1994). The ability to predict specific treatment choices based upon generally stated values and beliefs is not uniformly congruent for patients and their proxies (Emanuel & Weinberg, 1993; Schneiderman, Pearlman, Kaplan, Anderson, & Rosenberg, 1992).

Overall, however, studies show that, even if flawed, patients' wishes and decisions expressed by health care proxies more closely approximate the patient's own treatment preferences than do decisions of physicians or others. In general, patients' decisions seem to be fairly stable over time, especially among patients who have completed advance directives (Emanuel, Emanuel, Toeckle, Hummel, & Barry, 1994; Danis et al., 1994). There is some evidence, also, that patients expect physicians to exercise some latitude in overriding their living will instructions if the physician thinks it would be best for the patient (Jacobsen et al., 1994).

Providers are particularly hesitant to approach patients about directives when the issue of stopping or withdrawing treatment is imminent (Solomon et al., 1993). Many providers erroneously perceive that there is a legal difference between foregoing and discontinuing treatment. Physicians and nurses, for example, are unsure about a patient's legal right to discontinue nutrition and hydration (Olson, 1993). Under such circumstances, providers need to be concerned about the extent to which patients (and health care proxies) are correctly informed about treatment alternatives and consequences and know the relevant laws.

INFORMED CONSENT

Informed consent, albeit a legal requirement, is also a moral imperative. The legal requirement of informed consent is based on the value of patient autonomy and self-determination. Every human being of adult years and sound mind has a right to determine what shall be done with [their] own body (*Schloendorff v. Society of New York Hospital*, 1914). Accordingly, the fundamental goals of informed consent are patient autonomy and self-determination (In re *Farrell*, N.J. 1987). This goal is effectuated by allowing a patient to make their own decisions about their health care based on their own values for as long as they are able.

A second goal of informed consent is to empower patients to exercise their right to autonomy rationally and intelligently (Meisel, 1995). There is no guarantee that providing patients relevant information about treatment will result in patients making intelligent decisions nor does it guarantee that they will use the information provided; however, without such a requirement the likelihood of rational decision making diminishes (Meisel, 1995). The patient's right to consent presumes the fact that the patient has sufficient information to make a reasonable decision.

Consent to treatment is only valid when the patient has the capacity to consent (Meisel, 1995). Competence and incompetence are not the same yet they are frequently considered to be synonymous. Competency to make health care decisions is a legal term that is determined only by a court. The law presumes that all adults are competent and have the decision-making capacity (Applebaum & Grisso, 1988) to make health decisions and the assumption is ordinarily correct (Meisel, 1995). To be considered competent an individual must be able to comprehend the nature of the particular action in question and be able to understand its significance. One need not be adjudicated incompetent to lack the capacity to consent to medical treatment and one who is adjudicated incompetent does not necessarily lack the capacity to consent (Meisel, 1995).

Capacity, on the other hand, is determined not by the courts but rather by clinicians who assess functional capabilities to determine whether or not it is lacking. Incapacity is not determined solely by a medical or psychiatric diagnosis, rather it rests on the judgments that an informed lay person might make (Mezey, Mitty, & Ramsey, 1997).

The basic elements of a valid consent, the determination that a patient has sufficient decisional capacity to consent or refuse treatment are based on the observation of a specific set of abilities: 1) the patient appreciates/understands that he/she has the right to make a choice; 2) the patient understands the medical situation, prognosis, risks, benefits, and consequences of treatment (or not); 3) the patient can communicate the decision; and 4) the patient's decision is stable and consistent over a period of time (Roth, Meisel, & Lidz, 1977).

Not all health decisions require the same level of decision-making capacity in order to make a decision. Decision-making capacity is not an "on-off switch" (Mezey, Mitty, & Ramsey, 1997); you do not either have it or not. Rather, during the past 20 years during the "right to die" movement, bioethicists and lawyers suggested that capacity be viewed as "task specific" rather than in general terms (Mezey et al., 1997). An individual may be able to perform some tasks adequately, may have the ability to make some decisions, but is unable to perform all tasks or make all decisions. The notion of "decision specific capacity" assumes that an individual has or lacks capacity for a particular decision at a particular time and under a particular set of circumstances (Mezey et al., 1997). Most people have sufficient cognitive capability to make some, but not all decisions (Miller, 1995).

Nurses can make a valuable contribution in ensuring that the informed consent process is accurately met (Davis, 1989). Yet, nurses have little training in assessing decision-making capacity (Mezey et al., 1997). Nurses must become proficient in assessing decisional capacity and an active participant in discussions with other members of the health care team when determining decisional capacity. Those with the most knowledge of the patient should be asked to contribute meaningful and relevant information about the person. When nurses and other health care professionals learn how to objectively assess capacity, two types of mistakes will be avoided. First, mistakenly preventing persons who ought to be considered capacitated from directing the course of their treatment and, second, failing to protect incapacitated persons from the harmful effects of their decisions (President's Commission, 1982). Nurses at all educational levels should make efforts to meet their legal and ethical obligations so that patients will retain their rights to make decisions for as long as they are able.

INTRACTABLE PAIN LEGISLATION

All patients, not just the dying, who suffer from pain should be treated. The debate about patient-requested euthanasia and assisted suicide has drawn national and international attention to the fact that appropriate interventions can eliminate or drastically reduce the pain and suffering that many persons experience. The need for appropriate types and amounts of pain medications was made clear in the U.S. Supreme Court ruling in Vacco v. Quill (1997). There is a relationship between pain and symptom management and the requests for assisted suicide (Foley, 1991).

The federal government in 1974 through the Federal Intractable Pain Regulation clarified the federal law that prohibits physicians from prescribing opioids to detoxify or maintain an opioid addition. The regulation stated, in part, that the prohibitive regulations are "not intended to impose any limitation on a physician . . . to administer or dispense narcotic drugs to persons with intractable pain in which no relief or cure is possible or none has been found after reasonable effort" (IOM, 1997). Similarly, some courts explicitly recognize that a patient's "right to be free from pain . . . is inseparable from their right to refuse medical treatment" (Meisel, 1995), and have granted immunity to health care providers who treat pain with strong doses of analgesic medications that inadvertently end the patient's life (*McKay v. Bergstedt,* Nev. 1990). Moreover, several states have enacted intractable pain statutes to encourage those who treat terminally ill patients with intractable pain to manage the pain without threat of legal liability if the treatment results in the patient's death. Nurses should also be aware of the legislation involving the treatment of pain and should advocate to treat patient's pain and assist in the development of institutional policies that embrace the spirit of these laws.

The IOM report coupled with other palliative care literature asserts that change must occur at many levels if we are to improve care for the dying. The development of intractable pain statutes is a good first step to the undertreatment of pain. However, they are not the end all and be all. Problems associated with intractable pain statutes include:

1. [They] do not, in all cases, mark a clear area of medical practice in which physicians feel free to manage their patients' pain. The more specific laws, for example those that set out detailed prescription practices, may actually afford physicians less leeway in the practice of medicine. Additionally, by carving out an area of pain treatment that is immune from medical board discipline, there may be an implication that other forms of pain treatment should be subject to disciplinary review.
2. Even the strongest intractable pain law is still limited by the term intractable. Many cases are ambiguous, and physicians may believe that they must delay opioid treatment until pain is far enough along to be called intractable.
3. An additional problem arises when state laws define addiction without regard to pain management. As noted earlier, California defines addicts as "habitual users," which might include patients taking opioids for chronic pain. Such confusing definitions . . . expose physicians to the threat of medical board discipline.
4. Finally, legal affirmations in these laws of the importance of pain control do not, in themselves, correct practice patterns or improve physician training. Laws could, however, encourage patients to expect diligence in pain relief, including use of generally effective medications. Medical boards could consider disciplining physicians who fail to apply proven methods of pain control (IOM, 1997).

Thus, health care system changes are needed to improve access to care and to eliminate barriers to effective treatment. Nurses need to educate patients and families about their right to adequate palliative care. In states where there are intractable pain statutes, the PSDA requires all covered facilities to inform patients of their state law rights to adequate palliative care (Meisel, 2000). Health care providers need to "add the assessment of pain as the fifth vital sign" (Meisel, 2000), and national pain management standards ought to be followed (Pain Relief Promotion Act of 1999). However, central to all reform is the need for educated professionals to direct this change. Such direction came from The Mayday Fund and the Emily Davie and Joseph S. Kornfeld Foundation in 1995 and 1997 when they funded a project on pain management, and the American Society of Law, Medicine & Ethics (ASLME) worked to address legal and regulatory barriers to effective pain relief (Johnson, 1998). These projects have had significant impact on the problem. Several manuscripts addressed issues such as pain management and managed care (Hoffman, 1998); health care providers' liability for inappropriate pain management (Shapiro, 1996); pain management and disciplinary actions by medical boards (Hyman, 1996); and the clinical, legal, and regulatory barriers to appropriate management of pain (Lo, Rothenberg, & Vasko, 1996) all continue to influence the literature today.

Notwithstanding, there is current debate in the Congress regarding the Pain Relief Promotion Act of 1999, a bill to promote palliative care. Some argue that the proposed legislation will eradicate years of process in the field and others, including Senator Patrick J. Leahy (D-Vt.), argue that pain relief is a matter too complex for the federal government to rule on (H.R.2260). Nurses should be aware of legislative and political debates and should act upon them when they impact patient care.

ETHICS COMMITTEES

Ethical issues in clinical practice often involve life or death decisions and such decisions give rise to a host of emotions. Just as physicians and patients turn to medical specialists and subspecialists for advice and consultations on questions of medicine, physicians and patients may need to turn to ethics committees or ethics consultants to discuss today's perplexing ethical issues. Ethics consultations are more timely, less adversarial, and more flexible than court proceedings as a way to resolve disputes. According to one study in 1995 by Bernard Lo, twenty-one years post the New Jersey Supreme Court decision in the matter of Karen Ann Quinlan, between two-thirds and three-fourths of large hospitals have ethics committees. The Joint Commission of Accreditation of Healthcare Organizations (JCAHO) now requires institutions to have a mechanism to consider "ethical issues arising in the care of patients," such as an ethics committee or consultation service. Moreover, some suggest that individuals with special training in clinical ethics may be an alternative to ethics committees. For institutions such as Long-term Care facilities which are not subject to the JCAHO requirements, they too are establishing ethics committees or regional ethics networks in an effort to embrace the spirit of recent regulations and the need of health care providers to be knowledgeable and informed about ethical questions concerning life-sustaining treatments.

The goal of case consultations by ethics committees or consultants is to help resolve disagreements over ethical issues. Who serves on the committee is a most important question. The committee should look like members of the health care team. In other words, an interdisciplinary ethics committee is needed. The committee members should include physicians, nurses, house officers, social workers, clergy, lay people (community representatives), and members who have formal training in medical ethics, philosophy, religion, and law. The question about the relevance of lawyers being on the committee is mixed. However, if the hospital lawyer or risk manager is a committee member, it is essential that the potential legal risk to the institution does not dominate discussions and trump discussions that are ethically challenging and relevant to health care providers.

The Role Of Ethics Committees

The overall role of an ethics committee is threefold. One, the committee may educate itself, the hospital administration, and the hospital staff about medical-ethical issues occurring in our current health care environment. For example, providers' fear of legal intervention when life support systems are removed from a terminally ill (or even someone brain-dead) patient and fear of the ethics committee can be alleviated arguably through education. Second, the committee may participate in policy development. For example, an institution may draft a DNR policy, a determination of brain death statute, or an advance directive policy. Third, the committee has a role to participate in ethics consultation and to assist in the resolution of bioethical dilemmas. For example, a physician or family who are uncertain or unclear about whether it would be appropriate to discontinue therapy on a patient might consult with an ethics committee and the committee would assist by considering the issue(s), providing information to the physician and family, revisiting the physician's and family's previous decision, or it may move forward and decide the case itself.

Bernard Lo identified five (5) goals of ethics case consultations (Lo, 1995). First, the ethics committees can help the health care team identify and understand the specific ethical issues the case raises, for example, cases that involve questions about advance directives, surrogate decision making, and resolving disputes over life-sustaining treatments. Health care providers need to think carefully and critically through the ethical issues themselves before they try to resolve disagreements with the patient or family. Second, the ethics committees can suggest how health care providers might improve communications with the patient and family. Some committees will hold a meeting with the family and the heath care team and include the patient, if he or she is available. Nonetheless, poor communications and lack of communication among the health care providers and members of the team may be a problem that the ethics committee can identify and help resolve. Third, the committee may provide emotional support to the physician, the nurses, and other health team members in a case. Some members of the team may fear being sued and additional support is helpful and needed. Fourth, another role of the committee is to offer specific recommendations. Some committees or consultants help the health care team analyze the ethical issues and facilitate discussions with patients and families; however, they fall short of giving recommendations. Most committees or consultants do offer specific recommendations for resolving ethics dilemmas and this should be the role of all committees. Lastly, the committees or consultants have a role to improve patient care. They can prevent patient care decisions that contradict ethical guidelines. Patient care decisions do not necessarily need to change after consultations and there is no mandate for such. However, by participating in consultation, health care providers, patients, and families may feel that their concerns have been addressed and may better understand the rationale for the treatment decision that is being proposed.

Committee members should be respected by colleagues and peers for their clinical judgment and their interpersonal skills. They should be receptive to different ideas and points of view, and most important be able to deal with emotionally charged issues and interpersonal disagreements/conflicts, and be able to tolerate ambiguity and complexity (Lo, 1995). Ethics Committees, generally, have found that they serve institutions best in their role as educator. Through education policies are developed and people are willing to seek the committee for consultation. Committees also are more likely to be accepted if they are an advisory group, not a formal and binding court of appeal on pending substantive bioethics questions.

Ethics committees should be voluntary, educational, and advisory in purpose so as not to interfere with the primary responsibility and relationship between physicians and patients. Some view ethics committees as intrusive, claiming that they undermine the physician and result in loss of control and responsibility of the physician. Medical staff bylaws and institutional policy and procedures should delineate the functions of the committee and the parameters of the committee's activities. Again, the function of the ethics committee is to consider and assist in resolving unusual, complicated ethical problems involving issues that affect the care and treatment of patients within the institution and with concern for those who are responsible for their care and treatment. Typically, issues that involve quality of life, terminal illness, or life-sustaining treatments can give rise to disagreements that are often complex and emotionally charged. Values and belief stemming from cultural, ethnic, and religious customs play a pivotal role in these discussions. Emotional and psychological reactions to the decision-making process, and to the issue of treatment termination, can also cause disagreement. Although the distinction between withdrawing and withholding treatment has no legal or ethical significance, it nevertheless can have a profound emotional effect on the health care team. Similarly, despite, as set forth in Cruzan, widespread agreement that artificial nutrition and hydration are simply another form of life sustaining medical treatment, many people feel strongly that these forms of treatment are fundamental and owed to all people. Thus, patients and families are extremely resistant to suggestions to terminate them and the ethics committee may be the best forum to mediate such disputes.

In addition, disagreements that stem from uncertainty or miscommunications between patient and family may mandate that physicians consult with ethics committees. Uncertainty may arise because of the difficulty in determining the patient's medical condition or the effect of various treatment alternatives. Likewise, the patient's failure to state his or her treatment preferences explicitly can create uncertainty. A dilemma may result in miscommunication when the physician leader failed to convey clear and relevant information, when interested individuals do not have an accurate picture of the patient's treatment wishes, preferences, diagnosis, prognosis, and treatment options or of the concerns, hopes, and fears of other interested individuals. Accordingly, regardless of the source of the disagreement, health care providers should be sensitive to warning signs of a brewing disagreement. When a seemingly unresolvable treatment termination disagreement arises, an ethics committee must be consulted and physicians must not view it as intrusive, but rather as clarifying and strengthening the relationship between the parties.

There are times when disagreements concerning life-sustaining treatments give rise to litigation. Thus, the institution's lawyer is well suited to advise and educate the health care team about litigation and should be available to answer questions about the legal process that the staff may encounter during litigation. Discussions with the lawyer may ease some of the fears and dispel some of the misconceptions that health care providers have about the law and litigation in this area. In addition, discussion with the lawyer may address the potential liability for members of the committee and available immunities.

EDUCATION OF NURSES AND OTHER HEALTH CARE PROFESSIONALS REGARDING ADVANCE DIRECTIVES

Education can change nurses' comfort with and willingness to approach patients about advance directives. When they are well-informed and comfortable with their own feelings, they are more likely to initiate discussion about advance directives. Physicians who are educated about directives are more comfortable with such discussions, have more discussions with their patients, and their patients complete more advance directives than do patients of noneducated physicians (Greenberg, Doblin, Shapiro, Linn, & Wenger, 1993; Robinson et al., 1993).

Education of health care providers about advance directives must be multifaceted. For example, less than 50% of nursing homes in New York

City provide ongoing education about advance directives for nurses and fewer than one-third provide education for physicians (Mezey, Mitty, Bottrell, Ramsey, & Fisher, 2000). Much of the PSDA information available to institutions comes from legal departments, state departments of health, or from professional organizations (DHHS, 1993). The extent to which this information is sensitive to the needs of the institution, its subspecialty areas, or the cultural and socioeconomic differences of patients and families is unknown. Education requires more than a description of the law and the steps to be taken in formulating directives. Nurses and other health care providers need to learn how to: discuss advance care planning with patients and families; assess decisional capacity to execute a directive; identify methods to help patients analyze the benefits and burdens of decisions; and resolve conflicts among staff with different values and beliefs about end of life treatment. Education should also include the dissemination and discussion of treatment guidelines, attention to the psychology of decision making, and a dialogue between those who develop ethical recommendations and those who must carry them out at the bedside (Solomon et al., 1993).

Finally, it is important that providers review with patients how and with whom they should communicate that a directive has been formulated. People need to be encouraged to discuss their values and health care preferences with their health care proxy (if one is appointed), their family, and a personal physician, if they have one. A study of recently discharged hospital patients with advance directives documented that less than 15% were asked about existing advance directives during their hospitalization, 60% of patients did not disclose to the hospital staff that they had a directive, and only 35% informed their physician about their advance directives (Mezey, Kluger, Maislin, & Mittelman, 1996). While failure to communicate this information might be attributed to the patient's presumption that the directive would not be relevant for the hospital stay, selective disclosure may reflect a patient's misunderstanding and/or fear about their use.

CONCLUSION

Numerous factors make it likely that end of life decision making will continue to raise difficult issues for health care professionals, patients, and patients' families. The reasons that people do not complete advance directives and discuss end of life care, even after educational interventions, seem much more compelling than the reasons for completing them. Individuals who have completed living wills were often introduced to the concept through experience with the terminal illness of a friend or relative or were told about them by a friend or relative (Elpern et al., 1993). Health care providers often do not have enough regular ongoing contact with patients so that patients do not feel comfortable discussing end of life issues or completing advance directives. The most successful outreach programs had regular contact between health care providers and patients (Luptak & Bould, 1994). Many individuals do not execute an advance directive because they "do not feel their present perceived state of affairs urgently call for advance directives, and there is widespread confidence that they can rely on others" (High, 1993). Any effective educational intervention would have to address this belief, if only to note that the "others" need to know the person's values, beliefs, and desires.

Instead of focusing on the actual number of advance directives completed, we should look at whether our activities are encouraging discussions of end-of-life care with patients and families. The evidence, to date, indicates that simply providing information encourages patients to talk about their preferences with family members and friends (Emanuel & Weinberg, 1993) who are the people that will be making decisions in the event the patient loses decision-making capacity. Anything that encourages such conversations enhances patient autonomy and self-determination.

Advance directives, do-not-resuscitate orders, and court and legislative actions are all important mechanisms for nurses to consider when seeking ways to resolve the ethical dilemmas that exist when caring for patients at the end of life. Nurses must have opportunities to critically think and articulate their views and positions on dilemmas that they face as individuals and professionals. Ethics rounds, grand rounds, ethics colloquiums, courses in basic nursing education, continuing education offerings, and conferences all provide forums for nurses, students, faculty, and clinicians to enhance their ethical and legal awareness. The American Nurses Association Center for Ethics and Human Rights is one rich resource for nurses who seek consultation and ethics information.

Education Plan 6.1 Plan for Achieving Competencies: Legal Aspects of Palliative Care

Knowledge Needed	Attitudes	Skills	Undergraduate Behavioral Outcomes	Graduate Behavioral Outcomes	Teaching/Learning Strategies
Dilemmas in health care can be ethical or legal issues which must be addressed by nurses.	*Appreciate the difference between ethical and legal issues at the end of life. *Acknowledge nurses' role in legal aspects of end-of-life care.		*Discuss the relevant laws related to end-of-life decision making. *Apply legal principles in end-of-life decision making. *Collaborate with patients and health professionals in examining and resolving bioethical issues.	*Shape public policy regarding patient and surrogate participation in end-of-life decision making.	*Review the ethical/ legal issues of the Karen Ann Quinlan and Nancy Beth Cruzan cases. Discuss the rulings and the implications for nursing care at the end of life.

Education Plan 6.1 *(continued)*

Knowledge Needed	Attitudes	Skills	Undergraduate Behavioral Outcomes	Graduate Behavioral Outcomes	Teaching/Learning Strategies
The Law and End of Life Care: —The Right to Die; —Purpose of advance directives; —Types of advance directives.	*Affirm the patient's right to refuse life-sustaining treatments. *Emphasize the value of advance directives.		*Educate patients, families, and other health professionals regarding the purpose and value of advance directives, types of advance directives (including the type recognized by the state), the formalities for executing an advance directive, and limitations in honoring advance directives.	*Guide patients and families in implementing advance directives.	*Invite a guest speaker knowledgeable about the legal aspects of end of life care to discuss such issues. *Encourage students/nurses to complete advance directives, reviewing with them the completion of the forms.
The Patient Self-Determination Act: —Right to participate in medical decision making and formulate advance directives. —Provisions of the legislation	*Acknowledge the key provisions of the Patient Self-Determination Act.		*Inform patients about the provisions of the Patient Self-Determination Act.	*Insure compliance of the institution in informing patients regarding the provisions of the Patient Self-Determination Act.	*Review the Patient Self-Determination Act with students/nurses. Discuss how the act influences nursing practice.

Education Plan 6.1 *(continued)*

Knowledge Needed	Attitudes	Skills	Undergraduate Behavioral Outcomes	Graduate Behavioral Outcomes	Teaching/Learning Strategies
Nurses' Responsibilities regarding Do Not Resuscitate Orders.	*Acknowledge nurses' responsibilities regarding Do Not Resuscitate Orders. *Acknowledge that slow or partial codes are unethical.		*Seek a DNR order when resuscitation would be medically futile. *Institute CPR as a full code unless a DNR order has been written. *Communicate to other health professionals that a "slow or partial" code is unethical. *Advocate on behalf of the patient if the physician is unable to comply with the patient's request for a DNR order. *Confirm which patients have DNR orders and patient's preferences regarding DNR.	*Assist patients, families, and other health professionals in determining the appropriateness of a DNR order. *Educate health professionals of unethical behavior in performing a partial or slow code. *Review with health professionals the institutional policies and laws governing the use of DNR directives.	*Review the completion of the various forms for DNR orders recognized within institutions and in the community with students/nurses. *Explore students'/nurses' feelings and attitudes regarding DNR orders. Discuss the implications to palliative care.

Knowledge Needed	Attitudes	Skills	Undergraduate Behavioral Outcomes	Graduate Behavioral Outcomes	Teaching/Learning Strategies
Factors Influencing the Completion of Advance Directives: —Communication with health professionals; —Age; —Cultural values; —Concern about withholding of care or treatment; —Socioeconomic factors; —Education of nurses and health professionals regarding advance directives.	*Appreciate the emotional issues and factors influencing the completion of advance directives. *Acknowledge the responsibility of nurses and other health professionals in discussing advance directives with patients.		*Discuss the completion of advance directives with patients through multiple conversations and in advance of a life-threatening illness.	*Examine the institutional policies, or professional and patient behaviors related to the completion of advance directives. *Resolve conflicts among staff with different values and beliefs regarding end-of-life treatment. *Collaborate with members of the interdisciplinary team to implement strategies that will increase the completion of advance directives.	*Based on case studies, determine those factors that positively or negatively influence the completion of advance directives. *Invite a guest panel of speakers to class to discuss the completion of advanced directives from a personal perspective, and professional perspective.

Education Plan 6.1 *(continued)*

Knowledge Needed	Attitudes	Skills	Undergraduate Behavioral Outcomes	Graduate Behavioral Outcomes	Teaching/Learning Strategies
Informed Consent	*Acknowledge the legal responsibility of nurses in obtaining informed consent. *Consider the difference between competency and capacity in determining patient's decision-making ability.	*Demonstrate competence in assessing the decision-making capacity of patients.	*Insure that the informed consent process is accurately met in the provision of care. *Actively participate in discussions with other members of the health care team when determining decisional capacity of a patient.	*Coordinate interdisciplinary efforts to determine patient's decisional capacity. *Educate other health professionals regarding the difference between patient competency and capacity in determining decision-making ability.	*Role play patient caregiving situations to determine patient's decision-making capacity. Have students play the roles of interdisciplinary team members in determining capacity.

Education Plan 6.1 (*continued*)

Knowledge Needed	Attitudes	Skills	Undergraduate Behavioral Outcomes	Graduate Behavioral Outcomes	Teaching/Learning Strategies
Intractable pain legislation.	*Affirm the responsibility of nurses in alleviating intractable pain.		*Discuss intractable pain legislation. *Advocate for effective pain management for patients with intractable pain. *Seek referrals to specialists for the management of intractable pain.	*Participate in the development of institutional policies that support adequate pain management, including situations of intractable pain. *Educate health professionals regarding statutes, which encourage physicians and nurse practitioners to treat patients with intractable pain.	*Review case studies of patients experiencing intractable pain. Discuss pain assessment, and interventions in accordance with intractable pain legislation.

REFERENCES

AMA Council on Ethical and Judicial Affairs. (1991). Guidelines for the appropriate use of DNR orders. *Journal of the American Medical Association, 265,* 1868–1871.

American Nurses Association. (1991). Position statement on nursing and the Patient Self Determination Act, pp. 5–7. Washington, DC: Author.

American Nurses Association. (1992). Position statement on nursing care and do-not-resuscitate decisions, pp. 12–14. Washington, DC: Author.

Anderson, G. C., Walker, M. H., Pierce, P. M., & Mills, C. M. (1986). Living wills. Do nurses and physicians have them? *American Journal of Nursing, 86*(3), 271–275.

Annas, G. (1997). The bell tolls for a constitutional right to physician-assisted suicide. *NEJM, 337,* 1098–1103.

Applebaum, P. S., & Grisso, T. (1988). Assessing patient's capacities to consent to treatment. *New England Journal of Medicine, 319*(25), 1635–1638.

Black, H. C. (1990). Law Dictionary (6th ed.). St. Paul: West Publishing.

Burt, R. (1997). The supreme court speaks. Not assisted suicide but a constitutional right to palliative care. *NEJM, 337,* 1234–1236.

Caralis, P. V., Davis, B., Wright, K., & Marcial, E. (1993). The influence of ethnicity and race on attitudes toward advance directives, life-prolonging treatments, and euthanasia. *Journal of Clinical Ethics, 4*(2), 155.

Collins, F. J., Lombard, J., Moses, A., & Spitler, H. (1994). *Durable powers of attorney for health care directives* (3rd ed., Sect. 3. 01). Colorado Springs: McGraw-Hill, Inc.

Conn. Gen. Stat. Ann. '19A-571.

Covinsky, K. E., Goldman, L., Cook, E. F., et al. (1994). The impact of serious illness on patients' families. *JAMA, 272,* 1839–1844.

Covinsky, K. E., Landefeld, S., Teno, J., et al. (1996). For the SUPPORT Investigators. Is economic hardship on the families of the seriously ill associated with patient and surrogate care preferences? *Arch Intern Med, 156,* 1737–1741.

Cruzan v. Director, Missouri Dept. of Health, 497 U.S. 261 (1990), 110 S. Ct. 2841 (1990).

Danis, M., Garrett, J., Harris, R., & Patrick, D. L. (1994). Stability of choices about life-sustaining treatments. *Ann Intern Med, 120,* 567–573.

Davidson, R. W., Hackler, C., Caradine, D. R., & McCord, R. S. (1989). Physician attitudes on advance directives. *JAMA, 262,* 2415–2419.

Davis, A. J. (1989). Clinical nurses: Ethical decision making in situations of informed consent. *Advances in Nursing Science, 11*(3), 63–69.

Davis, A., Aroskar, M., Liaschenko, J., & Drought, T. (1997). *Ethical dilemmas & nursing practice* (4th ed.). Stamford, CT: Appleton & Lange.

Department of Health and Human Services, Office of the Inspector General. (1993). Patient advance directives: Early implementation experience, OEI 06-91-01130.

Elder, N. C., Schneider, F. D., Zweig, S. C., Peters, P. G., & Ely, J. W. (1992). Community attitudes and knowledge about advance care directives. *J Am Board Fam Pract, 5,* 565–572.

Elpern, E. H., Yellen, S. B., & Burton, L. A. (1993). A preliminary investigation of opinions and behaviors regarding advance directives for medical care. *American Journal of Critical Care, 2,* 161–167.

Emanuel, L. L., Barry, W., & Stoeckle, J. D. (1991). Advanced directives for medical care—A case for greater use. *NEJM, 324,* 889–895.

Emanuel, L. L., Emanuel, E. J., Toeckle, J. D., Hummel, L. R., & Barry, M. J. (1994). Advance directives: Stability of patient's treatment choices. *Arch Intern Med, 154,* 209–217.

Emanuel, E. J., & Weinberg, D. S. (1993). How well is the patient self-determination act working: An early assessment 95. *American Journal of Medicine, 95,* 619–627.

Fins, J., Miller, F., Acres, C., Bacchetta, M., Huzzard, L., & Rapkin, B. (1999). End-of-life decision-making in the hospital: Current practice and future prospects. *Journal of Pain and Symptom Management, 17,* 6–15.

Foley, K. (1991). The relationship of pain and symptom management to patient requests for physician-assisted suicide. *Journal Pain & Symptom Management, 6,* 289.

Furrow, B., Greaney, T., Johnson, S., Soltzfus, J. T., & Schwartz, R. (1995). *Health Law, 2,* 369.

Garger v. New Jersey, 429 U.S. 922 (1976).

Gazelle G. (1998). The slow code—Should anyone rush to its defense? *NEJM, 338,* 467–469.

Gordon, G. H., & Dunn, P. (1992) Advance directives and the Patient Self-Determination Act. *Hospital Practice, 27(4A),* 39–40, 42.

Greenberg, J. M., Doblin, B. H., Shapiro, D. W., Linn, L. S., & Wenger, N. S. (1993). Effect of an educational program on medical student's conversations with patients about advance directives. *Journal of General Internal Medicine, 8,* 683–685.

Haas, J. S., Weissman, J. S., Cleary, P. D., Goldberg, J., Gatsonis, C., Seage, G. R., & Fowler, F. J. (1993). Discussions of preferences for life sustaining care by persons with AIDS. *Archives of Internal Medicine, 153,* 1241–1248.

Haidet, P., Hamel, M. B., Davis, R. B., et al. (1998). For the SUPPORT Investigators. Outcomes, preferences for resuscitation, and physician-patient communication among patients with metastatic colorectal cancer. *Am J Med, 105,* 222–229.

Hall, J. (1996). *Nursing ethics and law.* Philadelphia, PA: W. B. Saunders Company.

Hamel, M. B., Phillips, R. S., Davis, R. B., et al. (1997). For the SUPPORT Investigators. Outcomes and cost effectiveness of initiating dialysis and continuing aggressive care in seriously ill hospitalized adults. *Ann Intern Med, 127,* 195–202.

Hamel, M. B., Phillips, R. S., Teno, J. M., et al. (1996). For the SUPPORT Investigators. Seriously ill hospitalized adults: Do we spend less on older patients? *J Am Geriatr Soc, 44,* 1043–1048.

Hamel, M. B., Teno, J. M., Goldman, L., et al. (1999). Patient age and decisions to withhold life-sustaining treatments from seriously ill, hospitalized adults. *Ann Intern Med, 130,* 116–125.

Hare, J., & Nelson, C. (1991). Will outpatients complete living wills? *Journal of General Internal Medicine, 6,* 41–46.

High, D. M. (1993). Advance directives and the elderly: A study of intervention strategies to increase use. *Gerontologist, 33,* 342–349.

Hoffman, D. (1998). Pain management and palliative care in the era of managed care: Issues for health insurers. *Journal of Law, Medicine, & Ethics, 26(4),* 267–289.

Hopp, F., & Duffy, S. (2000). Racial variations in end-of-life care. *J Am Geriat Soc, 48,* 658–663.

Hyman, C. (1996). Pain management and disciplinary action: How medical boards can remove barriers to effective treatment. *Journal of Law, Medicine & Ethics, 24(4),* 338–343.

IOM (Institute of Medicine). (1997). Approaching death: Improving care at the end of life, M. Field and C. Cassel, eds. Washington, DC: Committee on Care at the End of Life.

In re Westchester County Medical Center (O'Connor), 72 N. Y. 2nd 517, 531 N. E. 2d 607, 534 N. Y. S. 2d 886, rev'g 139 A. D. 2d 344, 532 N. Y. S. 2d 133 (1988).

In re Farrell, 108 NJ 335, 529 A. 2d 404 (N. J. 1987).

Jacobsen, J. A., White, B. E., Battin, M. P., Francis, L. P., Green, D. J., & Kasworm, E. S. (1994). Patients' understanding and use of advance directives. *West Journal of Medicine, 160,* 232–236.

Johnson, S. (1998). Introduction: Legal and regulatory issues in pain management. *Journal of Law, Medicine & Ethics, 24(4),* 265–266.

Kayser-Jones, J. (1990). The use of nasogastric feeding tubes in nursing homes: Patient, family and health care provider perspectives. *Gerontologist, 30,* 469–479.

Knaus, W. A., Harrell, F. E., Lynn, J., et al. (1995). For the SUPPPORT Investigators. The SUPPORT prognostic model: Objective estimates of survival for seriously ill hospitalized adults. *Ann Intern Med, 122,* 191–203.

Lo, B. (1995). *Resolving ethical dilemmas: A guide for clinicians.* Baltimore, MD: Lippincott Williams & Wilkins.

Lo, B., Rothenberg, K., & Vasko, M. (1996). Appropriate management of pain: Addressing the clinical, legal and regulatory barriers. *Journal of Law, Medicine & Ethics, 24*(4), 285–286.

Luptak, M. K., & Bould, C. (1994). A method for increasing elders' use of advance directives. *Gerontologist, 34*(3), 409–412.

McKay v. Bergstedt, 106 Nev. 808, 801 P. 2d 617 (Nev. 1990).

Meisel, A. (1995). *The right to die* (Vol. 2). New York: Wiley Law Publications.

Meisel, A. (2000). *The right to die* (Vol. 1 & 2). New York: Aspen Law & Business.

Mezey, M., Kluger, M., Maislin, G. A., & Mittelman, M. (1996). Life-sustaining treatment decisions by spouses of patients with Alzheimer's disease. *Journal of the American Geriatrics Society, 44*(2), 144–150.

Mezey, M., Leitman, R., Mitty, E., Bottrell, M., & Ramsey, G. (2000). Why hospital patients do and do not execute an advance directive. *Nursing Outlook,* (in press).

Mezey, M., Mitty, E., Bottrell, M., Ramsey, G., & Fisher, T. (2000). Advance directives: Older adults with dementia. *Clinics in Geriatric Medicine, 16*(2), 255–268.

Mezey, M., Mitty, E., & Ramsey, G. (1997). Assessment of Decision-Making Capacity: Nurse's Role. *Journal of Gerontological Nursing, 23*(3), 28–35.

Mezey, M., Ramsey, G., Mitty, E., & Rappaport, M. (1997). Implementation of the Patient Self-Determination Act (PSDA) in nursing homes in New York City. *Journal of the American Geriatrics Society, 45*, 43–49.

Miller, T. (1995). Advance directives: Moving from theory to practice. In P. R. Katz, R. L. Kane, & M. Mezey (Eds.), *Quality care in geriatric settings* (pp. 68–87). New York: Springer.

Murphy, D. J. (1990). Improving advance directives for healthy older people. *J Am Geriatr Soc, 38*, 1251–1256.

Murphy, P., Kreling, B., Kathryn, E., Stevens, M., Lynn, J., & Dulac, J. (2000). Description of the SUPPORT Intervention. *J Am Geriatr Soc, 48*(5), S154–161.

New York State Task Force on Life and the Law. (1995). A message about the Family Health Care Decisions Act of 1995. New York, New York.

Olson, E. (1993). Ethical issues in the nursing home. *Mt Sinai J Med, 60*(6), 555–559.

Orentlicher, D. (1997). The supreme court and physician assisted suicide. Rejecting assisted suicide but embracing euthanasia. *NEJM, 337*, 1236–1239.

Overcast, T. D., Bowen, L. E., Hoe, M. M., & Livak, C. L. (1984). Problems in the identification of potential organ donors: misconceptions and fallacies associated with donor cards. *JAMA, 251*, 1559–1560.

Pain Relief Promotion Act of 1999 (HR 2260).

Phillips, R. S., Hamel, M. B., Covinsky, K. E., & Lynn, J. (2000). Findings from SUPPORT and HELP: An Introduction. *J Am Geriatr Soc, 48*(5), S1–5.

Phillips, R. S., Hamel, M. B., Teno, J. M., et al. (1996). For the SUPPORT Investigators. Race, resource use, and survival in seriously ill hospitalized adults. *J Gen Intern Med, 11*, 387–396.

President's Commission for the Study of Ethical Problems in Medicine and Biomedical and Behavioral Research. (March, 1982). Deciding to forego life-sustaining treatment. *United States Government Printing Office: Washington D.C.,* pp. 55–68.

Pub. L. No. 101-508, '4206, 4751 [hereinafter OBRA], 104 Stat. 1388–115 to 117, 1388–204 to 206 (codified at 42 U. S. C. A. '1395cc(f) (1) & id. '1396a(a) (West Supp. 1994).

In re Quinlan, 70 N. J. 10, 355 A. 2d 647 (N. J. 1976).

Robinson, M. K., DeHaven, M. J., & Koch, K. A. (1993). Effects of the patient self-determination act on patient knowledge and behavior. *Journal of Family Practice, 37*(4), 363–368.

Roth, Y. L., Meisel, A., & Lidz, C. W. (1977). Tests of competency to consent to treatment. *American Journal of Psychiatry, 134*, 279–284.

Rubin, S. M., Strull, W. M., Fialkow, M. F., Weiss, S. S., & Lo, B. (1994). Increasing the completion of the durable power of attorney for health care. *Journal of the American Medicine Association, 271,* 209–212.

Sachs, G. A., Stocking, C. E., & Miles, S. H. (1992). Failure of an intervention to promote discussion of advance directives. *Journal of the American Geriatrics Society, 40*(3), 269–273.

Schneiderman, L. J., Pearlman, R. A., Kaplan, R. M., Anderson, J. P., & Rosenberg, E. M. (1992). Relationship of general advance directive instructions to specific life-sustaining treatment preferences in patients with serious illness. *Archives of Internal Medicine, 152,* 2114–2122.

Schloendorff v. Society of New York Hospitals, 211 N.Y. 125, 105 N.E. 92 (1914).

Schonwetter, R. S., Walker, R. M., Kramer, D. R., & Robinson, B. E. (1993). Resuscitation decision making in the elderly: The value of outcome data. *Journal of General Internal Medicine, 8,* 295–300.

Shapiro, R. (1996). Health care providers' liability exposure for inappropriate pain management. *Journal of Law, Medicine & Ethics, 24*(4), 360–364.

Smith, S. A., & Davis, A. J. (1980). Ethical dilemmas: Conflicts among rights, duties, and obligations. *American Journal Nursing, 80*(8), 1462–1466.

Solomon, M. Z., O'Donell, L., Jennings, B., Guilfoy, V., Wolf, S. M., Nolan, K., & Jackson, R. (1993). Decisions near the end of life: Professional views on life-sustaining treatments. *American Journal of Public Health, 83*(1), 14–23.

Stetler, K. L., Elliott, B. A., & Bruno, C. A. (1992). Living will completion in older adults. *Arch Intern Med, 125*(5), 954–959.

Swidler, R. (1989). The presumption of consent in New York State's do-not-resuscitate law. *New York State Journal of Medicine, 89,* 69–72.

Teno, J., Lynn, J., Phillips, R. S., et al. (1994). For the SUPPORT Investigators. Do formal advance directives affect resuscitation decisions and the use of resources for seriously ill patients? *J Clin Ethics, 5,* 23–30.

Teno, J., Lynn, J., Wenger, N., et al. (1997). For the SUPPORT Investigators. Advance directives for the seriously ill hospitalized patients: Effectiveness with the patient self determination act and the SUPPORT Intervention. *J Am Geriatr Soc, 45,* 500–507.

Teno, J. M., Licks, S., Lynn, J., et al. (1997). For the SUPPORT Investigators. Do advance directives provide instructions that direct care? *J Am Geriatr Soc, 45,* 508–512.

Vacco v. Quill, 521 U. S. 793, 117 S. Ct. 2293 (1997).

Washington v. Glucksberg, 117 S. Ct. 2258 (1997).

Wenger, N., Phillips, R., Teno, J., Oye, R., Dawson, N., Liu, H., Califf, R., Layde, P., Hakim, R., & Lynn, J. (2000). Physician understanding of patient resuscitation preferences: Insights and clinical implications. *J Am Geriatr Soc, 48*(5), S44–51.

PART 3

Psychological Aspects of Dying

June 18, 2000

Candy had a friend from the neighborhood over when I arrived today. This woman was very anxious to be of help to Candy and her family; apparently the whole neighborhood had rallied and were offering support by grocery shopping, preparing meals, house cleaning, and offering to watch the children. Candy's 5-year-old son was at his first sleepover and she was both pleased and sad that he felt comfortable leaving her to stay with a friend. She talked about how involved her husband was with her and the situation that they were in. She said they laughed about the sounds that came from her colostomy and how she could talk to him about the decisions she had to make regarding her care. Her therapist had talked with the children to determine their feelings and ideas about what was happening and help them to deal with their mother's illness. Candy did say that she has not talked to them about dying because she was not ready to talk about it herself. She was still struggling with her loss of function, and role changes, now that she did not have the energy to physically care for her children.

Yet, Candy was still hoping for a cure. As a nurse, I knew that at some point the hope would change from a hope of a cure to the hope for a comfortable death, free of pain, and surrounded by those who loved her. I could only imagine her feelings of loss and grief. I, too, pushed the

217

thoughts of death from my mind. Since I was close to her age, I became increasingly aware of my own mortality. As Candy told me how her children snuggled close to her in bed, I felt incredibly saddened by the thought of her death, and the idea that her children would lose their mother. I imagined the pain of my children, if I were to die.

7

Communicating With Seriously Ill and Dying Patients, Their Families, and Their Health Care Providers

Kathleen O. Perrin

AACN Competency

#3: Communicate effectively and compassionately with the patient, family, and health care team members about end-of-life issues.

> Mitch, he continued softly now, you don't understand, I want to tell you about my life. I want to tell you before I can't tell you anymore. His voice dropped to a whisper. I want someone to hear my story. Will you?
>
> —Albom, M. (1997), *Tuesday's With Morrie*, p. 63

Seriously ill or dying patients and their families want their health care providers to communicate with honesty (Furukawa, 1996) and caring (Czerwiec, 1996) prognoses and treatment options. The Study to Understand Prognoses and Preferences for Outcomes and Risks of Treatment (SUPPORT, 1995) demonstrated that this discussion does not occur as often as families and hospitalized patients would prefer. Since, most Americans still die in hospitals; the absence of such discussion is a major shortfall in the care of dying Americans. Moreover, even for patients who are cared for at home and referred to hospice, discussion and preparation for death are often avoided until hospice referral. Since most patients are not referred to hospice until the last weeks of their lives, this means that discussion of end of life care is often postponed until it is unavoidable.

According to Servaty, Krejci, and Hayslip (1996), health care providers with less anxiety about death are more likely to talk meaningfully with dying patients. In their study, nursing students were less anxious and more willing then other college students and beginning medical students to communicate with dying people. Thus, they reasoned, nursing students may be responsive to educational endeavors to promote honest, caring communication with patients and families at the end of life. This chapter will explore ways in which educators might encourage both undergraduate and advanced practice nursing students to facilitate communication with dying patients, their families, and their health care providers.

In addition to patients and their families benefiting from communication with nurses at the end of life, the nurses may also benefit. Stiles (1990) described seven types of personal growth that nurses dealing with dying patients felt that they experienced as "gifts" from their patients. These included: learning to confront their own mortality, learning about self, developing a faith in self and a higher being, transcending their limitations, learning realistic expectations, and clarifying personal responsibility. Although experienced nurses perceived these opportunities for personal growth as "gifts" from their patients, undergraduate nursing students may be more distressed by them. Ways in which nursing faculty members might assist undergraduate nursing students to enrich themselves by working with dying patients will also be explored in this chapter.

This chapter will be organized according to the phases of the therapeutic relationship since in many ways the phases of the therapeutic relationship, introductory, working, and termination parallel the dying trajectory. When appropriate in the phases, distinctions will be made between the roles and educational needs of the undergraduate nursing student, the nurse with an undergraduate degree, the advanced practice nursing student, and the nurse with an advanced practice degree.

INTRODUCTORY PHASE

During the introductory phase of the therapeutic relationship, the nurse and patient open the relationship, begin to clarify and define the problem that has brought the patient in contact with the nurse, and begin to define their relationship.

OPENING THE RELATIONSHIP

For the undergraduate nursing student, the components of this phase include: conveying respect for the dying patient and his/her family as well as establishing a trusting relationship. These constituents are no different from their establishment in any therapeutic relationship. The student should introduce her/himself to the patient and identify how s/he will be involved in the patient's care. The nursing faculty member ought to note if the student caring for a dying patient seems unusually reluctant to engage in care of that patient. If the student appears hesitant, the faculty member might demonstrate by introducing him/herself to the patient that this portion of the relationship is no different merely because the patient is dying. At this very early stage in the relationship, the student, or any health care provider, probably ought to avoid discussing the subject of death and dying unless the patient brings up the topic (Byock, 1997).

In contrast to the undergraduate nursing student or the nurse with an undergraduate degree, it may unfortunately be the responsibility of the advanced practice nurse to explain to a patient that s/he is severely ill and may be dying during one of their initial meetings. It would always be preferable that the advanced practice nurse and patient have had an opportunity to establish a trusting relationship before the advanced practice nurse is required to deliver such bad news to the patient. However, in today's fast-paced health care environment, especially in emergency departments and critical care units, that is not always possible.

Conveying such "bad" news requires thought and preparation. When preparing for the discussion, Buckman, Lipkin, Sourkes, and Tolle (1997) recommend that the health care provider ask the patient to have a family member or friend present, have all information available to explain to the patient, and practice what s/he is planning to say. Buckman et al. (1997) suggests that after any introductions are made to the patient and family that the patient be asked if it would be permissible to tape the interview. They state that taping the interview and providing the tape to the patient when the interview is finished enhances the patient's long-term adjustment. The steps recommended by Buckman (1992) for breaking bad news are listed in Table 7.1.

Buckman et al. (1997) recommends starting the interview by finding out what the patient knows or suspects. Often the patient has a preconception of the problem and it may be necessary not only to convey "bad" news but to counter the patient's and family's misconceptions of the situation. Since not all patients want to know the extent of their illness, it is also important for the advanced practice nurse to determine at this point in the interview how much information the patient desires.

TABLE 7.1   Steps in "Breaking Bad News" According to Robert Buckman (1992)

- Get the context right
- Find out what is already known
- Find out how much information the patient and/or family wants to know
- Share the information, starting from their viewpoint and step by step bring their understanding closer to the medical facts
- Respond to their reactions using an empathetic approach
- Explain the treatment plan and prognosis, summarize, and make a contract

Before actually stating the problem, Buckman et al. (1997) suggests foreshadowing the news in simple language such as "I'm sorry I have some bad news for you." Then they suggest that the bad news be explained in simple terms that are understandable to the patient. At this point, Buckman et al. (1997) recommends something that can be very difficult for the beginning practitioner, silence. During the period of silence, the patient will have an opportunity to absorb the information, react, and ask questions.

After the information is conveyed to the patient and the patient has had a chance to react, Buckman et al. (1997) suggest an empathetic approach. This implies that the advanced practice nurse should first identify the emotion that the patient is experiencing and identify the origins of the emotion. Then, the nurse should respond in a way that tells the patient that s/he understands what the patient is experiencing. This means the nurse should "reflect, name, and legitimize the patient's feelings" (Buckman et al., 1997, p. 63).

The final step in breaking bad news is providing an initial explanation of potential treatments and prognoses. Later in the therapeutic relationship, the advance practice nurse may become involved in empowering the patient to be an active participant in the decision-making process about his/her treatment and developing an agreement about care. At this stage, the possibilities are usually just described to provide the patient with an opportunity to begin thinking about goals of treatment. Before the interview is complete, the advanced practice nurse should summarize the discussion for the patient.

Tulsky, Chesney, and Lo (1996) recommend that a new practitioner (such as a resident or advanced practice nurse student) be observed several times and offered feedback before being allowed to discuss "bad" news without supervision. Emanuel (1998) suggests the new practitioner be provided with "talking points" so that all of the appropriate information is covered. Latimer (1998) describes criteria for ethical communication of information that might be used to evaluate the communication skills of a beginning practitioner. To be ethical according to Latimer, the communication should be timely and desired by the patient. The information must be accurate. The words should be understandable to the patient and family and the information must be conveyed in a gentle, respectful, and compassionate manner.

CLARIFYING THE PROBLEM

There are several components to the phase of clarifying the problem. They include: facilitating the patient's expression of her/his emotions, identification of what the patient and family believe are problems, and identifying and responding to the patient's and family's concerns about care. Nurses at all levels should be expert in assisting patients to clarify what they believe are their significant health care-related concerns.

It is not always easy for a nurse to identify if a patient has received "bad news" or when a patient is prepared to discuss such news. May (1995) suggests that if the nurse was present at the interview when the "bad" news was delivered, the patient will feel free to initiate a conversation when s/he is ready. If the nurse was not present during the interview, but suspects such an interview has occurred, s/he might say to the patient, "I noticed the physician (or advanced practice nurse) was speaking with you, what did s/he have to say?" May emphasizes that the nurse should not initiate such a discussion unless s/he is able to sit down and actively listen to the patient. Initiating a discussion of patient concerns or problems requires the nurse have strong facilitative communication skills and be able to put aside other competing demands for her/his time.

May (1995) warns that when a nurse asks a patient how s/he feels, the patient usually responds by describing her/his physical condition. Thus, if a nurse wants information about the person's psychological concerns, the question will need to be phrased somewhat differently. Byock (1997) began using the phrase, "How are you feeling within yourself?" after he had noticed that hospice workers in England successfully cut though defenses and learned how the patient was feeling when they asked that question. He suggests it is a way of getting immediately to the heart of the patient's concerns. Emanuel (1998) recommends several questions including: "During the last few weeks how often have you felt downhearted or blue?" What do you believe is bothering you? Who are you able to confide in?".

Wilkinson (1991) examined factors that influenced how nurses communicated with cancer patients. She concluded that in general, nurses had difficulty employing facilitative communication with patients with cancer. She noted that nurses frequently used blocking techniques when dealing with patients who had had a recurrence of their cancer. Since these blocking techniques prevented the nurses from identifying patient concerns, the nurses obtained only a superficial nursing assessment and planned nursing care based on assumptions rather then actual patient concerns.

Wilkinson (1991) identified three groups of nurses who used different methods to block patient communication. These were ignorers, informers, and mixed responders. Ignorers ignored patient cues to talk about specific problems or issues throughout the interview. These nurses changed the subject, engaged in conversation with the patient's relative, or began social chitchat to avoid emotionally laden conversations. Informers were nurses who gave elaborate explanations of procedures, offered inappropriate advice, or stated their opinions without being asked. These nurses indicated that providing such detailed, unasked for information allowed them to maintain control of the situation and avoid difficult or emotionally laden conversations (Wilkinson, 1991). Mixed responders were the largest group of nurses in Wilkinson's study. They utilized both facilitative and blocking responses, attempted to understand patient problems, and were more aware of their blocking behaviors when questioned about them.

Although they had been taught facilitative communication most of the practicing nurses in Wilkinson's 1991 study were unaware that they were blocking their patients' attempts to communicate important needs and concerns until they listened to an audio tape and discussed their responses. Undergraduate nursing students need experiences in communicating with dying patients with opportunities to have their interactions evaluated by a nursing faculty member in order to develop proficiency in communication with seriously ill patients. An audiotape allows the faculty member a complete, accurate record of the verbal component of the communication between the student and patient. The patient's consent for taping must be obtained and in some circumstances the Institution Review Board (IRB) of the facility may also need to provide approval. The faculty member then may use the tape as a tool to discuss the student responses as well as possible facilitative alternatives. Heaven and Maquire (1996) noted that demonstration with audiotaping and feedback improved nurses with an undergraduate degree's facilitative communication skills. However, since the improvement was not to a statistically significant extent, further study of this approach is warranted.

Moreover, taping is often not possible. On occasion, the faculty member may be present during the student's interview with the patient. This has the advantage of allowing the faculty member to observe the nonverbal behavior of the student and patient as well as the verbal. In many circumstances it permits the faculty member to provide immediate feedback to the student. If direct observation is not possible, then student journals or verbatim process recordings can be used to allow faculty to help students develop an ability to facilitate rather then block communication with seriously ill patients.

Slightly less then a quarter of the nurses in Wilkinson's 1991 study used primarily facilitative communication techniques when interviewing cancer patients. Nurses who used these techniques were able to do so no matter how ill the patient was or how emotionally laden the material s/he might divulge. By employing such standard facilitative communication techniques as active listening, use of open-ended questions, reflection or clarification of patient concerns, and empathy they were able to obtain a more in-depth understanding of their patients' problems and concerns. In "An interview" (1999), Farber states that patients and families most welcomed and remembered interactions with nursing staff that were personalized to the needs of the individual patient and family.

It is also important to realize that just because the topic is dying and the problems are serious, the talk does not always need to be solemn. Langley-Evans and Payne (1997) noted that lighthearted talk about illness, symptoms, bereavement, and personal mortality was quite valuable to outpatients in a palliative day care center. What was important was the nursing staff created an atmosphere that facilitated rather then blocked patients' disclosure of their concerns. Table 7.2 lists essential nursing communication behaviors for both the undergraduate and graduate nurse.

Advance practice nurses can do a great deal to encourage nurses with an undergraduate degree to communicate with dying patients. Studies by Wilkinson (1991) and Booth, Maguire, Butterworth, and Hillier (1996) found the major predictor of nursing staff's use of facilitative communication with patients with cancer or in hospice was the supportiveness of the nurses' supervisor. In the study by Wilkinson, the ward sisters (unit managers) who took assignments, cared for patients, and demonstrated facilitative communication with patients to their staff had staff who were more likely to communicate therapeutically with their patients. These same ward sisters also encouraged their nurses to work autonomously and make decisions about nursing care. They had negotiated with the physicians who admitted patients to their units to obtain permission for the nurses to talk truthfully with any patient who requested information about her/his prognosis or treatment.

Advanced practice nurses and students need to have excellent facilitative communication skills. They must be able to communicate with patients individually but they must also be able to demonstrate to staff member's ways to communicate with difficult patients and families. They may be asked to advocate for nurses with an undergraduate degree autonomy in patient communication before the institutional administration or physicians. The

TABLE 7.2   Essential Behaviors

Basic
Interpreting "bad" news
Listening to clients' and families' concerns about EOL care
Reviewing EOL treatment options
Assisting patients, families, and HCPs to make EOL decisions
Advocating for patient's choices at EOL
Implementing EOL treatment withdrawal
Preparing patient and family for physical signs of impending death
Smoothing the passage
Being with patient and family during the dying process
Consoling the bereaved family

Advanced
Conveying "bad" news
Initiating the discussion of EOL treatment options
Promoting a supportive unit environment
Determining with other HCPs that patient is dying
Initiating discussion of EOL treatment withdrawal
Establishing palliative care contract
Dealing with families in crisis after a sudden unexpected death
Presenting organ donation options

advance practice nurses' effort to create an environment where communication between patient and nurse is valued is essential to developing the communication skills of the nurse with an undergraduate degree. Although theory is important, it is practice with evaluation or supervision by a skilled practitioner that allows an advanced practice nurse to develop such a level of mastery of facilitative communication skills.

STRUCTURING AND FORMULATING THE CARE AGREEMENT

There are several components to this phase of the therapeutic relationship. In any therapeutic relationship, the nurse and patient should be continuing to develop trust during this phase, coming to an agreement about the frequency of meetings, and developing goals for care and the relationship. At this point in a dying patient's care, the advanced practice nurse might initiate a discussion of the patient's treatment goals. Murphy and Price (1995) emphasize the nurse should avoid using any phrase which resembles "There is nothing more that we can do." Although the phrase may be intended by the health care provider to convey that the patient's disease will progress and the patient will eventually die, to the patient and family, it often implies that the health care team will abandon the patient. Instead of focusing on what will not be done, the advanced practice nurse, patient, family and other members of the health care team should begin to identify goals for patient care.

Farber in "An Interview" (1999) identified a number of possible goals which a dying patient might choose. These included: living to the last possible second, living until the burden becomes too great, living at home with family avoiding medical interventions, living as comfortably as possibly until death, and avoiding medical treatments unless they will have meaningful outcomes. Once a goal has been identified, the health care team, patient, and family can begin to identify interventions that will achieve that goal.

Cotton (1993) noted that many physicians avoid initiating discussions about end of life treatment with their patients for fear that the patients will become depressed or distrustful of the physicians' willingness to care for them. Often physicians of dying patients will delay the conversation until the patient is unresponsive and the family must be consulted (Shmerling, Bedell, Lilienfeld, & Delbanco, 1988). In fact, patients, especially elders, want to identify goals and interventions for end-of-life care and are relieved when the subject is broached. Most Americans do not have an advance directive, yet it is their right, as long as they are competent, to have the deciding voice in the type of health care they receive. When the physician or advanced practice nurse avoids discussing the goals of end-of-life care until the patient is unresponsive, s/he deprives the patient of her/his right to determine appropriate end-of-life care.

The role of the nurse with an undergraduate degree is to interpret the medical information into terms the patient can understand and repeatedly explain the end of life treatment options to the patient. Patients and families often indicate that listening to the health care provider's explanation of a patient's prognosis and possibilities for treatment is like trying to understand a foreign language. In addition, most patients and their families experience stress when they receive "bad" news. Thus, they are unable to hear or retain much of what the physician or advanced practice nurse explained to them. Being able to repeatedly replay the taped information is one of the reasons why the tape recording of the initial interview recommended by Buckman et al. (1997) may be beneficial for some patients and families. However, most of the time, it is the responsibility of the nurse with an undergraduate degree to translate medical jargon into language that the patient can comprehend and to reinforce the information regularly.

WORKING PHASE

During the working phase of the therapeutic relationship, the nurse explores and understands the patient's feelings and expectations, elaborates on the goals of treatment developed in the previous phase, and facilitates or takes actions which the patient desires. In this case, the feelings and expectations explored relate to the dying process and the goals include defining what the patient believes considers as dying well.

EXPLORING AND UNDERSTANDING PATIENT'S FEELINGS AND EXPECTATIONS ABOUT DEATH AND DYING

Both the advanced practice and undergraduate nursing student should be able to assist a patient to define what s/he believes constitutes dying well or represents a good and timely death. One aspect of dying well may be attention to the patient's cultural and religious preferences. So, it is essential that the nurses identify and respect those end-of-life rituals which provide meaning to the patient and his/her family.

The nurse will need to identify with the patient which issues would be most important to address so that her/his particular patient might die well. Nurses at all practice levels should be involved in helping to identify the issues in the patient's life that require resolution. Some of the issues that may be important to patients at the end of life include: completing unfinished business; resolving relationship concerns with family and friends; and carrying out a life review. Once the issues are identified, members of the health care team may assist in addressing the issues.

Patients may have a wide variety of unfinished business. Often these issues are related to the patient's age and developmental level. For example, a teenager might want to graduate from high school or an older adult might want to witness the arrival of a first grandchild. To identify what, if any, business the patient would like to complete, the nurse might ask "If you were to die soon, what would be left undone?" or "Is there some event that would add a great deal of meaning to your life? What do we have to do so that event can take place?" Once the issue has been identified, rules might need to be bent (e.g., a child allowed to participate in graduation ceremonies without completing required coursework, a grandchild or pet allowed in an Intensive Care Unit), resources expended, or help mobilized to permit the event to happen.

Patients may need both time and assistance in resolving relationship problems with their family and friends. Emanuel (1998) notes that some patients seem to be able to postpone dying so that they can complete their family business. Often, deaths occur after important events such as birthdays or holidays. One woman who was dying from respiratory failure asked to have her life prolonged by whatever means necessary until her estranged daughter, who she had not seen in 10 years, arrived from across the country.

After the daughter's arrival, arrangements were made for counseling sessions for the mother and daughter. Two days later, the mother died with the daughter present holding her mother's hand.

Life review is an important part of both the aging and the dying process. According to Butler ("Roundtable discussion," 1996), "life review is a normal developmental task of the later years characterized by the return of memories and past conflicts. In some cases, this can contribute to psychological growth, including the resolution of past conflicts, reconciliation with significant others, atonement for past wrongdoing, personality integration, and serenity" (p. 42). Being present with the patient while the patient begins a life review means a commitment on the part of the nurse to listen actively and devote time to the patient. This is a skill that all nurses ought to have, although it does not require the presence of a nurse or even a professional for the patient to conduct a life review. Life review provides the patient with a powerful way to work out family relationships and gain a sense of inner peace.

TALKING WITH PATIENTS ACROSS THE LIFE SPAN AND THEIR FAMILIES ABOUT DEATH

A nurse caring for a dying child must establish a trusting relationship with the child and her/his parents. New graduate of undergraduate nursing programs and undergraduate nursing students should be especially aware of their emotions and though empathizing with the family should avoid burdening them with their own emotions (Buckman et al., 1997). Children want to know varying amounts of information about their illness. However, most children want to have an appreciation of how the illness will affect the way they will be able to live their lives. But, like adults, children vary in how much information they are able to understand and absorb even when it is presented at an appropriate level. Young children's verbalization about their potential death can vary across a continuum and may be fluid over time (Buckman, et al., 1997). At one end of the continuum, children will state that they are very sick or have a bad disease but will not mention death. Other children will mention an uncertainty about living but will not allude to dying. At the far end of the continuum, children will state that they could die from their illnesses. The advance practice nurse might utilize play therapy or drawing with various colors to help the child to express her/his emotions, fears, and realizations about death.

Parents of seriously ill, possibly dying children may have difficulty making sense of what is being said or experienced (Anderson & Hall, 1995). They may feel unable to make decisions, especially if they believe that both minor and major decisions are needed simultaneously. At times, according to Anderson and Hall (1995), the parents may feel they cannot differentiate the decisions that merely involve personal preference from the ones that have grave implications. They may need help from nurses untangling these concrete issues but also in dealing with more philosophical ones such as "How can we determine the line between what is best or right for our child and what is best or right for us?" Nurses can help these families by reminding them that "forced or hasty decision making may cause them to abrogate responsibility because they have not had an opportunity to understand the issues, their feelings or their roles" (Anderson & Hall, 1995, p. 16). Experienced nurses with an undergraduate education can assist the parents to understand the issues, express their feelings, and delineate their roles so that the parents can be actively involved in the decision-making process for their children.

Young or middle-aged adults who are dying may feel as though they have a great deal of unfinished business or many unresolved relationships. The dying patient may need professional assistance in dealing with anger at leaving so much undone. A parent who is dying and leaving young children behind may need assistance from a nurse to find ways to leave mementos or lasting words of wisdom for their children. Some dying parents pick out special Christmas mementos in July for their children. One mother made 12 audiotapes with words of love and encouragement for her only child, one for each year until he reached age 21.

Older adults are often perceived by health care providers as having lived a full life and being prepared to die. But, according to Cavendish (1999), nurses should assess all elders' quality of life prior to the illness and realize that many have the potential for additional healthy, happy years. Farber in "An Interview" (1999) states that adults over the age of 70 usually do not believe they have a choice in health care treatment. When asked, "How did you make decisions?", they answered, "What do you mean? The doctor told us what to do and we did it." Nurses, especially advance practice nurses, need to assist elders to participate in their treatment decisions whenever they appear to desire a decision-making role. Finally, life review is particularly important for the dying elder (Roundtable, 1996) so time and a compassionate listener should be allotted to this important activity. The nurse with an undergraduate degree might be this compassionate listener or s/he might delegate another individual for this task.

FACILITATING AND TAKING ACTION

There are several components of this phase. The first part is determining that the patient will die soon. The nurse with an undergraduate degree may be involved with other health care providers in deciding when the patient is entering the active dying phase. While, the advanced practice nurse, in some circumstances, may participate in the decision that further treatment is futile when the patient is clearly dying. According to Cassem (Stein, 1999), nurses are the people who guide patients along the path to a peaceful death by recognizing when the patient is suffering needlessly through the provision of inappropriate aggressive treatment. The physician, in some settings, may be the last to realize that the patient is dying. Therefore, it becomes incumbent on nurses to relay their impressions to the physician and possibly to the family. The SUPPORT (1995) study indicates that there are problems in the way that such information is communicated in hospital settings. Ways to improve the communication between nurses, physicians, and patients or their families when the patient's life is about to end are under investigation (Jezewski, 1996).

Determining and agreeing that the patient is dying is extremely important, since most deaths in the United States occur in hospitals and all patients in hospitals must receive cardiopulmonary resuscitation (CPR) unless the physician or advance practice nurse has written a Do-Not-Resuscitate (DNR) order. Once there is a determination that the patient is dying, the physician or advanced practice nurse should discuss a DNR order with the patient and family.

There are two common mistakes that inexperienced practitioners make when discussing a DNR order. The first is to ask "Do you want everything done?" Most lay people don't assume everything means compressing the chest of a person who has already died. They assume it means comfort, care, and support. So, they often answer "yes" when they really would not want CPR. The second mistake is to use the words "There is nothing more we can do." Although the patient is dying and medical interventions will not prevent the death, there is much that health care providers can do to help the patient to die well. The role of the advanced practice nurse is to initiate this discussion using Latimer's (1998) criteria for ethical communication described earlier and listed in Table 7.3. However, Tulsky et al. (1996)

TABLE 7.3   Criteria for Ethical Communication of Information from Latimer (1998)

- The communication should be timely and desired by the patient
- The information must be accurate
- The words should be understandable to the patient and family
- The information must be conveyed in a "gentle, respectful, and compassionate manner"

stress that new practitioners, such as residents and advanced practice nursing students should be evaluated by skilled professionals before being allowed to attempt such a discussion on their own.

The nurse with an undergraduate degree is usually the staff member to whom the patient and family turn to discuss exactly what a DNR order is and what the ramifications are likely to be for the patient. If that nurse was not present for the discussion, s/he might use the question, "I noticed the physician (advanced practice nurse) was speaking with you, what did s/he say?" The nurse might follow that with, "Many people have questions about what this means for them, what questions do you have?" Most people want reassurance that they are not forgoing an intervention that is likely to offer them benefit. Since only about 12% of all patients survive from CPR to hospital discharge, this reassurance is easy to provide.

As noted previously, the nurse is often the guide on the path to a peaceful death (Stein, 1999). This role is important because the decision to forgo CPR is merely the first of many decisions that the patient and family may need to make about end-of-life care. After deciding to forgo CPR, the patient and family might choose to forgo any further curative therapy or might opt to have only comfort measures provided for the patient. Palliative care decisions which involve the amount of pain medication the patient desires and whether or not the patient wishes to receive medical interventions for hydration and nutrition or even continue eating and drinking may need to be made. The nurse with an undergraduate degree who is caring for a dying patient should be able to describe the benefits and burdens of each of these therapies to her/his patient. They should also be able to facilitate patient and family decision making about these choices through effective communication.

The nurse may be responsible for advocating for the patient's wishes for end-of-life care and communicating them to the family and other health care providers. This is easier if the patient has verbally expressed a preference to the nurse and is willing to state that preference to the physician and family. It may be more difficult when the nurse, physician, and family are trying to interpret an advance directive that does not precisely fit the patient's situation, when the person who has the durable power of attorney for health care purposes is not clear about the patient's wishes, or when there is no advance directive. Harlow in "Family letter writing" (1999) recommends that the family or proxy consider the following:

1. What type of person was the patient?
2. Did s/he ever comment on another person's situation when they were incapacitated or on life support?

3. Did s/he relate those experiences to her own personal views for her/himself?
4. What vignettes can you recall from his/her life that illustrates her/his values and beliefs?

Harlow in "Family letter writing" (1999) then asks the family to write a letter incorporating the answers to these questions. He believes that the process is almost a spiritual one for the families which often brings them closer together. It helps them to review and clarify the person's life and understand what was meaningful to the person. Harlow notes that family letter writing may be "experienced by the family as a last act of commitment and caring toward their loved one." The nurse may be the person who encourages the family to begin such an activity. However, the ultimate decision on how to respond to the patient's and family's wishes rests with the physician or advance practice nurse.

Once a decision is made to limit further aggressive, curative treatment, the advance practice nurse may be involved in establishing a palliative care understanding with the patient and her/his family. This is an understanding of what the health care team will do for and with the patient and his/her family. Byock (1997) offers the following version of a commitment between the health care team and a dying patient:

"We will keep you warm and we will keep you dry. We will keep you clean. We will help you with elimination, and your bowels and your bladder function. We will always offer you food and fluid. We will be with you. We will bear witness to your pain and your sorrows, your disappointments and your triumphs; we will listen to the stories of your life and remember the story of your passing" (247).

Although the advance care nurse or physician may be the person who establishes this palliative care understanding, it is the nurse with an undergraduate degree who is responsible for assuring that it is carried out. It is imperative that the nurse demonstrates by her/his words and deeds that the health care providers will not abandon the patient after her/his end-of-life choices are made. That instead, nurses and other health care workers will provide the care the patient needs or will teach and assist family members or friends to provide the care and support that the patient requires as s/he dies.

TERMINATION PHASE

During this phase in the therapeutic relationship, the nurse, family, and patient prepare for the end of the relationship, accept the feelings of loss, and review or evaluate what has occurred. As a patient is dying this phase may entail: withdrawing medical interventions, preparing the patient and family for the physical signs of impending death, smoothing the passage, consoling the bereaved family, exploring personal reactions, and evaluating nursing responses.

WITHDRAWING MEDICAL INTERVENTIONS

During the termination phase, medical interventions, such as ventilators, IV fluids and nutrition, or dialysis may be withdrawn. The nurse reassures the family that withdrawing such aggressive medical interventions from the dying patient is acceptable to most of the major religious and ethical traditions. The nurse demonstrates that despite the withdrawal of curative measures, the health care team will remain present and will provide aggressive comfort measures and respect the patient's individuality.

PREPARING THE PATIENT AND FAMILY FOR PHYSICAL SIGNS OF IMPENDING DEATH

Both the nurse with an undergraduate degree and the advanced practice nurse will need to be able to explain the final stages of the dying process to the patient and family. A family that does not understand the dying process may become anxious and feel unable to cope with the patient's care. The nurse may initiate the discussion by stating, "There are some common signs and symptoms that identify when a person's life is coming to an end. Not all of the signs occur in every person nor do they happen in the same sequence in each person. But, it might be helpful if we talk about what may be occurring soon and what you may need or want to do."

SMOOTHING THE PASSAGE

As death approaches, patients may display a variety of typical behaviors. Nurses educated at the undergraduate and graduate levels should be able to explain these behaviors to family members and assist families and dying patients to communicate with each other during the patient's last days and hours. According to Callanan (1994), when a patient is approaching death, s/he may begin to speak in symbolic language. The patient might say "Oh, here are my mother and brother-in-law, they've come to get me. We have to catch the train." Or, the patient may say, "It's a beautiful place that I'm going to now." Callanan cautions that the family may fear the patient is "losing his/her mind" or believe s/he is reliving her/his past. In actuality, it is believed that the patient is preparing to detach from this life. Callanan suggests nurses should help the family to listen to the patient's statements and respond with gentle open-ended questions such as "When does the train leave?" The family should be discouraged from trying to reorient the patient ("Your mother died years ago.") or contradicting the patient ("You're not going anywhere!").

Close to the moment of death, the patient may appear more withdrawn, almost detached from her/his surroundings. The nurse should inform the family that although the patient may appear unresponsive, they should still communicate verbally with the patient because the patient can probably still hear what people in the room are saying. The family may want to say "Good-bye" or "I love you" if they have not done so already. This might be a time for the family to recount some favorite memories that illustrate what the dying person meant to them. A member of the family might say "We will miss you, but we will always love you and we understand that it is time for you to go." Or, a family member or close friend might simply be present with the dying patient, sitting nearby, holding her/his hand or lying next to the patient and embracing her/him.

It is the role of the nurse to help the patient and families find an appropriate way to express their feelings and to smooth the patient's passage from this life. A person takes her/his own time dying and each death occurs at its own pace. The nurse may need to help the patient's family to understand how idiosyncratically and sometimes how slowly the final moments may pass.

CONSOLING THE BEREAVED FAMILY

Nurses educated at all levels of practice will need to be able to console families through the bereavement process. If the family has not been present during the death, the nurse will want to prepare the body and attempt to create a peaceful environment for the family to view the deceased. Because the nurse is often the professional present at the death or the one who views the body with the family, the nurse will need to demonstrate an acceptance of death and display respect for the deceased. If the family was not present for the death, the members may want a description of the patient's last moments. The nurse should respond both tactfully and truthfully. If it is true, saying to the family, "She was not alone" or "He seemed to be at peace" may be a great source of comfort to the family.

Although students in undergraduate programs and the recent graduates of these programs are often worried about what they ought to say to the family at this time, bereaved families usually are more in need of someone to listen to them. Thus, one of the major roles of the nurse at this time is active, compassionate listening. Short statements like "I'm sorry" and "I'll keep you in my thoughts or prayers" may be helpful but the nurse usually does not need to say much. Trivializing statements such as "S/he is better off now" or "I know just how you feel" are inappropriate. Depending on the nurse's relationship with the family, a hug might be helpful to both the family and the nurse. The nurse's expression of emotion through tears is not unprofessional when it is an expression of the attachment between the nurse and the patient.

When the death is sudden and unexpected it is often more difficult for both the health care providers and the family to understand. It is usually the physician or the advance practice nurse who conveys the fact of the death to the family. Buckman et al. (1997) recommend a simple unequivocal statement that the patient (her/his name should be used) has died and the cause stated. Then the health care provider should remain silent and allow an opportunity for the family to respond and ask further questions. A truthful statement that the advance practice nurse is sorry helps some families. While some people prefer a human touch at this point, others may withdraw in grief. When the initial response has subsided, Buckman recommends focusing on the needs of the family, determining if they need to phone anyone or if they would like an opportunity to view the body. If there is a possibility of organ donation, the advance practice nurse would broach the subject at this time.

REVIEW OF THE RELATIONSHIP, EXPLORATION OF PERSONAL FEELINGS, AND EVALUATION OF NURSING RESPONSES

Although not a specific step in the therapeutic relationship, it is always wise following the termination of a relationship for the nurse to review the process to explore her/his feelings and evaluate her/his behavior. An undergraduate nursing student encountering her/his first experience with death may need to explore the experience with the faculty member after the patient and family has been cared for. In most circumstances, it is helpful for the student to be involved in preparing the body and talking with the family. For the first experience with death, it is helpful if a nursing faculty member or an experienced nurse prepares the body with the student. While preparing the body, most undergraduate nursing students find it helpful if the faculty member provides simple factual statements of how the body changes after death. Many students will remark how different the deceased seems once the suffering is over and life has departed.

Undergraduate nursing students often state that listening to the family helps them to find some meaning in the dying experience. If the death has been anticipated, the family will frequently discuss how the patient felt in the last few days and weeks and will often convey a sense of relief that the patient is no longer struggling. The family may review the person's life and help the student to realize that it had reached its natural end.

When the death is sudden and unexpected, undergraduate nursing students often are distraught. This is especially true if the patient was close to their own or their parents' ages. A review of what happened to the patient with an emphasis on how the health care team responded may at least help the student to realize there was no way in which the health care team could have prevented the death. Later, many undergraduate nursing students and new graduate nurses question why this person had to die at this time in their life. Active listening by the nursing faculty member or perhaps the hospital chaplain is most likely to assist the student to come to some understanding of the death.

Undergraduate nursing students may idealize death; they may want each experience to be mystical and transcendent. However, death, like birth, is both messy and difficult as well as beautiful and transcendent. Learning to live and care within the realm of what is possible for people at the end of their life is often difficult for the undergraduate nursing student and the new graduate of an undergraduate nursing program. Nursing faculty should help the student to recognize the realities that shaped the way in which this particular patient died and identify factors that s/he would want to modify when caring for future patients.

CONCLUSION

When nurses communicate with their dying patients and the families, they have a clearer understanding of their patients' needs and goals at the end of life. Once these goals are established, the nurse may assist the patient in dying well. That death might include limited technology, symptom relief, life review with resolution of past uncompleted business, and the presence of loving family and friends. Or, it might involve fighting for the last breath, remaining alive until the last possible second using the latest medical technology. However, without thoughtful communication with the patient and family, the nurse cannot be sure which course to take to help the patient to die well.

Education Plan 7.1   Plan for Achieving Competencies: Communication With Patients, Families, and Health Care Providers

Knowledge Needed	Attitude	Skills	Undergraduate Behavioral Outcomes	Graduate Behavioral Outcomes	Teaching/Learning Strategies
Importance of communication for patients, families, and health care providers at the end of life.	*Affirm the value for communication at the end of life, for patients, family, and health care provider. *Appreciate the benefits of communicating honestly with the dying patient and family. *Acknowledge own level of death anxiety.	*Communicate with the dying patient and family in an honest and empathic manner.	*Effectively and compassionately communicate with patients and families at end of life. *Clarify information presented by health care providers to the patient and family. *Communicate patient/family wishes and preferences to members of the interdisciplinary team.	*Serve as a role model for effective and compassionate communication with patients and families at the end of life. *Create an environment where effective and compassionate communication is a goal of care.	*Use a death anxiety instrument to measure nurses' own level of death anxiety, and discuss their death experiences in post-conference or seminar. *Have students describe experiences of personal or professional growth related to end-of-life discussions. *Have students write a letter to a member of their family, describing their end-of-life wishes (not to be shared in class).

Education Plan 7.1 *(continued)*

Knowledge Needed	Attitude	Skills	Undergraduate Behavioral Outcomes	Graduate Behavioral Outcomes	Teaching/Learning Strategies
Phases of a Therapeutic Relationship: Introductory Phase: —Opening the relationship; —Breaking or reinforcing bad news; —Clarifying the problem by effective communication skills; —Structuring and formulating the care agreement and goals of care.	*Convey respect for the dying patient and family. *Recognize the patient's right to participate in and determine end-of-life care and treatment goals. *Appreciate the need for information based on personal preference and culture.	*Demonstrate effective and compassionate communication skills. *Demonstrate by words or actions that the patient/family will not be abandoned. *Initiate discussion with patient and family regarding end-of-life issues.	*Develop a trusting relationship with dying patients and families. *Facilitate patient/families expression of feelings, needs, and concerns. *Assist the patient/family to discuss what he/she believes is dying well. *Facilitate the completion of unfinished business.	*Convey bad news, including diagnosis, prognosis, or death using an empathic approach. *Guide patients and families in determining the goals of care. *Communicate effectively and compassionately in complex and difficult family systems. *Assist patients and families in resolving interpersonal conflicts/issues.	*Role play and critique communication in the following situations: —Delivering bad news; —Reinforcing bad news; —Determining goals of care; —Clarifying information; —Reassessing previous decisions; —Individuals presenting interpersonal conflicts.

Education Plan 7.1 (continued)

Knowledge Needed	Attitude	Skills	Undergraduate Behavioral Outcomes	Graduate Behavioral Outcomes	Teaching/Learning Strategies
Working Phase: *Exploring and understanding patients feelings and expectations about death and dying —dying well —unfinished business; —life review —talking with patients and families about death as it is experienced throughout the life cycle.	*Acknowledge the difficulty of patient and family in making end-of-life decisions. *Accept the patient/family's level of readiness for information related to decision making. *Acknowledge patients' and families' feelings as valid. *Value nursing presence during the dying process for patient and family and the importance of compassionate care.	*Use effective and compassionate communication skills to deliver information, establish a plan of care, and console the patient, family, and other health professionals. *Act in accordance with state statutes and institutional policies regarding end-of-life decision making. *Teach families impending signs of death.	*Provide the opportunity for patients to conduct a life review. *Describe the benefits and burdens of various treatments at the end of life. *Provide patient and family with assurance of aggressive palliative care to provide comfort during the dying process. *Interpret medical information to patient and family in terms that they can understand. *Convey a change in patient's status to APN, MD, and family.	*Facilitate patient, family, and health care provider communication to determine the goals and plan of care, and affirm end-of-life decisions. *Coordinate health care team activities aimed at achieving the patient's goals and wishes. *Prepare the family and staff for patient's imminent death. *Convey the fact of death to the family. *Present organ donation options to the family, when appropriate.	*Use video taped interviews with patients and families, exemplifying therapeutic communication skills, i.e., "Before I Die," and "Cancer Evolution or Revolution." *As faculty, model therapeutic communication for student in introductions to patients and families. *Conduct an exercise in which one student actively listens to another student regarding a transition in their life without speaking for 5

Education Plan 7.1 *(continued)*

Knowledge Needed	Attitude	Skills	Undergraduate Behavioral Outcomes	Graduate Behavioral Outcomes	Teaching/Learning Strategies
*Facilitating and Taking Action: —DNR orders and other advanced directives. —Family letter writing —nurses' reassurance of comfort and non-abandonment. Termination Phase: Withdrawing medical interventions; Preparing patient and family for signs of death; Aggressive comfort measures at the end of life; Consoling the bereaved;	*Express an acceptance of death. *Express respect for the deceased. *Acknowledge feelings of loss and grief expressed by patient, family, and health care providers. *Consider patients' and families' values and beliefs related to the end-of-life care.	*Explain the detachment of the patient in the dying process. *Assist families in expressing their feelings to the patient.	*Console the bereaved. *Seek support and an opportunity for exploration of students'/nurses' feelings and responses related to caring for a dying patient and their family.	*Provide a supportive environment for review of nurses' feelings and behaviors in caring for the dying patient and family.	minutes. Discuss the experience of active listening, and the experience of being heard. *Perform a life review with a selected patient in a clinical setting. Describe the initiation of life review, the strategies that enhanced communication and barriers to communication as it relates to the patient, nurse, and environment. *Reconstruct a conversation that the nurse found difficult.

Education Plan 7.1 *(continued)*

Knowledge Needed	Attitude	Skills	Undergraduate Behavioral Outcomes	Graduate Behavioral Outcomes	Teaching/Learning Strategies
Reviewing the relationships for personal feelings and evaluation of nursing responses.					Evaluate the communication skills, and recommend an alternative communication strategy. *Critique a case study of communication with patient and family at the end of life. *Have students attend a support group for bereaved families to identify bereavement issues, observe the role of the group leader, and identify barriers or facilitators to effective and compassionate communication.

REFERENCES

Albom, M. (1997). *Tuesday's with Morrie.* New York: Doubleday.

Anderson, B., & Hall, B. (1995). Parents perceptions of decision making for children. *Journal of Law, Medicine & Ethics, 23*, 15–19.

An Interview with Dr. Stuart Farber, Living with a serious illness: A workbook for patients and families. *Innovations in end of life care: An international on-line forum for leaders in end of life care* (1999). [on-line] Available: http://www2.edc.org/lastacts/featureinn.asp.

Booth, K., Maguire, P. M., Butterworth, R., & Hillier, V. F. (1996). Perceived professional support and the use of blocking behaviors by hospice nurses. *Journal of Advanced Nursing, 24*, 522–527.

Buckman, R. (1992). *How to break bad news: A guide for health professionals.* Baltimore: Johns Hopkins Press.

Buckman, R., Lipkin, M., Sourkes, B., & Tolle, S. (1997, June 15). Strategies and skills for breaking bad news. *Patient Care,* 61–66.

Byock, I. (1997). *Dying well: Peace and possibilities at the end of life.* New York: Riverhead Books.

Callanan, M. (1994). Farewell messages. *American Journal of Nursing, 94*(5), 19–20.

Cavendish, R. (1999). Improving care for the elderly. *American Journal of Nursing, 99*(3), 88.

Cotton, P. (1993). Talk to people about dying—They can handle it, say geriatricians and patients. *Journal of the American Medical Association, 269*(3), 321–323.

Czerwiec, M. (1996). When a loved one is dying: Families talk about nursing care. *American Journal of Nursing, 96*(5), 32–36.

Emanuel, E. J. (1998). The promise of a good death. *Lancet, 351* (9114, Suppl. Cancer), S1121–1126.

Family letter writing: An interview with Nathan Harlow (1999). *Innovations in end of life care: An international on-line forum for leaders in end of life care* (1999). [on-line] Available: http://www2.edc.org/lastacts/featureinn.asp.

Furukawa, M. M. (1996). Meeting the needs of the dying patient's family. *Critical Care Nurse, 16*(1), 51–62.

Heaven, C. M., & Maguire, P. (1996). Training hospice nurses to elicit patient concerns. *Journal of Advanced Nursing, 23*(2), 280–286.

Jezewski, M. A. (1996). Obtaining consent for Do-Not-Resuscitate status: Advice from experienced nurses. *Nursing Outlook, 44*(3), 114–119.

Langley-Evans, A., & Payne, S. (1997). Light-hearted death talks in a palliative day care context. *Journal of Advanced Nursing, 26*, 1091–1097.

Latimer, E. (1998). Ethical care at the end of life. *Canadian Medical Association Journal, 158*(13), 1741–1745.

May, C. (1995). To call it work somehow demeans it: The social construction of talk in the care of the terminally ill patients. *Journal of Advanced Nursing, 22*, 556–661.

Murphy, P. A., & Price, D. M. (1995). ACT taking a positive approach to end of life care. *American Journal of Nursing, 95*(3), 42–43.

Roundtable discussion: Part 2 (1996). A peaceful death: How to manage pain and provide quality care. *Geriatrics, 51*(6), 32–42.

Servaty, H. L., Krejci, M. J., & Hayslip, B. (1996). Relationships among death anxiety, communication apprehension with dying and empathy in those seeking occupations as nurses and physicians. *Death Studies, 20*, 149–161.

Shmerling, R. H., Bedell, S. E., Lilienfeld, A., & Delbanco, T. L. (1988, July/August). Discussing cardiopulmonary resuscitation. *Journal of General Internal Medicine, 3*, 317–321.

Stein, C. (1999, March 14). Ending a Life. *Boston Globe Magazine, 13*, 24, 30–34, 39–42.

Stiles, M. K. (1990). The shining stranger: Nurse-family spiritual relationship. *Cancer Nursing,* *13*(4), 2235–245.

The Support Principal Investigators (1995). A controlled trial to improve care for seriously ill, hospitalized patients: The study to understand prognoses and preferences for outcomes and risks of treatments (SUPPORT). *Journal of the American Medical Association, 274*(20), 1591–1598.

Tulsky, J. A., Chesney, M. A., & Lo, B. (1996). See one, do one, teach one? House staff experience discussing do-not-resuscitate orders. *Archives of Internal Medicine, 156*(12), 1285–1289.

Wilkinson, S. (1991). Factors that influence how nurses communicate with cancer patients. *Journal of Advanced Nursing, 16,* 677–688.

8

Caring for Families: The Other Patient in Palliative Care

*Suzanne K. Goetschius**

AACN Competency

#5 Demonstrate respect for the patient's views and wishes during end-of-life care.

> It is curious how sometimes the memory of death lives on for so much longer than the memory of the life it purloined.
>
> —Roy, 1997

The nursing care of any patient is planned with an understanding of the system or family in which the person functions. Family can mean direct blood relatives, relationship through an emotional commitment, or the group or person with which someone feels most closely connected (Field & Cassell, 1997). Family can be brothers, sisters, parents, children, cousins, nieces, nephews, aunts, uncles, or grandparents. Family can be spouse, partner, or significant other. Family can be best friends, colleagues, neighbors, or even caregivers. A nursing assistant who gives personal care everyday may have a significant personal tie with a patient. Understanding these roles and relationships is critical to both thorough assessment and effective care

---

*This chapter is written in the memory of Albert T. Tremblay, RN, MSN who died as I was writing this chapter. The lessons I learned from him and his family would fill a thousand pages.

planning in nursing. Knowing who is providing home support for a patient is key to developing a successful discharge plan. Knowing who prepares meals is key to doing nutrition teaching. Knowing whose presence is the most comforting to a patient is key to maintaining their sense of well-being during stressful times. In end-of-life care (EOLC), this is especially true and yet, takes on even greater importance. Nurses must consider not only how the family can help the patient, but how the nurse must help the family—the other patient—face what may be their most difficult challenge: the death of a loved one.

As families struggle to be caregivers of the dying, they must also struggle with their impending loss, their changing roles and relationships, watching a loved one suffer-both physically and emotionally, and dealing with their own concerns about their ability to be a caregiver. Key nursing competencies in end-of-life care include assisting families to develop skills in effective communication, identify their roles, cope with all that is happening emotionally, use available resources, and provide direct care (AACN, 1998). Teaching nursing students the "how-to" of the palliative care of families is a challenge. Undergraduate students are overwhelmed with their own issues around death and dying, their limited knowledge base about "how-to" themselves, and the incredible fear of "saying the wrong thing." They are in the position of needing to let the family "do for" and empowering the family at a time in their own role development when their focus is on "doing" themselves. Advanced practice nursing students may have to correct concepts learned from their undergraduate programs and their own experiences with patients, families, and death: leaving families alone or not getting involved in EOLC.

In this chapter, the interventions and suggestions for palliative care for families will include care in a variety of settings—and along the continuum of care that people may traverse as they approach the end of life. Caring for the families of children who are dying and young children in end-of-life care is not part of this author's expertise and will not be addressed here.

FAMILIES AND END-OF-LIFE CARE

One of the fundamental principles of palliative care is that the patient and family together are the unit of care (Reimer, Davies, & Martens, 1991). As the health care system and society have shifted their expectations about EOLC from an institutional setting where professional caregivers are in charge to a home setting where the family is in charge, so must nursing refocus its efforts in addressing the needs of families in EOLC. Family has been the focus of much research both in terms of how they are affected by the EOLC process and how their needs can be met.

Joanne Lynn (1997) notes that suggested domains for measuring quality at the end of life should include patient and family satisfaction and family burden, including financial and emotional burden. Patient and family satisfaction should include the patient's piece of mind, the family's perception of the patient's care and comfort, the decision-making process, the care received—both by the patient and the family, and the extent to which opportunities were provided to complete life in a meaningful way. The time spent by patient and family should be treasured and not simply tolerable. According to Donaldson (1998), assessment of quality in EOLC is focused on patient and family caregivers, but could also include a social network and their support. Survivors' memories of a loved one's death are important in their own right because dying is not only what the patient experiences but what the survivors remember (Jacobson, 1998). The survivor's experience of EOLC is examined to assess quality and outcome of interventions in EOLC. If the family is essential to measuring quality and positive outcomes in EOLC then what do nurses who provide EOLC need to know to meet their needs?

Field and Cassell (1997) noted that general nursing curricula should address the variations in dying related to clinical conditions and family circumstances, mental states, and other factors that may require alternate nursing strategies. They also noted that students receive limited exposure to dying patients and limited guidance in handling their personal reactions to the dying and their bereaved families. Curricular foci should include clinical knowledge, interpersonal skills, ethical awareness, and other aspects of care with case-based learning, role playing, and experiences in different settings.

A study by Emanuel et al. (1999) found that 96% of primary caregivers of the terminally ill are family members and 72% are women. Less than 3% of all patients received any volunteer assistance and paid caregivers are used less than 20% of the time. Patients with cancer seemed to fair better than others, having fewer unmet needs, fewer caregiving needs, and less reliance on paid caregivers than those with an illness like heart disease or emphysema. The researchers noted that more attention has been focused on the terminal care needs of cancer patients than other disease processes. Support services may exist for cancer patients and their families that do not exist for others.

Families experience both physical and emotional distress while experiencing the death of a loved one. According to Sherman (1998), there is a "reciprocity of suffering" that can occur for family members. Family members may suffer physical, psychosocial, emotional, and spiritual distress during EOLC. Not only are they experiencing their own pain as they deal with the impending death but they suffer as they try to fulfill new roles as caregivers. They fear being unable to relieve the suffering and pain of their family member. It is necessary to cope with the disruption of their lives, abandonment by friends, and with anticipatory grief. They face financial burdens, loss of employment, and loss of their major source of income. Patients may fear their own suffering and death less than they fear being a burden to their families.

Reimer et al. (1991) noted that the EOL process for cancer families could be seen as a passage they referred to as "fading away." The process of fading away starts with "ending," when the family perceives the final decline of the patient is occurring. Families have two tasks during this time: redefining themselves and dealing with burden. Nursing interventions during this phase include being aware that each person will process the change differently and that change will take time. Nurses can provide opportunities for discussion, assist with keeping the patient as independent as possible, provide resources, and tailor interventions to the individual's need to process change. Once the ending has been realized, the family moves from their old way of living with cancer into a neutral zone, where they struggle with the change from their pre-decline life, contend with change, and search for meaning. Here, nurses can serve as a sounding board to validate feelings, to help the family explore options, and to identify the limits of their tolerance. The nurse must also be aware of their own feelings, recognizing the importance of their response to the well-being of the family. Finally, the family moves to their new beginning of living day-to-day in the present and preparing for death. The nurse needs to be able to discuss the inevitability of death and all its implications. By focusing not only on death but also on the life that will go on, nurses can affirm for families their ability to manage and grow from the experience by encouraging life review and the completion of unfinished business. How the family copes with these changes is colored by past coping styles and past experiences with death and loss.

Several authors have noted that families want a few basic interventions from nurses (Hull, 1989; Lewandowski & Jones, 1988; Sherman, 1999; Waltman, 1990). First, families want honest, open communication and the sharing of accurate, straightforward information about the patient's condition and the process their loved one is to undergo. False reassurances, false sympathy, and overzealous attempts to show empathy are not welcome by families. Second, they want skilled nursing interventions aimed at the care and comfort of the patient. They want to be physically near and sometimes alone with their family member, but not abandoned. Research with 40 families by Lewandoski and Jones (1988) showed that families tend to stay focused on the needs of the family member who is dying and fail to consider their own needs. Assurance that a loved one is comfortable and cared for and having access to information was cited as essential nursing interventions. According to Lewandowski and Jones (1988), families go through three phases of living with cancer—initial, adaptation, and terminal phases. Families in the initial phase were interested in information and hope. In the second phase, they continued to focus on information. In the third phase, they no longer focused on hope but expressed a need to ventilate feelings, spend time alone, and continue to receive information. Across all three phases, families felt the need for the focus of nursing care to be the patient's care and comfort and not the family. The authors felt it was important for nurses to be knowledgeable about family dynamics and that care planning must focus on the patient as a part of the family system. They emphasized that the family is capable of change and growth even during a terminal illness. Key to family growth was teaching and giving the family information.

Nursing has begun to look at what could be provided to families once basic patient care needs are met. McCracken and Gerdson (1991) noted that the nurse must assess the family members as well as the patient. An interdisciplinary team should provide EOLC. The family should be taught about the physical EOL process, the completion of relationship issues, and how to begin letting go. Information regarding the physical, emotional, and spiritual signs of impending death such as withdrawal, visions, unusual communications, and saying good-bye should also be included in the teaching plan.

Based on interviews with 10 nurse educators and 10 experienced palliative care nurses, Degner, Gow, and Thompson (1991) noted seven critical behaviors in the care of the dying including responding to the needs of the family. The critical behaviors included: responding to the family's need for information; reducing the potential for future regrets; and including them in the care or relieving them of the responsibility depending on their needs. Negative behaviors towards families included not providing information, refusing to discuss dying or spiritual issues even when the family indicated they wished to, and passing judgment on family decisions and behaviors.

Cutillo-Schmitter (1996) recommends four strategies for managing the "ambiguous loss"; a loss which accompanies decline from a terminal or a dementing illness and in which the patient's and family's roles and relationships have changed. The path to EOL may be prolonged and uncertain. Family members may have a wide range of responses from denial to anger, helplessness and guilt. Nursing strategies with ambiguous loss include being present and acknowledging what can and cannot be done; identifying the loss as ambiguous and clarifying what is lost and what remains of relationships. The nurse can provide family with the opportunity to share their perceptions of the loss, and educate and support the family regarding disease progression and resources.

The five relationship completion tasks of EOL as identified by Byock (1997) are important to explore with family and patient. Such tasks include saying forgive me; I forgive you; I love you; thank you; and good-bye. Knowing where the caregiver is in completing these tasks with the patient may help them to define ways to achieve some of the personal growth and sense of mastery that can occur at the end of life (Byock, 1997).

Czerwiec (1996) interviewed families who experienced death in hospitals. She found that actions directed at patient comfort were important to families, as well as the nurse's attitude while performing the action. The families saw nurse's actions directed towards their needs as a sign of extraordinary caring. Presence, the time the nurse spent with them, was noted as influential. She recommended assessing how long and how well the family and patient have been coping with the illness, the family member's status as caregiver and their health, how well they understand the illness, and their relationship with the health care team. Recommended interventions included being able to discuss difficult issues, providing for the physical needs of the family, creating a safe environment for the family, offering spiritual care, and learning about the person who is dying. Nursing diagnoses associated with families and EOLC included " . . . hopelessness, anticipatory grieving, spiritual distress, fear, caregiver role strain and altered family processes" (Czerwiec, 1996, p. 35).

Wilson and Daley (1999) found the following aspects for families experiencing EOLC in the institutional long-term-care setting to be important: caring staff behaviors, participation in the dying process, presence at the time of death, and provision of spiritual support. A study by Furukawa (1996) revealed that families in critical care have similar needs from nursing such as: assurance that the patient is cared for; proximity or access to their loved one; and information. Implications for nursing care of the family in the critical care setting included unrestricted, flexible visiting policy, early social service intervention, realistic hope, facilitation of communication between families and physicians, and sending sympathy cards to families.

CARING FOR FAMILIES ACROSS THE HEALTH CARE CONTINUUM

Nurses interact with families in a variety of settings from primary through palliative care. Despite both evolving societal expectations of where EOLC should occur and increasing numbers of persons who choose to die at home, the majority of people in the United States still die in an institutional setting, though this varies somewhat regionally (Meier & Morrison, 1999). While the demographics of where nurses practice continues to change, it is likely that many nurses will experience a patient's death for the first time in an institutional setting. In acute care, the opportunity to develop rapport with families is fleeting and events can occur quickly. A hospitalized patient whose heart failure was stable yesterday may be actively dying today. Nurses must learn palliative care skills to use in these fast-paced settings where they are likely to find themselves dealing with dying patients and their grieving families—not just in a hospice setting. The family of a patient who dies in the ICU should have the same opportunity to experience a "good death" despite the limitations the setting may impose. It is important to improving *all* end-of-life experiences to teach nurses how to help families across diverse health care settings.

Understanding why death occurs and the dying process is important in preparing students for EOLC. Much of what we teach about EOLC is based on experiences with oncology patients and their families. However, cancer is not the most common fatal illness in this country. Heart disease continues to be the number one cause of death in this country (Smith, Martin, & Ventura, 1999). In fact, the majority of people who die are older adults dying of chronic illnesses such as heart disease, cancer, cerebrovascular disease, chronic obstructive pulmonary disease, and Alzheimer's disease (Brock & Foley, 1998). The trajectory of illness and decline is different for most progressive fatal diseases when compared to cancer. The SUPPORT study (The SUPPORT Investigators, 1995) found the common course at the end of life is a seemingly sudden, unpredictable change in a chronic fatal illness. Yet, we still have very little evidenced-based information about meeting the EOLC needs of anyone but cancer patients and their families (Meier & Morrison, 1999). Nurses need palliative care experience and education to provide care to patients and families coping with all fatal illnesses and to assist them in making end-of-life decisions.

Nurses can begin to develop the skills needed for more intensive end-of-life care in every setting from the doctor's office to the long-term care setting. It is critical for nurse educators to use these opportunities as they arise. For instance, a nurse may encounter a woman in a well-baby clinic, and in the course of her assessment, find out that she is also the caregiver for her dying father. The educator could support the nurse in identifying the issues the woman may have and assessing how they influence her other roles—like new mother—and what interventions may be necessary. Perhaps the family could benefit from a hospice program and the nurse could discuss this option and provide a referral. The new mother may also need referral to a counseling service, some extra assistance with child care at home, referral to a home care agency's maternal child health services to offer in-home support, or other holistic interventions.

Advanced practice nurses in a long-term-care setting may offer support to the nursing assistant during the death of a favorite patient; a situation where the patient and the nursing assistant may have a true "family" relationship (O'Hara, Harper, Chartand, & Johnston, 1996). Advanced practice nurses (APN) may also be in the position of having to tell or be a partner in telling a patient and family about a poor prognosis. This may be the true beginning of a family's education about end-of-life care and can set the tone for the rest of the family and patient's experience. APNs often bring with them a great deal of experience with EOLC and can begin to answer questions for the family and patient. A nurse's skills in therapeutic communication are critical at those moments and may make the APN the best person to have such a discussion, especially if a sound relationship exists.

Nurses will be caring for patients and families when they are diagnosed, admitted with an acute exacerbation of a chronic problem, during their active treatment and during palliative care. The need for components of palliative care can occur at any time over the course of an illness. In a recent communication (Listserve communication, October 22, 1999), Joanne Lynn noted that trying to identify an exact point when palliative care should be initiated might not be appropriate.

> Quite simply, I think that such a transition is largely a social construction made to keep us all more comfortable, and it neither serves the patient well nor helps us structure our care system optimally. It would be better, generally, to develop new models of care that combine palliation, treatment (and rehabilitation, prevention, informing, etc.)—in the mix that regularly serves patients of certain sorts. AND [*sic*] to be able to tailor the fine points of such systems of care to the individual circumstances and preferences of the patient.

Assessing the family and patient over the course of an illness trajectory can be an opportunity to educate nurses about the changes that occur in relationships as the family tries to cope. With a new terminal diagnosis, for example, the patient may be keeping details from the family to protect them—or vice versa. As a family struggles with the impact of treatment on their lives, the nurses can examine how the roles and values within the family may be changing and how to facilitate skill development for a new role. A nurse in home care may observe that a husband needs assistance with learning how to prepare meals if his elderly wife is no longer able. The nurse may develop a plan of care that begins to examine with the husband what other roles are going to change as the illness progresses and how to begin to prepare. A patient and family choosing palliative care may need education about physical care as well as the changes associated with the dying process. Spiritual support or respite information is also important.

The nursing student will need to have the resources to deal with these deficits. Gaining experience in these areas can facilitate managing the more intense clinical needs of an actively dying patient.

ASSESSING FAMILIES DURING END-OF-LIFE CARE

Palliative care is a holistic approach to care for patients and their families during life-threatening illness. The focus of care is the entire family unit as it is altered by the illness of one of its members. Assessing the family as a system and determining appropriate interventions are important in EOLC. As a system, the family is made up of elements (family members) with their own separate traits, who are interdependent, but who also function as a whole. The system/family and the individual elements are constantly impacted by changes from inside the system or outside influences such as nursing care. Systems strive to achieve equilibrium and stability. When that stability is threatened by an impending loss of a member, the family/system may need some assistance to return to or maintain its stability.

Nurses can assess the individuals and relationships within the family system. The nurse can then begin to develop interventions to counter the influences that have upset the balance of the family system. Families are capable of learning, evolving, and developing through the course of a loved one's illness (Lewandowski & Jones, 1988). In the case of families, understanding how the dying and death of one member impacts each individual and their relationships to each other, as well as the family as a whole allows the nurse to plan interventions to meet the needs of the family. Families identify the care and comfort of their family member as their number one priority (Lewandoski & Jones, 1988). Nurses must also help family members identify what their *own* needs are in EOLC.

Assessing the family is the first step in developing a plan of care. The important areas for assessment include: family structure, roles and relationships, modes of communication, strengths and weaknesses, knowledge deficits, and available resources (Cutillo-Schmitter, 1996; Czerwiec, 1996; Lewandowski & Jones, 1988; Sherman, 1998). The care setting can be a barrier in the EOLC assessment process. In an acute care setting, the student may have very little time to gather information from the family. In long-term care, the student may have the time—but little access to family. In hospice, time may or may not be short and access to family may be occurring at a time when they are feeling the burden of care already.

Educators will need to be creative in providing the student assessment opportunities with an EOLC focus. If time is an issue, interdisciplinary assessments by social workers, counselors, pastoral care providers, or nursing staff may give the student access to the information needed or provide validation. Case studies are valuable in developing skills and communication techniques and promote an opportunity for discussions about difficult issues that the students may encounter when caring for patients and families during EOLC. Conducting home visits may also be of benefit in following a family over the course of the dying process and across various settings.

Family assessment requires an adjustment of the perspective from the patient alone, to the system the patient functions in, and its components in relation to one another. Families are reluctant to see their needs as vital and may resist any focus on themselves. It is important to assure them that their loved one's needs are being met and that addressing their needs is equally as important in promoting their health and well-being. Through the assessment process, family members and the patient may be able to identify their goals, expectations, and preferences, and share what outcomes are critical to them. These outcome measures can assist the nurse in identifying measurable goals and objectives and the appropriate interventions to achieve them. Important points in assessing families include:

1) Family structure:
   a) Names, sex, and age of each family member
   b) Their relationship to the patient
2) Roles and expectations about roles:
   a) Pre-EOLC roles if known
   b) Patient's roles and EOLC goals
   c) Members roles at present and EOLC goals
   d) Cultural/ethnic/spiritual influences on roles and goals
   e) Lines of communication and how they share information
   f) Life span issues
   g) Gender issues
3) SWOT Analysis (strengths, weaknesses, opportunities, and threats):
   a) Identify factors that may enhance or inhibit family system
      i)   Issues related to the site of care
      ii) Family members who have health care training
      iii) The frail health of the spouse
      iv) Other family members to call on
      v)   Dependent care benefits at work
4) Knowledge Deficits:
   a) Past death experiences—positive and negative experiences
   b) Understanding the terminal state and prognosis
   c) Awareness of disease progression
   d) Knowledge of caregiving skills
   e) Legal/financial choices

f) Resources available such as palliative care consultation in acute care, hospice programs in the community, spiritual resources, and respite care. (Field & Cassell, 1997; McCracken & Gerdson, 1991; Sherman, 1998)

FAMILY STRUCTURE

Family structure includes all members of the family as identified by the patient and may include "informal" family such as friends or co-workers who provide care or support. Identifying roles may come from interviews and observations of a family over time. The assessment can be documented using a narrative or a family genogram with data filled in beside each individual's name.

If possible, the nurse should identify how the family functioned before the illness. This information can be helpful in understanding problems or planning interventions. A man whose wife had made all of her treatment decisions before her illness progressed may be unsure and hesitant when the role of decision maker becomes his. Without knowing why he was hesitant, the nurse might assume he did not understand the treatment plan. The intervention based on this information might be to talk with the husband about how his wife made decisions and to identify her priorities. This intervention may help him develop confidence in his new role.

ROLES AND EXPECTATIONS

Both family structure and roles will evolve over time as family member's abilities and experiences determine their degree of involvement in EOLC. The nurse may have the greatest impact in supporting or educating a family member who wishes to have a role they don't feel prepared for or finding ways to support their usual roles while they focus on their EOLC role. Family members may not know how to support an ill loved one or what they can do to be a part of the process. For example, in one family, the son was withdrawn and uncommunicative when visiting his father. The nursing student learned that he did not know what to do when he was visiting and felt as if he had nothing to offer. The student showed him how to get his father ice chips and fluids from the kitchen and invited him to go there as needed to help his father. The son was able to offer this service to his father independently and felt relieved to have something concrete to do that helped his father.

Some roles are long-standing and historical like the authority figure of a father. It is difficult for family members to change roles—for a mother to allow a daughter to be her caregiver. The concept of role reversal is often used to describe changes in role but can be a harmful way to frame the switch in tasks that are occurring. Clarifying this is sometimes important in helping families adjust. While some parents are comfortable being cared for by their child, they may express concern about the discomfort of losing that role and relationship as parent and child. In the film "One True Thing," a husband and daughter are caring for the terminally ill mother. In a moment of anguish that makes this issue clear, she shouts at her caregivers, "I'm still the mother in this house." The nurse can reframe these "role reversals" as something more positive—an opportunity for the children to honor their mother and her role and giving them the opportunity to experience the joy she felt when she cared for them.

Other roles may be brought about by EOLC situations. In one family, the son had difficulty being in the room while his mother was dying and spent most of his time pacing the halls, telling the nurse about how bad he felt that he couldn't "be in there." He became the family chauffeur for all the relatives who could not drive, bringing them back and forth to visit. While he could not be there himself, he made sure there was someone who could be. He developed a role that helped the family but was in his "safe zone." The nursing intervention in this case may be to help him and the rest of the family "see" his role and its value to the system.

Roles may be altered artificially by the environment of care. A caregiver may unwillingly relinquish their role as physical caregiver if an unobservant nurse takes over these tasks. The nurse needs to assess whether this is the wish of the caregiver before intervening. The authority figure of the nurse, even a student, may intimidate the caregiver and weaken his/her confidence in his/her caregiving abilities.

The well-being of primary caregivers must also be carefully assessed. The success of a given plan of care often rests on the shoulders of this individual and the ability of the family system to support their role. The health and functional ability of the caregiver may be compromised by caregiving; knowing the caregiver's limitations in advance can allow the nurse to address potential problems. The primary caregiver's coping skills and support systems are also important. What are the caregiver's needs in the process of EOLC? Do they want to be present at all times? Are they counting on other family members to take on certain tasks and roles that they will need to communicate? Perhaps they see their role as it has always been, a loving partner and spouse but they do not want to take on the physical caregiver role. It is important to have the significant other's goals and expectations identified, especially as it relates to the patient's.

Knowing the patient's roles and goals are critical for planning family interventions because the patient has a significant impact on the family as a whole and each person in it. For the most part, the patient's preferences and wishes become the outcomes that direct the plan of care and guide family decisions. Assessment should also include how the patient fits in the family traditionally and currently; how they handle their role as patient; are they still making their own decisions; and are they worried about being a burden to the rest of the family? If being a burden is a concern, they may resist their family's attempts to care for them, thwarting the family's role as caregivers. Roles of other family members may be impacted when the patient is unable to fulfill their usual roles. When a patient, who has been the financial support for the family can no longer work, someone else may have to start working to support the family or maintain insurance coverage. If this someone is also the primary caregiver, it may sabotage a plan for home caregiving.

Understanding cultural, ethnic, and religious influences may help define family roles in EOLC (Pickett, 1993). For example, current American culture espouses that a good death occurs at home with loved ones as caregivers (Jacobson, 1998; Pickett, 1993). A wife, who feels that to be a "good wife" she must care for her husband at home, may experience great distress at the prospect of bringing him home if she is not able to provide his physical care. How will she feel if she makes the choice to care for him in a nursing home? Is she still a "good wife"? The guilt and dissonance may be too painful for her to reveal and cause great issues if it is not resolved. If the focus of the nursing care plan was on caregiving skills without identifying and addressing the wife's concerns, the EOLC experience could be a painful one for the wife. In assessing roles, it is important for the student to maintain a culturally sensitive approach in dealing with all potential caregivers. Even dominant cultural beliefs may be the source of issues for family so it is critical that nurses carefully identify subtler or less well-known cultural influences during assessment.

Lines of communication are often related to role. Knowing how information is shared within a family both before and during an illness is important, especially as it pertains to planning interventions. The family spokesperson may be the only one who talks to health care providers while the others wait for feedback from the spokesperson. Clear communication is the key to avoiding role conflicts and confusion. For example, in one family, the daughter asked all the questions about her mother's physical care as she was planning to be the primary caregiver. The father sat quietly by and asked no questions. Rather than assuming this was lack of concern by the husband, the nurse spoke to him to assess how he felt about what was occurring. From this discussion, she recognized that he was going to continue his role as husband and supportive partner while his daughter did the physical care. Their communication style gave clues as to how they were defining their roles.

Gender and developmental stage may also influence roles and relationships. Older women are more likely to have a limited support network. Often, their spouse has already died, they are living alone, and they may be reluctant to impose on their adult children (Administration on Aging, 1999). They may already have endured significant loss or change of many roles. Older persons are less likely to have a large network of coworkers and friends who can offer tangible support because of their own health problems or limited resources. In these instances, the student may want to look for other types of "family": paid caregivers, religious affiliations, social groups, etcetera. The number of friends and family who want to be involved in EOLC may overwhelm a younger adult. The student may help them identify which roles and relationships are critical and help the family find ways for others to be involved more appropriately. Developmental tasks of all family members need to be assessed. Providing EOLC may alter certain developmental tasks: completing an education, marriage, starting a family, or job-related advancement.

SWOT ANALYSIS

Strengths, weaknesses, opportunities, and threats can be traits of either the family or the environment that potentially imperil or enhance the EOLC process. Strengths might be a facility that has a palliative care consultation service or a family that has a dependent caregiver benefit at work. Weaknesses may be a community with no respite services or a family caregiver who is an alcoholic. Opportunities may be the presence of three daughters who will take turns providing care for their mother at home or an ICU that has developed a new family-centered care policy for the families of terminal patients. Threats may be a health care provider with limited experience in EOLC or the declining health of the spouse who is the primary caregiver.

KNOWLEDGE DEFICITS RELATED TO EOLC

Assessing knowledge deficits in EOLC is also extremely important. Nurses must understand that after seeing to the comfort and care of the patient, information is the next concern of families (Lewandowski & Jones, 1988). The disease process and its variable trajectory will influence what families need to know and when they want to know it. A patient who is just diagnosed may not be ready to discuss terminal care in detail. In diseases like congestive heart failure, it may be difficult to identify a time frame for initiating palliative care. The nurse must be attuned to the goals of the patient and family rather than the process of the illness itself to develop a plan of care. Assessing the family's understanding of EOLC will require a more direct discussion and strong therapeutic communication skills, since talking about death directly is still a taboo among many people. Fear of upsetting someone, causing them to cry, and not knowing what to do are often concerns nurses bring up when beginning to work in EOLC. Often nurses want to avoid any discussion of death or terminal illness directly for fear of saying something wrong.

Framing discussions about EOLC as therapeutic offers a different perspective. Anxiety about the unknown and the mysteries that surround the end of life add to the impending loss of a loved one and can be overwhelming. Families need to have a "safe place" to begin discussions regarding end-of-life care. The nurses can model for the family that it is appropriate to talk about this process and ask questions. The nurse educator may take the lead in beginning some of these discussions for the novice nurse; pairing them with an APN or staff nurse may be helpful. Working with other care providers, such as social workers and chaplains may also give guidance to nurses.

Asking about past death experiences can also contribute valuable information. Nurses can glean information about what the person understood about the experience and process at the time, what was the overall impression of the experience, and what the family might have wanted to be different. Do they have regrets about past choices? What is the one thing they would like to change? Was there a role they had that they wished they could have fulfilled or managed differently? This is often a good starting place for developing a teaching plan.

Skills in fostering therapeutic communication about past death experience should be practiced in advance. The nurse educator may do this as a group exercise to help nurses develop comfort with the process. Interviewing each other and presenting what they gleaned may offer the educator an opportunity to model interviewing techniques. It is also important to receive feedback from one another. It is important for nurses to have discretion in sharing their own experiences with death and dying with families though it may serve a critical function in establishing rapport. Nurse educators might also arrange for a panel of family members to share their experiences with the students—what went well, what they disliked, what nursing interventions helped, and what interventions were not helpful. Support groups may be an excellent resource for this type of group and may be helpful for a family member who wants to have an impact on the care of others because of their experience.

Advanced Practice Nurses are probably best able to assess a family's understanding of the terminal state and prognosis due to their nursing experience. Nurses should develop an understanding of the specific disease process before meeting with families. Understanding how each disease progresses toward death is important in preparing families for what is to come. A diagnosis of Alzheimer's disease may involve an 8–20 year disease trajectory before death and can be unpredictable in its progression. Cancer is more predictable but varies from type to type. Information about what a family understands about prognosis and disease progression may be obtained from both questioning and observations. Nurses may learn from role playing some of the difficult situations that might arise during this part of an assessment. Questions about how much time is left, the efficacy of experimental treatments, use of alternative therapies in symptom relief, or telling or not telling family/patient about a poor prognosis could be used to stimulate discussion and identify supportive interventions. It may be within the scope of the APN to discuss options for care with the family/patient such as pursuing further therapy or clinical trials. The level of information needed is most likely beyond an undergraduate student because of the various factors involved in making treatment choices.

Many families focus on physical care skills as their first learning objective. Their key concern is their ability to manage comfort and pain. Experiences with EOLC may reinforce the need to learn technical care skills, especially if family members felt unable to relieve suffering in previous experiences. The role a family member feels comfortable with may depend on their confidence in physical caregiving. Often, what a family knows and what they can learn determines the options for where care at the end of life can occur. Nurses can reassure family members that they will be taught the skills needed and explain how support will be provided while skills are developed. Nurses need to validate their knowledge and skills to insure they are current and up-to-date. This is especially true for pain medication and issues such as hydration in EOLC.

The nurse should also address a family's accurate understanding of legal and financial implications of EOLC. Novice nurses as well as APNs should assess a family's understanding of the implications of the presence or absence of an advanced directive or a "do-not-resuscitate" order. Johns (1996) found that patients may hesitate in discussing advanced directives. They prefer that health care providers begin such discussions and often wish to have family members as their surrogates. The trusting quality of nurses' relationships with patients and families may facilitate discussions about advanced directives. Johns notes, "Nurses, because of their insights into patients' preferences and their role as patient advocates, have a legitimate role in monitoring compliance of treatment with patient's preferences as expressed in advanced directives . . . " (p. 152). Nurses should also know how to access resources such as an ethics consult for both their own or the patient/family's sake if issues are identified during an assessment of the family.

Assessing what the family knows about community or institutional resources is critical in planning care. The presence or absence of resources will influence where EOLC is delivered. A family may be unsure about what resources are available to them in making care decisions, which may limit what they can do for their family member. If families believe they have only one option for care, they can be forced into a decision they may regret.

There are several barriers to completing a successful assessment of a family needing EOLC. As mentioned earlier, the site of care may be a barrier; there may not be enough time to talk with the family. In an acute care setting, the patient's condition may be deteriorating so quickly that nurses have limited time to intervene in all aspects of care. Limited options for family involvement may be a source of frustration. In this case, nurses should identify what would be needed to meet the family/patient's needs.

The issue of care versus cure may also arise. It may be unclear to the family or staff what the goals of care are. Some family members may be working towards a cure while others are preparing to care; nurses may need some guidance with this type of family discord. Advanced Practice Nurses may be able to work with the family to help identify gaps in communication and facilitate resolution.

A nurse's personal issues may also threaten assessment. While nurses may have had limited exposure to death in their personal lives, they are not immune to its impact. Other nurses may have had a variety of both personal and professional experiences that influence their perceptions and observations regarding death and patient/family responses. It is the nurse educator's role to prepare nurses to achieve clinical competency in EOLC. Experiential exercises such as role-playing may be useful in identifying those students who need extra guidance and clinical support.

GOALS AND PLANS FOR CARE

The process of assessment can delineate a number of possible goals and objectives. Validating the goal that family members view as most important is the first step in developing a plan of care that is family-centered and collaborative. Based on the assessment of family roles and knowledge about EOLC, nursing diagnoses can be made and measurable objectives can be developed for short-term goals. Often, the family member's most important goal is identified from past experiences and something they wanted to change. Some examples may be, "I don't want her to die alone," "I want him to be home in his own bed," "I don't want him to be in pain," or, "He wants to have the family with him." Objectives can then be developed to meet that goal. For instance, if the goal is to have their loved one die at home, the student may need to teach the family how to administer medications, involve other family members in providing respite for the primary caregiver, and educate them all about the hospice program available in their community.

It may be difficult for a nurse to distinguish between the family's needs and the patient's needs in care planning. It is valuable to write two separate care plans based on the assessment—one for the family and one for the patient. Comparing the goals and objectives can reveal areas of overlap or conflict that need to be addressed. The nurse can begin to see how each intervention influences the family system and its members. The pain management plan for the patient supports the family's objective of keeping the patient comfortable. For example, a plan to teach a daughter physical care may fulfill the patient's wish to have some time alone with her daughter. Conversely, the patient may be interested in pursuing a clinical trial but the family wants to take him home to die. The nurse may have learned from the assessment that the patient felt it was important to do one last good thing for others through a clinical trial, while the family wanted to spend as much time with the patient as possible before he dies. With this information, interventions can be developed to resolve this difference and lead to a positive outcome.

BARRIERS TO DEVELOPING AN EFFECTIVE PLAN OF CARE

In helping nurses plan care for families at the EOL, it is important to be aware of how values and assumptions influence practice. First, this experience may be the nurse's first close contact with death and dying. It can be as traumatic for the nurse as for the patient and family. The nurse educator must assess the nurse's skill level and prior experiences with EOLC. They need to prepare nurses for how it may feel not to be able to fix everything for the family. Death is ultimately unavoidable despite the best care plan. It will be important for the educator to frame the outcomes of care so that the student can see successes.

Death is a painful experience, under the best of circumstances. Cutillo-Schmitter (1996) notes that while we cannot take away a family's grief, we can provide our caring presence. Listening is a difficult but valuable way of being present with families. What to say to families after death is even more challenging. Role-playing may be helpful in identifying therapeutic verbal and nonverbal behaviors. Practicing responses and actions such as how you would greet them, should you hug them, what if you feel like crying, and what about contact with the family after the death may be helpful. Articles by Miles (1993), Brown (1994), and Czerwiec (1996) offer simple, straightforward information about how to speak with families and loved ones. Examining what has been learned in the past is beneficial. Interviewing surviving family members on a panel may be useful to nurses. A family member who is comfortable with their experiences may be a good speaker with undergraduate students.

The educator must be cognizant of the nurse's own end-of-life experiences and their effect on interaction with the family. In undergraduate and graduate nursing education, knowing student concerns about the clinical assignment to provide EOLC may be useful in planning orientation or pre/post conference discussions. The students can write a paragraph early in a clinical rotation about their concerns. The nurse educator could ask questions like, "What do you worry might happen during this rotation?"; "Do you have any concerns about talking with families?"; "What worries you most?"; "What are you looking forward to?"; "What are your strengths in this setting?" which may help students verbalize their concerns.

It is important to avoid provider bias in developing any care plan and this is true with patients and families at the EOL. The prevailing sentiment today seems to be that all good deaths occur at home and any death in a hospital is a "bad death." This belief can lead to great distress if families are led to believe that they are *expected* to care for their family member at home. Care at home needs to be presented as a choice in a continuum of care that is available at the end of life without a value attached. Good deaths do occur in institutions and nursing care is a vital part of any positive EOL experience. What is critical is that a sound assessment be used to match the patient, the family, and its resources to the care that best meets their goals. With our current culture's emphasis on families taking loved ones home for care, families who cannot or who try and have to revert to a formal care setting often experience guilt and a sense of failure. Rather than expecting all families to provide EOLC at home, nurses must assess the family and identify their strengths and weaknesses in order to identify the setting and resources that fit the family. Arblaster, Brooks, Hudson, and Petty (1990) found that patients and families want responsive nursing care that enables them to bring their own resources to the dying process rather than having nurses impose care which they decide is appropriate. Nurses should be encouraged to provide quality end-of-life care independent of the setting where the care is provided.

As much as understanding a family member's past experiences is useful to the nurse in developing appropriate goals of care, it is important that the nurse understand that they cannot wholly compensate for the past. If a family member has significant issues around past EOLC, the nurse may need to refer them to another member of the interdisciplinary team to assist in resolving the issues, such as a pastoral counselor, a social worker, or a bereavement counselor.

The reality of EOLC is that, sometimes, even the best plan needs to be abandoned and rewritten for any number of reasons. Nurses may need support if a plan to send someone home to die does not occur when this was the family's crucial goal. While any care plan can fail, EOLC carries such emotional overtones that the failure to execute a plan can be devastating. It is important to consider an alternate plan—at least in discussions—to prepare patients, family, and staff for the possibility that their plan may not work out.

Debriefing time is critical in formal EOLC clinical settings. The issues of death and dying effect nurses on both a personal and professional level. A patient that reminds them of their mother, facing the family after medicating someone for pain and having them die within minutes of the dose; or providing postmortem care with the family can be stressful for less experienced nurses. It is critical to explore student's thoughts and feelings before and after clinical experiences. In addition, it is important to be aware of resources available to assist the nurse in continued learning regarding palliative care.

INTERVENTIONS: FACILITATING ROLE DEVELOPMENT FOR FAMILY

After assessing the family and developing goals and objectives, the nurse can begin to plan interventions to assist family members in achieving the roles they desire in EOLC. First, the nurse should validate roles desired by the family member. Communication is directed at encouraging the family member to describe what it is they want. Questions about how they see their role, what their concerns are about the role, what they need to do it, and what barriers exist will help the nurse decide what interventions are necessary. For example, if a daughter has children, a job, and a husband, yet wants to care for her dying mother in her home, the nurse will need to find out what resources are available to help her with child care, what her home is like, what experience she has in providing care, what her fears are, what resources are available in her workplace, and if she is aware of her Family Leave program at work. From these answers, the nurse can begin to help plan interventions.

Access to information about available resources to meet the family's needs is critical and nurse's participation in interdisciplinary teams assisting the family will be important. Nurses can benefit from spending time with other team members as they interact with family members, if appropriate. Collaborative efforts can be initiated with pastoral care staff, social services, mental health counselors, respite providers, and support groups. While the planning for a goal of home care can be largely a staff issue, the nurse should work with the care team and family to achieve some of the objectives needed to facilitate care at home. For instance, the nurse could begin to teach the daughter about physical care, nutrition, or medications.

The nurse should be assessing how the family's plan coincides with the patient's plan. If the nurse notes the mother is uncomfortable with the daughter providing the physical care, she might want to validate her perceptions and then discuss how to proceed with the interdisciplinary team. It is important for the nurse to communicate the plans to staff so they do not inadvertently interfere with the family's plan. If a family member wants to do the bathing, the nurse needs to be sure that the staff member who is responsible for that task knows the plan and can support it. Documenting objectives and clear interventions in the patient's care plan is often overlooked since the interventions are actually family focused.

The primary caregivers may have clearly defined roles and responsibilities and have received much guidance in developing their role. The nurse can then reinforce teaching and provide support and positive feedback. In addition, the nurse can focus on other family members whose role may be undeveloped. Developing roles for other family members may be subtler but blends well with the novice nurse's limited technical knowledge base in EOLC. The nurse's intervention of showing the son how to get ice and fluids for the father helped a family member without a role to identify something he could do independent of everyone else. The nurse can encourage family members to teach others the skills they learn as a means of developing possible respite resources.

One source of conflict for less experienced nurses can be their need to learn new tasks at the same time the family is learning. In this scenario, the use of an APN, nurse educator, or staff to teach a task while the nurse and family observe might be best. Sometimes, family members feel better about their relative inexperience when they see that novice nurses have to start with the basics. This has to be assessed carefully since some families may experience more anxiety as a result of this knowledge. Feedback is necessary for family members to successfully develop their role. The nurse can offer positive feedback to the family as they acquire new skills and explore new knowledge.

Nurses must be as supportive of families who continue to serve in their traditional family roles as those who choose new roles in EOLC. A son who can visit the nursing home and hold his mother's hand for a few hours at a time is fulfilling the role he has always had as a loving son. The nurse can acknowledge his role and provide encouragement to continue. Clarifying how the son wants to be involved when death seems imminent, identifying other family members who may be available to keep vigil and support the son, and documenting the information for the staff are important nursing interventions. The nurse can attempt to provide more information about EOLC and the dying process, reassure the son about all that is being done to care for his mother, and ascertain his understanding about any further interventions.

TEACHING PLANS

Teaching families about EOLC includes education about community or institutional resources, the skills they need to perform their roles, what they can expect from the health care team, and what the process of EOL entails. A complete education plan for families in EOLC may be beyond the experience of the novice nurse. The role of the novice nurse may be to identify the knowledge deficits and then obtain the resources to address them. More advanced nurses may be comfortable with teaching skills. Experienced APNs may have had experience in all areas but should validate that their current knowledge base is appropriate, especially regarding topics such as hydration, pain management, and ethical/legal issues.

Teaching plans need to be considered in light of the urgency of the impending death. A nurse working with a newly diagnosed patient with a terminal prognosis will need to focus on one set of priorities while a nurse in an ICU with a family who has just chosen to stop treatment will have a very different focus. In the first setting, the nurse may need to teach the family about support systems, community resources, and any treatments needed such as pain management, nutritional support, wound care, etcetera. In the second setting, the nurse must quickly assess the family's understanding of the plan of care and their expectations. The nurse could provide information about the support the team will offer, provide them with privacy if they desire, describe what the EOL process will be like, and what types of care will be provided such as pain management, mouth care, and skin care, etcetera. At this point, the nurse may ascertain what roles the family wants to play and begin to facilitate this. The nurse may invite a spouse to provide or participate in personal care if they seem hesitant, help them arrange how to be contacted within the hospital so they can go to get food or rest as needed, and arrange for pastoral care if desired.

The trend of dying in institutions means that the average person has never seen death personally. Many families believe death will be as it is on television: the patient talking one minute and quietly dying in the next. Novice nurses themselves may believe this. The reality that death is not likely to follow this scenario and the lack of correct information can make it difficult for family to cope with the terminal process. Rather than focusing on the technical aspects of dying, the nurse can relate the process of EOL as "sharing what I see." The phrase, "I might see" or "I might expect" followed by a description of a finding or change can help the family to begin to assess the process for themselves.

Nurses can further assess the family's potential needs at the time of death. The death process can be difficult to experience. Some families want to be alone; others prefer the presence of someone—nurse, minister, other family. The nurse will need to determine if they or someone else can provide this caring presence when the time comes. It may be simply being in the room during the last minutes, talking actively with the family about how the process is progressing, and what the various symptoms indicate or "checking in" at predetermined intervals as requested by the family. The plan should be documented and communicated with other staff to assure continuity. As noted earlier, the novice nurse may not be able to intervene alone and may need support from the interdisciplinary team. The nurse should be clear about what her level of involvement will be with the family. Nurses should let family know when they will be available, when they will return, and how any plans will be communicated and carried out when the nurse is not available.

CONCLUSION

The value in preparing nurses to meet the needs of families during end-of-life care seems as obvious as preparing them to manage pain or provide skin care. As outcome tools are developed and tested, the impact of educational preparation on the ability of the nurse to meet those needs will be delineated. Until then, the words of Dr. Joanne Lynn (1993, p. 42) offer a humanistic outcome measure,

> "How can this work be other than rewarding? This family so obviously thrived, and this patient had so many good times in our care. . . . This family can look back on the good time that they shared under the shadow of death. The experience will illuminate and deepen their experiences over each lifetime. The caregivers involved can be confident that lives were made better by their efforts. What more can we ask of our work?"

Education Plan 8.1   Plan for Achieving Competencies: Caring for Families

Knowledge Needed	Attitude	Skills	Undergraduate Behavioral Outcomes	Graduate Behavioral Outcomes	Teaching/Learning Strategies
Identifying family structure and relationships.	*Accept as family, all individuals identified by patient as family.	*Elicit a family history to identify members and relationships.	*Document a history that identifies family structure and relationships.	*Communicate family structure and relationships to members of the interdisciplinary team.	*Create a genogram to identify family members' relationships. *Assign students to interview a patient to obtain a family history and compare data to chart documentation. *Present a family history at an interdisciplinary team meeting.

Education Plan 8.1 *(continued)*

Knowledge Needed	Attitude	Skills	Undergraduate Behavioral Outcomes	Graduate Behavioral Outcomes	Teaching/Learning Strategies
Research relevant to family caregiving.	*Value research related to family caregiving in developing evidence-based practice.	*Use research findings to establish plans of care for family members.	*Critique family caregiver research. *Utilize research findings in practice. *Identify needs for research in the area of family caregiving at the end of life.	*Collaborate in research related to family caregiving at the end of life.	*Critique 5 research articles relevant to family caregiving at the end of life and present the findings for future research to peers in post-conference or seminar. *As a class, document future areas of research in family caregiving.

Education Plan 8.1 (*continued*)

Knowledge Needed	Attitude	Skills	Undergraduate Behavioral Outcomes	Graduate Behavioral Outcomes	Teaching/Learning Strategies
The need for family care across the health continuum and health care settings.	*Perceive the need to provide care to family members across the health continuum and health care settings.		*Provide care to family members across the health care continuum and health care settings.	*Educate other health professionals regarding the needs of family caregivers across the health care continuum and health care settings.	*Develop a case history that identifies the changing needs of family members across the illness trajectory and health care settings. *Analyze a selected case history to determine unanticipated, or unmet family caregiver needs.

Education Plan 8.1 *(continued)*

Knowledge Needed	Attitude	Skills	Undergraduate Behavioral Outcomes	Graduate Behavioral Outcomes	Teaching/Learning Strategies
Family assessment	*Value the importance of a comprehensive family assessment.	*Assess a family using comprehensive assessment guidelines to identify roles, functions, and expectations of family members.	*Perform a comprehensive family assessment to determine basic family caregiver needs.	*Perform a comprehensive family assessment to determine complex family caregiver needs.	*Select a patient in the clinical setting or role play to conduct a family assessment. Report assessment findings in post-conference or seminar. *Use a movie or video to assess family caregiver needs at the end of life and discuss the assessment in class or seminar, i.e., "Fried Green Tomatoes or "Philadelphia."

Education Plan 8.1 *(continued)*

Knowledge Needed	Attitude	Skills	Undergraduate Behavioral Outcomes	Graduate Behavioral Outcomes	Teaching/Learning Strategies
Goals and Plans of Care	*Value the difference between families' and patients' needs at the end of life. *Recognize students'/nurses' own attitudes, beliefs, and past experience in developing a plan of care.	*Separate families' vs. patients' needs and provider bias in developing a plan of care.	*Develop a separate plan of care for family members.	*Develop an interdisciplinary plan of care for family members.	*Utilizing the family assessment above, identifies family members' goals of care, and develops a plan of care to address their needs.
Interventions: Facilitating Role Development for Family	*Be respectful of diverse feelings and attitudes toward end of life caregiving by family members.	*Guide the family in determining their roles and way of performing them. *Teach family members related tasks.	*Assist family members in the performance of caregiving roles.	*Collaborate with members of the interdisciplinary team to facilitate role identification and performance of family caregivers.	*Analyze a family caregiving situation, where roles are unclear or conflicts exist. Role plays interventions to facilitate role acceptance and development. *Develop a teaching plan based on identified family needs.

REFERENCES

Administration on Aging (1999). Profile of older Americans: 1999. [On-line].Available:http://www.aoa.dhhs.gov/aoa/stats/profile/profile99.html

American Association of Colleges of Nursing (AACN) (1998). Peaceful death: Recommended competencies and curricular guidelines for end-of-life nursing care. [On-line]. Available: http://www.aacn.nche.edu/education/deathfin.htm

Arblaster, G., Brooks, D., Hudson, R., & Petty, M. (1990). Terminally ill patients' expectations of nurses. *Australian Journal of Advanced Nursing, 7*(3), 34–43.

Brock, D. B., & Foley, D. J. (1998). Demography and epidemiology of dying in the U.S. with emphasis on deaths of older persons. In J. K. Harrold & J. Lynn (Eds.), *A good dying: Shaping health care for the last months of life* (pp. 49–60). Binghamton, NY: The Haworth Press, Inc.

Brown, M. A. (1994). Lifting the burden of silence. *American Journal of Nursing, 94*(9), 62–63.

Byock, I. (1997). *Dying well: The prospects for growth at the end of life.* New York: Riverhead Books.

Cutillo-Schmitter, T. A. (1996). Managing ambiguous loss in dementia and terminal illness. *Journal of Gerontological Nursing, 22*(5), 32–39.

Czerwiec, M. (1996). When a loved one is dying: Families talk about nursing care. *American Journal of Nursing, 96*(5), 32–36.

Degner, L. F., Gow, C. M., & Thompson, L. A. (1991). Critical nursing behaviors in care for the dying. *Cancer Nursing, 14*(5), 246–253.

Donaldson, M. S. (1998). The importance of measuring quality of care at the end of life. In J. K. Harrold & J. Lynn (Eds.), *A good dying: Shaping health care for the last months of life* (pp. 117–138). Binghamton, NY: The Haworth Press, Inc.

Emanuel, E. J., Fairclough, L., Slutsman, J., Alpert, H., Baldwin, D., & Emanuel, L. L. (1999). Assistance from family members, friends, paid care givers, and volunteers in the care of terminally ill patients. *New England Journal of Medicine, 341*(13), 956–963.

Field, M. J., & Cassel, C. K. (Eds.) (1997). *Approaching death: Improving care at the end of life.* Washington, DC: National Academy Press. [On-line]. Available: http://www.books.nap.edu/books/0309063728/html/R13HTML

Furukawa, M. M. (1996). Meeting the needs of the dying patient's family. *Critical Care Nursing, 16*(1), 51–57.

Hull, M. M. (1989). Family needs and supportive nursing behaviors during terminal cancer: A review. *Oncology Nursing Forum, 16*(6), 787–792.

Jacobson, A. F. (1998). Can hospital patient's have a "good death"? *American Journal of Nursing, 98*(9), 24.

Johns, J. (1996). Advanced directives and opportunities for nurses. *Image, 28*(2), 149–153.

Lewandowski, W., & Jones, S. L. (1988). The family with cancer: Nursing interventions throughout the course of living with cancer. *Cancer Nursing, 11*(6), 313–321.

Lynn, J. (1993). Travels in the valley of the shadow. In H. Spiro, M. G. McCrea Curnen, E. Peschel, & D. St. James (Eds.), *Empathy and the practice of medicine* (pp. 40–53). New Haven: Yale University Press.

Lynn, J. (1997). Measuring quality of care at the end of life: A statement of principles. *Journal of the American Geriatric Society, 45*(11), 526–527.

McCracken, A. L., & Gerdson, L. (1991). Sharing the legacy: Hospice care principles for terminally ill elders. *Journal of Gerontological Nursing, 17*(12), 4–8.

Meier, D. E., & Morrison, R. S. (1999). Old age and care near the end of life. *Generations, 23*(1), 6–11.

Miles, A. (1993). Caring for the family left behind. *American Journal of Nursing, 93*(12), 34–36.

O'Hara, P., Harper, D., Chartrand, L., & Johnston, S. (1996). Patient death in a long-term care hospital: A study of the effect on nursing staff. *Journal of Gerontological Nursing, 22*(8), 27–35.

Pickett, M. (1993). Cultural awareness in the context of terminal illness. *Cancer Nursing*, *16*(2), 102–106.

Reimer, J. C., Davies, B., & Martens, N. (1991). Palliative care: The nurse's role in helping families through the transition of "fading away." *Cancer Nursing*, *14*(6), 321–327.

Roy, A. (1997). *The god of small things.* New York: Random House Corp, p. 17.

Sherman, D. W. (1998). Reciprocal suffering: The need to improve family caregivers' quality of life through palliative care. *Journal of Palliative Care*, *1*(4), 357–366.

Sherman, D. W. (1999). Training advanced practice palliative care nurses. *Generations*, *23*(1), 87–90.

Smith, B. L., Martin, J. A., & Ventura, S. J. (1999). *Births and deaths: Preliminary data for July 1997–June 1998* (DHHS Publication No. (PHS) 99-1120). Hyattsville, Maryland: National Center for Health Statistics.

The SUPPORT Principle Investigators (1995). A controlled trial to improve care for seriously ill hospitalized patients. *Journal of the American Medical Association*, *274*(20), 1591–1598.

Waltman, N. L. (1990). Attitudes, subjective norms, and behavioral intentions of nurses toward dying patients and their families. *Oncology Nursing Forum*, *17*(3) supplement, 55–62.

Wilson, S. A., & Daley, B. J. (1999). Family perspectives on dying in long-term care settings. *Journal of Gerontological Nursing*, *25*(11), 19–25.

9

Loss, Suffering, Bereavement, and Grief

Mertie L. Potter

AACN Competency

#11: Assist the patient, family, colleagues, and one's self to cope with suffering, grief, loss, and bereavement in end-of-life care.

> ... weeping may endure for a night, but joy cometh in the morning.
> —Psalm 30: 5 KJV

LOSS AND SUFFERING

Two deaths stand out in my mind from my early childhood: my grandmother's and a little bird's. I was 6 years old. My sister and I were doing our nightly routine. My mother came into our room and sat down on my bed. Mom was crying. She had just received a phone call from way far away (my 6-year-old mind's concept of distance) in Canada that my grandmother had died. Although I only had seen my grandmother a few times in my young life, I felt very connected to her. I loved her very much, because I felt cherished by her. I also knew my Mom and Dad loved her greatly, and that Grammie had been sick for a long time. Mom answered our questions and prayed with my sister and me. After my mom and big sister left the room, I remember that I "talked to" Grammie out my bedroom window. I said, "I don't know if you can hear me, but I love you a lot and will miss you." I felt sad and cried. I waited, half-expecting to hear an answer from her. It was even okay when I did not. It was our little "good-bye" with one another. I felt secure that she was in Heaven and that Heaven seemed like a good place for her to be if she were dead and no longer "on earth." I felt at peace.

The other striking memory I have related to death occurred at the same period of time. My sister and I were playing in one of our favorite pine needle–laden spots on our farm. We came upon a dead robin. We were horror-struck to see this beautiful creature lifeless on the ground. We ran and got a dustpan and gently scooted the bird onto it with a little pine branch. We dug a hole, wrapped the bird in a paper towel, respectfully placed it in a shoebox, and laid the bird to rest in its grave. We read Scripture, sang a hymn, and prayed for the bird. I was very grateful I had an older sister who knew how to conduct a proper funeral service for this dear little creature. We were both sad and cried. That also was the first time I remember questioning if animals have souls and where they go when they die.

Loss and suffering are major experiences along life's journey. How one learns to accept, adapt to, and advance through these experiences determines how the individual will move through life itself. Are loss and suffering perceived as natural, functional, growth-promoting, and normal dimensions in and transitions through life or are they perceived as unnatural, dysfunctional, harmful, and abnormal circumstances to be avoided?

LIVING WITH AND DYING FROM TERMINAL ILLNESS

Is living with and dying from a life-threatening illness "normal?" Viorst (1987, p. 3) suggests that "losing, leaving, and letting go" are normal processes that help individuals grow. Loss and suffering, in fact, are inescapable dimensions of life. How an individual transitions through loss and suffering is what remains variable.

When planning the patient's care, it is important for the nurse to note how the patient with a terminal illness and his significant others view loss, suffering, and living with and dying from a terminal illness. It also is important for the nurse to examine her own beliefs related to these life experiences. Developing awareness of each person's perspective is key to formulating successful interventions.

The living-dying interval often is a time of great uncertainty and questioning. Patients may question, "Why? Why me? Why now?" Patients often seek answers to questions related to the meaning of life, the meaning of suffering, the meaning of death, and the meaning of loss. This may be a time of opportunity for the patient to grow and sense a greater wholeness than ever before in spite of an acute awareness of loss, suffering, and grief. Patients living with and dying from a terminal illness need to focus on what they are able to do rather than on what they cannot do.

THE NURSE'S ROLE

Nurses meet individuals across the life span and often, at the crossroads of their suffering and loss. Regardless of the setting, nurses are in a unique position to help individuals and their significant others who may be in physical, emotional, social, and/or spiritual pain related to suffering and loss. The nurse has a broad-based background in providing competent nursing care to individuals across the health/illness continuum. The breadth and depth of each nurse's skills in the specific area of giving care to those living with and dying from terminal illness will be dependent upon numerous factors. Some of these include the nurse's personal beliefs and values, life experiences (professional/non-professional), level of comfort with death and dying, educational level, licensure(s), and interest in this area.

Every nurse must be committed to providing patients, either directly or indirectly, with quality care at the end of life. Critical to helping the nurse fulfill this obligation is a degree of comfort in dealing with death and dying. Knowledge of the process of dying and the degree of comfort in dealing with others who are experiencing death and dying are two important areas in which the advanced practitioner's education, experience, and expertise will provide more depth in discerning the special needs of the patient. Furthermore, the advanced practice nurse's skill level is more appropriate for dealing with high risk and complicated situations.

Communication may be impaired or even unintelligible in the dying patient. In such circumstances, the nurse needs to inform the patient that she is attempting to understand. It also is important that the nurse convey understanding of how difficult it must be for the patient not to be able to communicate and that she will do her best to try to meet his needs.

Each patient must be allowed to live with and die from his terminal illness in his own way. The patient may need help in expressing what "his way" is. Quality of life issues that are important to dying patients are more apt to be peace of mind, comfort, and spiritual understanding rather than functional ability and psychological well-being (Stewart, Teno, Patrick, & Lynn, 1999).

Fostering patterns that are health-promoting and positive for individuals is the ideal in nursing care. Unhealthy patterns need to be identified, as well. Furthermore, patterns usually are established early in life.

EXPERIENCE OF LOSS AND SUFFERING ACROSS THE LIFE SPAN

At birth, an infant is thrust or pulled into his/her new environment through expulsion and separation from the mother's womb. S/he has no control over this experience. A fairly traumatic transition takes place; they no longer find themselves in the safe and warm environment that has nourished and protected them during this critical developmental stage. The infant now has to adjust to a new "home." This new environment includes the experiences of suffering and loss.

Nearing the sixth month, the infant usually develops an acute awareness of separation from the mother or mother-figure. This state is referred to as separation-anxiety. This keen awareness of loss may initiate a rudimentary development of death awareness (Backer, Hannon, & Gregg, 1994). This hypothesis is based on Bowlby's (1980) model of attachment between mother and infant and the infant's experience of separation from the mother. As the individual continues to develop, suffering and loss continue to occur. Generally, this occurrence causes the individual to move from a dependent state to an interdependent state and then to an independent state. In some cases, usually due to more loss and suffering, the individual may return to a dependent or interdependent state prior to death. Thus, life often involves a rhythm of change, interfacing with suffering and loss, from the time an individual is born.

Children under the age of 2 usually have a sense of separation but little understanding of the concept of death. For children between 2 and 5 years of age, death is seen as a transient state but not a permanent event. Between 6 and 10 years of age, children begin to grasp the reality of death (McIntier, 1995). Adolescents conceptualize death in a way similar to adults; namely, they are mortal and will eventually die. As the adolescent comes to terms with his individuality and increasing independence, he becomes more aware of his own mortality. Although death is considered as a future event to adolescents and young adults, death anxiety is more evident than at earlier ages. Middle-aged adults and older adults are more aware and accepting of death. However, no assumptions can be made concerning any age group. The above are generalizations. Each individual's response to death is unique (Rando, 1984) (see Table 9.1).

THEORETICAL UNDERPINNINGS AND THEORIES ON DEATH AND DYING

As reviewed below, Freud (1957), Lindemann (1944), Engel (1964), Glasser and Strauss (1965), and Kubler-Ross (1969) developed classical work related

TABLE 9.1   Developmental Views of Death

Age	Stage of development	Task/Area of resolution
Birth–2 years	Infancy	Sense of separation; no concept of death
2–5 years	Early childhood	Death is transient, not permanent state
6–10 years	Late childhood	Beginning awareness of the reality of death
13–25 years	Adolescence—Young adulthood	Similar to adult view—realization of mortality and eventual death; death anxiety more evident; death perceived as a future event
26–65 years	Middle-aged and older adults	More aware and accepting of death

(Adapted from McIntier, 1995 and Rando, 1984)

to dying and death. Pattison (1977), Bowlby (1980), Worden (1991), and Rando (1984) broadened knowledge in the field with their work. More recent writings by Corr (1992), Buckman (1993), Evans (1994), Copp (1997), and Mallinson (1999) have challenged, as well as added to, previous theoretical information. New information relevant to theories on death and dying is expanding rapidly. Contemporary research on death and dying views the time frame for grief resolution in a less restrictive way than earlier writings. Although different in some ways, most of the authors demonstrate a similar thread and core knowledge related to grief work that is helpful to both the beginning clinician and the advanced practitioner.

Freud (1957) brought the concept of grief work to the forefront after examining his personal feelings and societal observations following the mass losses brought about by World War I. Freud saw grief as a necessary process to assist an individual in adapting to loss. He also felt an individual needed to free him/herself from attachment to the "lost object."

Lindemann (1944) studied bereavement in individuals who were: 1) survivors of the Coconut Grove Hotel fire in Boston (as well as their close relatives); 2) patients who lost a relative while in treatment; 3) relatives of members of the service; and 4) relatives of patients who died while in the hospital. He determined that common physical symptoms, affective symptoms, behavioral manifestations, and physiological changes accompanied each grief experience. Lindemann also first alluded to anticipatory grief in relation to women anticipating the potential death of significant males in their lives during World War II.

Engel (1964) cited three stages through which one progresses in uncomplicated bereavement: 1) shock and disbelief; 2) developing awareness; and 3) restitution and recovery. Engel pointed out that denial predominates initially and helps prevent the individual from being totally overwhelmed. During the second stage, the individual may express guilt and cry. Finally, thoughts and memories of the deceased are discussed and behaviors of the deceased may be displayed by the bereaved.

Glasser and Strauss (1965) examined different contexts related to caregivers and patients in relation to knowledge about the patient's dying. They suggested that there are four awareness levels of dying: closed awareness, suspicion awareness, mutual pretense awareness, and open awareness. In the first context, closed awareness, caregivers are aware that the patient is dying but keep that information from the patient. In suspicion awareness, the caregivers know that the patient is dying, but the patient only suspects he is dying. The patient is ambivalent about wanting to know and not wanting to know that he is dying. In the mutual pretense context, both the caregiver and the patient act as though they do not know the patient is dying, but both know that he is. Within the context of open awareness, there is a sharing of knowledge, information, and communication about the patient's dying between the caregiver and the patient (Glasser & Strauss, 1965; Rando, 1984).

Kubler-Ross (1969) studied over 200 patients diagnosed with terminal cancer. Her work was pivotal in theorizing that individuals move through (not necessarily sequentially) five phases when trying to cope with pending death. These five stages are: denial and isolation, anger, bargaining, depression, and acceptance. In the denial and isolation phase, an individual experiences shock and disbelief. A comment such as, "I don't believe this is happening," may be made during the anger phase, the individual questions, "Why me?" Anger is often displaced. The individual may try to rationalize during the bargaining phase by pleading or regretting, "Yes, me, but . . ." Bargaining is an attempt to postpone death and extend life. It involves self-imposed deadlines. During the depression phase, the individual may express feelings of guilt or sadness, such as, "Yes, this is happening to me." There often is an awareness of great loss for the patient. In the acceptance stage, the struggle is over. The individual has come to accept his imminent death and is ready to let go and move on. A comment such as, "My time is close; it's all right now" may be made.

Pattison (1977) was the first to focus on a model that examined the "living-dying interval." Pattison defined that interval as existing between knowing that death was imminent and the actual point of death. He incorporates three clinical phases within the living-dying interval: acute crisis phase, chronic living-dying phase, and the terminal phase. During the acute crisis phase, the patient is confronted with the knowledge that a process beyond his control influences his death. The chronic living-dying phase involves an acute awareness of living and dying simultaneously. Lastly, the terminal phase commences when the patient starts withdrawing from the outside world. There is an internal awareness that he must conserve his energies for himself.

Bowlby (1980) described four phases of bereavement: 1) numbness; 2) yearning and searching; 3) disorganization and despair; and 4) reorganization. His theory is based on an attachment model in which the child must separate from the mother. The process includes: 1) shock and disbelief related to the loss (numbness); 2) protest involving an attempt to regain the lost object (yearning and searching); 3) an intense sense of despair in which the individual tries to regain the lost object (disorganization and despair); and 4) completion of the mourning when the individual stops searching and develops new relationships (reorganization) (Evans, 1994).

Worden (1991) refers to four tasks of mourning: 1) accepting the reality of the loss; 2) experiencing the pain of grief; 3) adjusting to an environment in which the deceased is not there; and 4) emotionally relocating the deceased and moving on with life. Mourning may become complicated, dysfunctional, or unresolved if the natural grieving process is delayed, obstructed, or chronic (Bateman, Broderick, Gleason, et al., 1992).

Rando (1984) cites six processes of mourning or grief work: 1) recognizing the loss; 2) reacting to the separation; 3) recollecting and re-experiencing the deceased and the relationship in a realistic way; 4) relinquishing old attachments to the deceased and the assumptive world; 5) readjusting to move adaptively in the new world without forgetting the old; and 6) reinvesting. Rando (1984) considers that complicated grief may exist if there is compromise, distortion, or failure of one or more of the six "R" processes occurring after consideration of the amount of time since death.

As mentioned, Corr (1992), Buckman (1993), and Copp (1997) developed more contemporary theories. Corr (1992) expanded the theoretical premise of task work postulated by Pattison (1977) and Kalish (1979) to include four major areas of task work in coping with dying, specifically physical, psychological, social, and spiritual loss. Addressing physical tasks involves meeting bodily needs satisfactorily and minimizing the individual's physical distress. Working through psychological tasks maximizes the individual's psychological security, autonomy, and richness of living. In order to meet social tasks, interpersonal attachments of significance must be sustained and enhanced, as well as assisting the individual to explore social implications of dying. In addition, spiritual task work involves determining and affirming sources of spiritual energy that, in turn, stimulate hope.

Buckman (1993) promoted the concept that grief is more characteristic of the individual than of an individual's progression through particular grief stages. The second major point made by Buckman is that an individual's movement during the grieving process is dependent upon resolution of various issues related to emotions rather than changing from one emotion to another, as in Kubler-Ross's model. Additionally, Buckman addressed other responses to dying, such as fear of dying, guilt, hope, despair, and humor (Buckman, 1993).

Copp's (1997) work with dying individuals and the nurses caring for them examined two additional dimensions which seem to occur within the dying individual: readiness to die and a body-person split. Copp observed many direct and nondirect actions between patients and nurses: protecting and letting go, watching and waiting, and holding on and letting go. Copp further noted a distinct reference by nurses and patients to the body as separate from the self in relation to patients who were nearing death. A dying individual's personal acceptance of imminent death and physical condition determined his/her readiness to die. The states of readiness included: 1) person ready, body not ready; 2) person ready, body ready; 3) person not ready, body ready; and 4) person not ready, body not ready). A major thrust of Copp's (1998) work is that the dying experience impacts everyone who is involved with the dying patient.

DIMENSIONS OF LOSS, SUFFERING, GRIEF, AND BEREAVEMENT

DEFINITIONS

Loss

Loss is defined as "the condition of being deprived of someone or something that one has had" (*The American Heritage Dictionary*, 1992, p. 1063). Losses can be actual, potential, physical, or symbolic. Loss related to health, function, roles, relationships, and life itself is the central focus of this book. Losses other than the death of the loved one are referred to as secondary losses (Rando, 1984).

Mitchell and Anderson (1983) describe six types of loss: 1) materialistic, 2) relational, 3) intra-psychic, 4) functional, 5) role, and 6) systemic. Material loss involves separation from a physical object or surroundings. In relationship loss, an individual no longer has the ability to relate to another individual. Intra-psychic loss impacts an individual's self-image through loss of what might have been, changed perceptions, lost emotions (i.e., faith, hope, or courage), or emotions that result when a major task has been completed successfully. Functional loss occurs through bodily decline or deterioration in illness or aging. Role loss results when an individual changes or loses (e.g., healthy person to terminally ill person) a customary role or acquires a new role (e.g., patient). Systemic loss involves the loss of contact with customary behaviors or functions within a system, such as absence from a usual work environment or home environment.

Loss can be primary or secondary. Primary loss refers to the initial loss (whether of health for the patient or possibly loss of the patient through death for the significant others). Secondary losses stem from the initial loss. For example, the patient as a result of his diagnosis with a terminal illness may also experience secondary losses of roles, job, income, etcetera. Significant others may experience secondary losses of roles, income, their own health, etcetera.

Suffering

Suffering is defined as "the condition of tolerating or enduring evil, injury, pain, or death or the source of pain or distress" (*The American Heritage Dictionary*, 1992, p. 1995). Suffering impacts a patient's body, mind, and spirit. Cassell (1991, p. 33) defines suffering as "the state of severe distress associated with events that threaten the intactness of person." Cassell recognizes the importance of human suffering within any of the human dimensions, such as body, mind, and spirit. He also advocates asking individuals about the presence or absence of suffering since suffering is a very individualized experience and may result from treatment, as well as from the disease process or a number of other events.

According to Georgesen and Dungan (1996), the presence of pain compounds suffering and results in spiritual distress. Pain is a frequent companion of terminal illness. Suffering can be present with or without the presence of pain. Suffering, however, cannot be "treated" or "managed" like pain. Suffering is a personal experience. Framing suffering in a religious, philosophical, or personally meaningful perspective can help patients endure it better (Rando, 1984).

Suffering can be acute or chronic. Acute suffering occurs when the patient is in crisis and confronted with an immediate loss. Chronic suffering results from the longer-term realization and impact of a loss that carries a great deal of significance for and meaning to the patient. The patient with a terminal illness may experience only one type of suffering, both types at different times, or both simultaneously. Intervention involves trying to understand the patient's suffering and trying to help the patient cope effectively with his suffering. Key to helping the suffering patient is attempting to understand the meaning of their suffering and attempting to comfort and sustain them through it.

Similar to chronic suffering is the middle-range nursing theory of chronic sorrow introduced by Eakes, Burke, and Hainsworth (1998). Chronic sorrow is viewed as normal in response to the recurrent experience of ongoing, significant loss that may be actual and/or symbolic. Major concepts within this theory relate to the following: losses, disparity between reality and idealism, trigger events or milestones, and an individual's internal and external means of managing reoccurring grief that accompanies chronic sorrow. One of the key antecedents to chronic sorrow, namely disparity between the individual's current reality and idealized reality, is what differentiates chronic sorrow from chronic suffering. An individual experiencing chronic suffering does not necessarily face disparity with chronic suffering.

Grief

Grief is defined as "deep mental anguish, as that arising from bereavement" (*The American Heritage Dictionary,* 1992, p. 796). Rando (1984) describes grief as a normal reaction to the perception of loss. Grief is generally a transitory, acute state in response to loss with the possibility that the individual's ability to function may be disrupted temporarily. In addition, the individual may be distracted, disoriented, and/or distressed (Mallinson, 1999). Feelings that may accompany grief include anger, shame, helplessness, sadness, guilt, despair, relief, peacefulness, calm, and release (McCall, 1999).

Common grief responses are listed (see Figure 9.1). These responses may involve physical, psychological, and/or spiritual responses. The impact of grief can be extensive and pervasive. Anticipatory grief, feelings of grief experienced prior to an expected loss, has been thought to assist individuals in: working through depression related to the upcoming death, rehearsing of the death, attempting to adjust to the consequences of the death, and having an increased concern for the terminally ill (Fulton & Fulton, 1971). Rando (1984) views anticipatory grief as also including allowing for gradual absorption of the reality of the loss, helping resolve unfinished business, changing assumptions about life and identity, and making future plans.

Evans (1994) challenges the belief that anticipatory grief experienced prior to death is the same process as the conventional grief experienced in the post-death period. Evans proposes use of the label "terminal response" to describe the process which occurs between diagnosis of terminal illness and death. Differences noted between pre- and post-death grieving include:

Physical	Psychological	Spiritual/Sociocultural
• Shortness of breath	• Depression	• Spiritual pain and suffering
• Insomnia	• Anxiety	• Spiritual loneliness
• Loss of appetite	• Guilt	• Fear of God, the unknown, and/or the future
• Loss of sleep	• Anger and hostility	• Feelings of failure and guilt
• Energy loss	• Anhedonia	• Feelings of unfairness and anger
• Greater susceptibility to illness	• Self-reproach	• Loss of transcendence
• Sighing	• Low self-esteem	• Hopelessness[1]
• Nervousness and restlessness	• Helplessness and hopelessness	• Search for meaning
• Sensation of something in the throat	• Sense of unreality	• A need for love and hope
• Feelings of emptiness or heaviness[1]	• Suspiciousness	• A sense of forgiveness[2]
• Heart palpitations	• Interpersonal problems	• Participation or lack of participation in formal religious group
• Crying	• Imitation of the deceased's behaviors	• Views related to use of "extraordinary" life-prolonging measures
• Psychomotor retardation	• Idealization of the deceased	• Beliefs related to afterlife
• Decreased libido or hypersexuality	• Ambivalent feelings about the deceased[1]	• Handling of the body after death
• Weight loss[2]		• Rituals performed after death[3]

FIGURE 9.1 Grief responses.

Physical—
   [1]taken from Lindemann (1944)
   [2]taken from Rando (1984)

Psychological—
   [1]taken from Lindemann (1944)

Sociocultural—
   [1]taken from Stuart & Sundeen, 1991, p. 154
   [2]taken from Pritchett & Lucas, 1997, p. 203
   [3]taken from Kazanowski, 1999, p. 176

1) anticipatory grieving ends at the time of death, whereas conventional grieving can go on indefinitely; and 2) anticipatory grieving increases as death draws nearer, but conventional grieving usually diminishes in intensity with time.

Bereavement

Bereavement is defined as the condition of being left "desolate or alone, especially by death" (*The American Heritage Dictionary*, 1992, p. 175). Rando (1984) describes bereavement as the state of having suffered a loss. McCall (1999) describes bereavement as the "overall reaction to the loss of a close relationship" and sees it as a description of various "patterns, phrases, and/or stages that an individual goes through when grieving" (p. 42). Mallinson (1999) depicts bereavement as the long-term process of the survivor's accommodating his life without the loved one.

Mourning, grief, and bereavement often are used interchangeably. Mourning often encompasses a sociocultural dimension and involves customs and rituals that are influenced by sociocultural and religious beliefs and values. Rando (1984, pp. 15–16) differentiates between the three in the following ways: 1) grief is the response to the perception of loss and is a transitional phase in the overall process of mourning; 2) mourning is the intra-psychic processes initiated by loss; and 3) bereavement is the state of having suffered a loss.

SIGNIFICANCE AND MEANING OF THE RELATIONSHIP TO LOSS AND SUFFERING

The intensity of loss for the dying patient and their significant others relates directly to each individual's perceptions of how close the relationship is and how great the loss of this relationship will be. The significance of the relationship impacts how the individual will interpret his loss and the accompanying suffering. The meaning which the patient, significant others, and nurse assign to loss and suffering also will determine how each individual faces the patient's dying and death. Interpretation of loss and suffering is unique to each individual and to each individual's particular circumstances.

Relationships fall into three categories: social, intimate, and therapeutic (Brady, 1997). Social relationships incorporate the everyday contacts individuals have, such as work colleagues and casual friends. Both individuals in this type of relationship are attempting to have their needs met. There is no particular goal within this relationship. Intimate relationships imply commitment by both individuals to one another. Therapeutic relationships involve goal-directed interaction with the purpose of helping one individual obtain an anticipated outcome to meet an identified need and facilitate growth.

The degree of intimacy and involvement within a relationship is not necessarily dependent upon the relationship's being a long-term one versus a short-term one or a blood relationship versus a non-blood relationship. Many factors determine how an individual will view his relationship with another individual. Some of these factors include respect, responsibility, commitment, compatibility, values, biases, beliefs, and time.

The stage of growth and development of the individual with terminal illness influences their ability to cope with the loss, suffering, and grief related to his/her terminal illness. The stage of growth and development of significant others and the nurse also determine their ability to cope with the loss, suffering, grief, and bereavement related to the patient with a terminal illness. In addition, the stages of growth and development for all three groups (patient, significant others, and nurse) significantly impact how each will deal with the other.

Two of the most difficult aspects of a terminal illness are the accompanying uncertainty and unpredictability. These two factors may stress the relationships between the patient, the significant others, and the nurse. For some individuals, not knowing what is going to happen to the patient and when it might happen are difficult and unbearable aspects of coping with the patient's terminal illness.

Some terminal conditions, such as HIV/AIDS, may not be discussed by the patient or significant others due to fear of stigma or repercussions. In such situations, it is imperative the nurse accept, understand, and be ready to assist the patient and significant others in sharing the pain associated with these conditions.

Nurses, patients, and caregivers assigned similar meaning to pain in a study of patients with cancer (Ferrell, Taylor, Sattler, Fowler, & Cheyney, 1993). Although both nurses and patients viewed pain as a challenge, nurses saw the challenge to eliminate pain, whereas, patients saw the challenge to live with the pain in order to obtain vitality. Caregivers greatly empathized with the patient's pain and experienced personal suffering and grief. Grief was triggered by pain, as it represented death to the caregivers.

Furthermore, an individual's view of change itself will help determine how that individual will accept loss and suffering related to his terminal illness. Has the individual's pattern been to welcome and embrace change or resist and fear change? The answer to that question can assist the nurse in implementing care that will help the patient and his significant others to grow through the loss and suffering associated with the patient's terminal illness. Knowledge of change theory can help the advanced nurse facilitate

acceptance of and growth through loss and suffering for the patient, his/
her significant others, and the nurse herself/himself. Knowing the benefits
and risks of change, change strategies, and resistance to change, can help
the nurse maximize the many changes within the patient's life.

ASSESSMENT—WHERE AM I (THE NURSE) ON THE JOURNEY?

In order to be an effective caregiver to the dying patient and his significant
others, the nurse must come to terms with his or her own mortality and
views on dying and death. Death is an inevitable outcome of life for each
individual. The death of a patient with a terminal illness forces the nurse
to acknowledge that a cure cannot always be achieved. Fear related to death
and dying is normal. Likewise, issues related to grief and bereavement during
the death and dying process also are normal and even necessary for healthy
adaptation to the preceding loss and suffering.

In American culture, individuals generally believe that explanations or
solutions for dying always should be given. Furthermore, Americans feel
options to deal with the dying process always should be available (Kazanowski, 1999). This widely held belief impacts the nurse, as well as the patient
and his or her significant others, in relation to high expectations of treatment, care, and even cure or illness.

Nurses are encouraged to maintain their composure when caring for
patients. However, professionalism for the nurse within this context does
not require that the nurse deny emotional engagement with the patient
and significant others during the dying process and bereavement period.
It does require, however, that the nurse's needs be subordinate to the needs
of the patient and significant others. Constructive self-disclosure by the nurse
of feelings may role model to others a healthy process of acknowledging and
resolving the suffering of loss. The nurse may or may not actually cry with
the patient and significant others. If crying occurs, the nurse needs to be
able to direct this situation into a meaningful and positive one for the
patient and/or significant others. Empathy appropriately shared in this
manner may well be described as a "therapeutic tear."

Lewis (1998) describes a strategy used to assist nursing students in working
with patients and significant others who are experiencing loss and grieving.
The learning activity is called "Culture and Loss: A Project of Self-Reflection."
Student nurses are requested to examine how their culture handles loss, to
prepare a creative presentation for a small group of peers on how their
culture responds to loss, and to describe to their class the meaning of their
project and how it connects to their culture. Goals for implementing this

strategy are: 1) identifying personal responses to loss; 2) recognizing differing responses to loss and the influence of individual and cultural factors; and 3) learning skills related to supporting individuals who are grieving.

Spencer (1994) examined what strategies were helpful to nurses in dealing with their own grieving. The most significant strategy noted was the nurse's informal network of peer group support. In addition, the nurses also recommended formal group support and increased grief resolution training. There are numerous other health-promoting strategies to help the nurse cope with caring for dying patients. These include: regular exercise, good nutrition, diversional activities, focus on caring rather than curing, emphasizing the positive dimensions of the nurse's role, and recalling positive experiences with families (Pritchett & Lucas, 1997).

Advances in technology have prolonged dying and death in our culture. As a result, advance directives have taken on greater significance in relation to end-of-life care. Studies have indicated that patients who have prepared advance directives select palliative care more frequently, are more accepting of death, and have less expensive care and less aggressive treatment (Danis, 1998).

There are incongruencies between the ideal and reality in end-of-life care. First, clinicians are expected to be able to predict the expected time of death for a terminally ill patient; however, this involves a great deal of uncertainty. Goals of care may need to change quickly as the patient's condition changes or therapeutic trials fail. Second, it is expected that the patient's clinicians know his wishes concerning his dying and death. In reality, organizational factors may impact the patient's care more than the patient's wishes during the end-of-life process. Third, it is thought that the patient's care is well-coordinated. Often this is not the case since some intensive care facilities are staffed with their own primary care providers who may not know the patient admitted with a terminal illness. Therefore, it is important for the nurse to work closely with the patient and his or her significant others concerning the patient's priorities and wishes. Finally, the measurement of goals and outcomes may not be congruent. Measures of care for dying patients usually focus upon frequency of do not resuscitate orders and lengths of time a patient spends on life support or in a coma. It may be more important to patients and significant others to examine issues related to pain management and satisfaction with care (Danis, 1998).

Confronting death with a terminal illness is difficult, painful, and complex. Nurses need to be strong advocates for satisfactory pain management. Keeping abreast of the patient's treatment wishes (which may change during the dying process) and coordinating care between facilities and providers also are important.

PERSONAL EXPERIENCES WITH DEATH

Personal experiences with dying and death influence how nurses give care to those who are dying and their significant others. For example, examining one's personal experiences can help nurses understand their own fears and anxieties related to dying and death. Understanding the meaning and significance of relationships helps put the loss in perspective. Articulating what the nurse feels determines a good or bad death is important when working with individuals who are dying. Exploring individual values and biases can enhance the nurse's competence; this helps the nurse better understand individual's health care attitudes and behaviors (Warren, 1999).

Use the following exercises to help you expand your self-understanding in relation to loss and suffering, dying and death, and grief and bereavement.

SELF-REFLECTIVE QUESTIONS

- What experiences have you had with death? Describe your earliest memory of death. Was anything positive about it? Was anything negative about it? Have you experienced what you would call a "good death?" Have you experienced what you would describe as a "bad death?"
- Can you picture yourself helping someone who is dying? How? What do you have to offer that is special and unique?
- Relate what you believe happens when someone dies. What do you fear about death? What do you fear about your own death?
- Assume you have just received news that you have been diagnosed with a terminal illness. What would be the most difficult things for you to have to give up during this time?
- How do you feel about cultural attitudes or behaviors that may be different from your own?

ASSESSMENT—WHERE IS THE PATIENT ON THE JOURNEY? THE LIFE CYCLE CONTINUUM—ACROSS THE LIFE SPAN ON THE JOURNEY

Living with and dying from a terminal illness can best be understood within the context of a continuum. One generally does not remain on a fixed point along the continuum. Like one's view of health and illness, living with and dying from terminal illness is a dynamic and fluid experience in which the individual moves back and forth across the continuum.

Reactions to dying and death vary across the lifespan. They also are dependent upon physical, psychological, spiritual, and sociocultural factors impacting the individual's sense of wellness. Physiological change can lead to a whole sequelae of loss: function, body image, self-esteem, sexuality, and role competence. The living-dying interval occurs from the time death is acknowledged as imminent to the point of the actual death. A difficult task during this period is continuing to treat the individual as still living and as a person and not just a patient. Tasks that the individual needs to attend to are: arranging his affairs; coping with loss (loved ones and self); attending to future care needs; planning remaining time; confronting loss of self and identity; facing his own death encounter; deciding whether to succumb to or resist the dying process; and struggling with the psychosocial problems of dying. Some of the issues for the individual during this period of time include: treatment choices, remissions and exacerbations, expression of sexuality, financial pressures, employment concerns, struggle for control, and suffering (Rando, 1984).

Depending upon the patient's level of maturity, s/he may be confronted with the meaning of life, relationship with God and others, and the reality of death (Georgesen & Dungan, 1996). In addition, the patient may face losses related to independence, control, work, physical comfort, a sense of normalcy, sexual activity, and usefulness when living with a life-threatening condition (Ferrell et al., 1993).

Once rapport has been developed, the nurse may suggest that the patient and/or his significant others consider attending a support group. Support groups have been found to be particularly helpful for significant others facing traumatic (e.g., loss of a child) or stigmatized (e.g., acquired immuno-deficiency syndrome) deaths, as well as for individuals who themselves are dying (Callanan & Kelley, 1992; Goodkin et al., 1999; Rando, 1984).

INDIVIDUAL NEEDS

During the illness/dying trajectory, the nurse needs to assess the patient's immediate and specific needs. Certain simple pleasures may be more important to the patient than a nurse-perceived need for oxygen. For a peaceful death, a patient may need the comfort and joy that a treat, such as food or music, may represent to him. Asking the patient (or his significant others if he is unable to respond) what the patient's immediate and specific needs are may bring insight as to what intervention is needed to help the patient be more comfortable.

Maintaining some control is especially important for the patient during this time, as they may have had to relinquish control in many areas. Moreover, having control over pain is critical. Patients with a terminal illness and their significant others fear lack of pain control during end-of-life care (Danis, 1998).

Having a sense of order and a sense of closure in personal affairs are important aspects to address with the patient also. Sharing what one needs to say to others, through direct contact (e.g., in person or phone) or indirect contact (e.g., written communication), may help the patient have a more peaceful death. Sensitivity to the patient's leading in this area is critical.

Areas of Assessment

Use the following questions to assess the patient on his journey living with and dying from a terminal illness in relation to loss and suffering, dying and death, and grief and bereavement.

- How do you view your illness?
- What is the meaning of your illness to you?
- What fears or concerns do you have regarding your illness?
- In what ways are you experiencing loss and/or suffering?
- Are there any unresolved issues or business that need to be resolved?
- Do you have any specific fears about dying and death in general? About your own dying and death?
- What concerns do you have for others now and after your death?
- What helps you maintain a sense of hope during difficult times?
- What specific needs do you have at this time?
- In what ways might I be most helpful to you in meeting those needs?

ASSESSMENT—WHERE ARE THE SIGNIFICANT OTHERS ON THE JOURNEY?

Healthy spouses of terminally ill cancer patients were studied (Siegel, Karus, Raveis, Christ, & Mesagno, 1996). Males were found to be more at risk for depressive symptoms than females if they were parents of school-aged children. Part of this could be due to their having less of a social network than females in general, and part may be due to their having to assume additional parenting responsibilities as the result of their spouse's illness and subsequent death. Overall adjustment was better for well spouses and inversely proportionate to the number of children in the household. Work was perceived as both a stressor due to the demands of the job and as a stress buffer due to the potential emotional support, sense of control, and predictability it may provide for the significant other. Elderly males have been found to be at increased risk for suicide after the death of a spouse (McCall, 1999).

Sherman (1998) refers to the reciprocal suffering inherent in being a family member or significant other of a patient diagnosed with a terminal illness. This results from the expectations and responsibilities placed upon the significant other to care for the patient, the mutual experience of intensified needs brought about by the patient's illness, and the often rapidly changing needs for both the patient and the significant other. Quality-of-life issues arise for the family members and significant others, as well as for the patient.

Koop and Strang (1997) reviewed a number of studies to determine correlates of greater satisfaction in families of patients with a terminal illness. They found higher satisfaction in families in which there had been psychosocial support from the nurse, fulfillment of basic needs, high frequency of home visits, support at night, connection to other services, visits to the bereaved caregiver, choices in treatments, privacy during hospitalizations, treatment of respiratory symptoms, the presence of professional caregivers (especially if the patient is at home), and participation in a hospice program.

There is interdependence between the patient, their significant others, and the nurse in relation to providing optimal care for the patient with a terminal illness. The nurse can maximize the positive aspects of this interdependence by recognizing and affirming the patient's significant others, incorporating them into the patient's care as desired by the patient, and assisting the significant others in their loss, suffering, and grief related to the patient's dying and death. In addition, the patient's significant others will experience bereavement issues once the patient dies.

How does one know when the patient is ready to die? Four types or stages of death occur, usually in the following order: social death, psychological death, biological death, and physiological death (Sudnow, 1967). Social death marks the narrowing of the patient's world, as he has known it. This is a highly individualized stage that is dependent upon the patient's level of involvement versus detachment in his social world. Psychological death is a death of the patient's personality. Relationships change. The patient withdraws and distances himself from others. Terminal illness places demands that result in the patient's becoming regressed and dependent. Biological death involves the loss of consciousness and awareness on a self-sustaining basis; the patient may be on life-supports at this point. Finally, physiological death occurs. All vital organs cease to function (Rando, 1984). At this point, a nurse or physician (depending upon state law) pronounces death. The moment of finality has arrived. Life as the patient and his significant others knew it for him has ceased.

RELATIONSHIPS

Support from significant others can aid in decision making and acceptance of death for a patient with a terminal illness. Patients and their significant others may determine together if they want to pursue life-sustaining procedures or to forgo them in light of the uncertainty and potential trauma which surround the situation. Close communication with the nurse during end-of-life care is essential since the needs of the patient and care planned for him are apt to change rapidly. Patients and their significant others may change their minds concerning treatments depending upon the patient's level of consciousness, the patient's pain level, both the patient's and significant others' fear levels, additional troublesome symptomatology for the patient, failure of therapeutic trials, and the level of support and contact between the patient and his significant others (Danis, 1998).

Significant others who care for a terminally ill patient are faced with increased feelings of powerlessness, anger, and grief when the patient's pain is unrelieved (Ferrell et al., 1993). Danis (1998) found that families of deceased patients indicate that more attention should be given to analgesia and communication in end-of-life care. The significant others may or may not provide direct care to the patient. They may have other resources, hired or voluntary, to provide caregiving to the patient. If the significant others are providing care, they will be at risk for burnout or fatigue. A proactive approach in order to prevent this should be in place in the patient's care plan.

AREAS OF ASSESSMENT

- Determine with significant others what they perceive as the patient's needs.
- Provide education in pain assessment and pain management strategies.
- Assess how the significant others feel they are doing and what degree of loss and suffering they currently are experiencing.
- What types of secondary losses are being experienced or anticipated as a result of the primary loss (i.e., anticipatory death or actual death of the patient)?
- Determine the level of emotional support needed.
- Ascertain if spiritual support is desired.
- Assure significant others that they are not an imposition to professionals who also are providing care for the patient.
- Identify available resources to help significant others' care for the patient.

- Encourage significant others to grieve in whatever ways are best for them.

NORMAL GRIEF

Grief is a normal response to loss. Grief may become manifest in feelings, physical sensations, cognition, and/or behaviors (see Figure 9.1). Psychological, sociocultural, and physical factors influence the grief reaction. The nurse needs to assess which factors are influencing the significant others. Rando (1984, pp. 43–57) addresses these influences as follows:

Psychological factors—

- Significance of the loss.
- Attachment level.
- Family role of the deceased.
- Individual coping behaviors, such as avoidance, distraction, preoccupation, impulsivity, rationalization, intellectualization, prayer, and connection with others.
- Intelligence and maturity levels.
- Previous experience with death and loss.
- Conditioned sex-roles.
- Age of the individual grieving.
- Age and characteristics of the deceased.

  - The death of a parent represents loss of the past.
  - The death of a spouse represents loss of the present.
  - The death of a child represents loss of the future. The death of a child may be the most difficult death to handle.

- Unattended business between the griever and the deceased.
- Perception of fulfilled life for deceased.
- Circumstances related to death including location, type, reason, and preparedness.
- Timing of the death. (Is the death psychologically acceptable?)
- Perception of death's prevention.
- Sudden or anticipated death.
- Chronic versus acute illness.
- Impact of anticipatory grief on the relationship with the dying patient.
- Impact of secondary losses.
- Additional stresses or crises.

Social factors—

- Level, acceptance, timing, and duration of support.
- Religious, sociocultural, ethnic, and philosophical backgrounds.
- Bereaved's educational, economic, and occupational status.
- Positive or negative funeral rituals.

Physiological factors—

- Positive and negative impact of medications.
- Need for nutrition, sleep and rest, exercise, and physical health.

CHILD'S EXPERIENCE OF LOSS

The death of a parent impacts a child greatly. Family life and daily routine are disrupted permanently. A child may have a depressed mood, cry, be sad or irritable, withdraw, or have sleep disturbances during the first 4 months after the loss of a parent. The child's reaction may be impacted by: individual personality factors, sociocultural factors, the child's age, child's history, child's religious beliefs, family dynamics, family's socioeconomic status, sex of the child and the remaining parent, additional stress in the child's life, parental substitutes, nature of the death, and how the child was notified (Geis, Whittlesey, McDonald, Smith, & Pfefferbaum, 1998).

If the child loses a sibling, other issues, such as, guilt, ambivalence, denial, increased vulnerability, and fear for his own well-being may arise. Parental response to the surviving siblings helps determine the child's adjustment. Similar responses may occur for adolescents with possible reframing of the adolescent's self-concept, self-identity, and family role (Geis et al., 1998). Tasks that occur for all siblings of a deceased child, regardless of age, include: grieving the deceased sibling, coping with family changes, realigning relationships, and attempting to understand the meaning of the tragedy within the family (Kiser, Ostoja, & Pruitt, 1998).

AREAS OF ASSESSMENT

- How is the child functioning socially according to his/her developmental level? What is the child's involvement in relationships, recreation, and routines?
- Is the child exhibiting any changed behaviors?

- What is the child's predominant mood (sad, withdrawn, hyperactive, angry?)
- How does the child express his/her suffering or "pain" related to the loss?
- What does the child feel might help make the "pain" better (besides the return of the lost loved one)?

FAMILY CAREGIVING—PARENTAL EXPERIENCE OF LOSS

Living with dying can tax a patient and his significant others economically, as well as physically, spiritually, and psychologically. Often the patient or his significant others lose work time due to the patient's care requirements. Additional expenses may arise with treatments, hospitalizations, or other hidden expenses, such as transportation, childcare, out of home food purchases, lodging, etcetera. Dying patients often experience much stress because of the financial burdens that fall upon his/her significant others (Rando, 1984). If the nurse feels unprepared to counsel the patient and his significant others in this area, it is imperative that s/he refer them to someone who can.

The loss of a child often is devastating to the parents and to the family. It is an unexpected and unacceptable reversal of roles. Parents feel responsible for their child's health, well-being, and safety. Parents usually do not expect their child to die. Grief related to the loss of a child is apt to be severe and complicated. Anniversary events and developmental milestones for the deceased child reopen the grief experience throughout the parents' lifetime (Kiser et al., 1998). Acknowledging that their lives have changed forever is part of the grief resolution that takes place for parents; however, recovery from the death of a child is a lifelong process (Geis et al., 1998). For the single parent, aloneness may be magnified (Backer et al., 1994).

In the case of a newborn with a serious condition, there is accompanying parental blame and guilt for the infant's condition. Parents must grieve the healthy, "normal" child that they lost in addition to the anticipated death of the infant.

AREAS OF ASSESSMENT

- How has your loved one's illness impacted your life?
- In what ways will you remember your child who died?
- What is the most significant type of suffering you are experiencing right now?

• What are your specific needs at this time and how can I help you meet them?

RISK FACTORS FOR COMPLICATED GRIEF

Predicting bereavement outcomes is difficult since the subjects are considered to be a vulnerable study population. A balance between the need for protection and the benefits of participation must be attained. Studies increasingly suggest that the greatest predictor of well-being during bereavement is prior well-being (Koop & Strang, 1997).

Although each individual's grieving is unique, the bereavement process may be functional or dysfunctional, adaptive or maladaptive. The time for grief resolution has varied from peaks at 4 months to as long as 3 years (Lev & McCorkle, 1998). Prolonged reactions occur in approximately 15% of the bereaved. These prolonged reactions range from exaggerated normal reactions to abnormal grief reactions.

Backer et al. (1994) describes three basic types of complicated grief reactions: 1) delayed, 2) inhibited, and 3) chronic grief. In delayed grief, the grief is triggered by the loss of someone or something else. There is minimal impact in this situation. For example, someone whose father has recently died may experience delayed grief related to the death of her mother 10 years prior to the father's death. The individual has never experienced full grief for the death of her mother until the death of her father. His death triggers the deeply felt but unexpressed loss of her mother.

Inhibited grief occurs when an individual never grieves. It also may occur if the individual feels great distress related to a lost relationship. This type of grief becomes complicated if another condition develops related to the unfelt grief.

Lastly, chronic grief exists when the grieving is unending, and the intense yearning for the lost relationship continues. A cause for this type of grief could be unspeakable deaths, such as those due to AIDS or suicide. Rando (1984) includes absent grief, conflicted grief, unanticipated grief, and abbreviated grief in his list of complicated grief types. A study reported in 1997 (Prigerson et al.) identifies grief involving trauma and separation as traumatic grief and indicates that psychiatric sequelae, such as traumatic grief, puts bereaved individuals at risk for complicated grief.

There are a number of individuals at risk for complicated grief after the death of an individual with a terminal illness. These include spouses; parents; those experiencing the loss of loved ones through unspeakable deaths; and those with a psychiatric history. Male spouses are more at risk than female spouses due to their more limited social networks. Single parents are at higher risk due to less support. Depression is the psychiatric condition causing the highest risk for complicated grief (Kurtz, Kurtz, Given, & Given, 1997).

Work done by Pennebaker, Mayne, and Francis (1997) indicates that language usage can help to positively impact bereavement outcomes. Encouraging individuals to talk about traumatic events forces a disorganized event and emotions to become more organized, coherent, and insightful. Over time, the use of insight and causation words in relation to the event and its accompanying emotions helps cognitively reframe the experience that results in more adaptive outcomes.

Frank, Prigerson, Shear, and Reynolds (1997) postulate that individuals experiencing elongated periods of distress (for several months) and exhibiting criteria for major depressive episodes are undergoing traumatic grief reactions. They advocate treatment interventions that involve re-experiencing the moment of death, saying good-bye to the deceased while still retaining special memories of him, and gradually being exposed to situations that the bereaved has avoided since the deceased's death. The outcome of this traumatic grief treatment has been reduced subjective distress. They do not advocate for pathologizing or treating brief periods of bereavement-related distress.

A number of factors were examined in a study attempting to predict depressive symptomatology in the post-bereavement period (Kurtz et al., 1997). Pre-bereavement depressive symptomatology scores, levels of support from friends, and caregiver optimism, predicted post-bereavement depressive symptomatology best. The link between pre-bereavement and post-bereavement depressive symptomatology scores was anticipated. The role of optimism is important for nurses to capitalize upon and strengthen when working with significant others. The connection between high social support in the pre-bereavement period from friends and post-bereavement depressive symptomatology was strong. This phenomenon could be caused by altered or lost relationships due to the dying and death of the spouse. Possibly friends experience a social death before the physical death of the bereaved's spouse.

Poor bereavement outcomes are apt to occur if the death is unexpected, untimely, or traumatic for the bereaved. Moreover, if the significant other had an ambivalent or dependent relationship with the deceased, perceives their social networks as unsupportive, and is experiencing concurrent loss, maladaptive grieving may occur. Family coping styles that negatively impact outcomes are: 1) hostile (high conflict, low cohesiveness, and poor expressiveness); 2) sullen (limited but less in comparison with the hostile group); and 3) intermediate (intermediate cohesiveness and low control and achievement orientation). Additional correlates for poor outcome include use of medications or alcohol, concern for self, level of contentment, and not viewing the deceased's body. Positive bereavement outcomes are more apt to occur in families who are supportive (high cohesion) and resolve conflict well (Kissane, Bloch, & McKenzie, 1997).

In more dysfunctional grieving situations, the advanced nurse practitioner must treat symptoms of pathological grief. Three major symptom categories of pathological grief would be intrusion, denial, and dysfunctional adaptation (Horowitz, Bonanno, & Holen, 1993). Spending long periods of time idealizing the memory of the deceased is a sign of an intrusive thought process. Living as if the deceased were still alive for more than 6 months is evidence of denial. Minimal dysfunction is evidenced in having difficulty making decisions, whereas major dysfunction is evidenced in more severe impairments. Such severe dysfunctional parameters would involve: extreme fatigue or somatic symptoms that last more than 1 month; inability to resume work, other interests, routines, and other responsibilities after more than 1 month; and reluctance to develop new relationships after 13 months of grieving (Lev & McCorkle, 1998, p. 147).

Use the following exercises to help you expand your understanding of helping the patient's significant others on their journey with the patient's living with and dying with a terminal illness in relation to suffering and loss, death and dying, and grief and bereavement:

Exercise I—Discuss how you might feel and what you might do if you were the nurse to walk into a patient's room just as he has died and his family and/or significant others are there.

Exercise II—A family member who has been estranged from the dying patient on your floor is in the room as you come in to check on the patient who is unconscious. The family member says, "He wasn't a very good father. He abused my sister and me. I'll be glad when he's dead." How would you respond to this family member?

Exercise III—You are the clinical nurse specialist heading up the first meeting of nursing staff since a patient on your floor died from terminal CA. What would be your objectives for the meeting?

CONTEXT OF CAREGIVING AND RELATED INTERVENTIONS

Working with the patient who is living with and dying from a terminal illness and his significant others requires compassion, skill, energy, sensitivity, and patience. Compassion promotes a positive connection between the nurse and the patient and his significant others. Skill gives the nurse credibility in working with them. Energy, often in the form of providing hope for the moment, moves the patient and his significant others forward when they feel like giving up. Sensitivity enhances understanding and rapport in the relationships. Patience allows each individual the time needed to face and plan for an uncertain and unpredictable future.

The nurse attempts to help meet the needs of the patient and his significant others. Addressing immediate needs may take on greater significance with the patient experiencing a terminal illness than addressing either short-term or long-term needs. Values, control issues, and goals of both the patient and his significant others need to be taken into consideration, addressed directly, and handled tactfully and sensitively.

The nurse has a unique window into the patient's circumstances. Depending upon the setting, nurses may provide 24-hour care. Even if nursing coverage is not for 24 direct-care hours, nursing care may be accessible for that period of time. Generally, it is the nurse who gets the most consistent, current, and constant view of what is actually happening with the patient and his significant others. With few exceptions, the nurse usually is the most readily available and informed team player to help coordinate the patient's care.

Developing goals with the patient and his significant others can provide some stability and security during this time. It can empower the patient and their significant others to take an active role in planning the patient's remaining earthbound journey, uncertain and unpredictable as it may be. Furthermore, it helps set the stage for the continuing connection between the nurse and the patient's significant others during their bereavement after the patient's death.

NURSE

Nurses care for themselves by seeking support from colleagues, assuring time for themselves by maintaining healthy boundaries with the patient and significant others, and tending to their own physical, emotional, sociocultural, and spiritual needs. After a patient's death, nurses may meet grieving needs by attending the memorial service for the deceased patient if this is deemed acceptable by the nurse's employing agency policy and the deceased patient's significant others. Sending a sympathy card to significant others, doing follow-up bereavement work with significant others, and reminiscing about the deceased patient with empathic colleagues usually help nurses in dealing with their own grief.

NURSING INTERVENTIONS

Nurses are accustomed to action-oriented, "doing for" interventions with curative results. Intervening with the patient with a terminal illness, however, the nurse's role may be less action-oriented. Nurses may need to adapt to interventions that are focused more on "being with" the patient and "caring" instead of "doing for" the patient and "curing" (Rando, 1984).

Given that so many American deaths occur in hospitals, the nurse is most apt to be with the patient and significant others at the exact time of death. Becoming comfortable with viewing the dying and death process, touching the deceased's body, talking with significant others about the death and their feelings, and dealing with the patient's death among staff are important aspects with which the nurse will be confronted.

The nurse's relationship with the patient will be critical in determining how she handles her grieving and bereavement in relation to the patient's dying and death. Was it a short-term nurse-patient relationship or did the nurse have a professional relationship with the patient for an extended period of time? In addition, how comfortable does the nurse feel sharing feelings, and how appropriate is it to share feelings with the patient? The nurse needs to answer for herself what the goal of sharing her feelings is and what the expected outcome of doing so is before proceeding.

Level of intervention by the nurse will be based on professional skills, theoretical background, and clinical setting. The nurse will develop therapeutic relationships, ensure the patient's physical comfort to maintain function, explore the meaning of physical suffering and loss with the patient and significant others, reframe the patient's limitations to identify areas of value that will enhance the patient's quality of life, encourage patient and significant others' attendance at support groups, and identify and maximize prior coping skills of the patient and his significant others. Advanced nurses will offer more intensive and extensive interventions for grieving and bereavement needs, be involved in more complex research studies, and be more directly involved with intensive treatment interventions. For example, the advanced practice nurse may prescribe various medications, offer individual or family counseling, lead a bereavement group, or conduct research on quality of life and quality of dying outcome measures.

PATIENT

Each patient who is living with and dying from a terminal illness is unique. His/her experiences living with and dying from his/her terminal illness also are unique. A critical factor in promoting good nursing care of this patient and his/her significant others is affirming this uniqueness. Affirming the individual's growth and wholeness during this difficult living-dying interval is critical (Georgesen & Dungan, 1996). Empowering the patient to integrate the living-dying experience and optimize his/her quality of life will further affirm the patient.

The patient is affirmed when the nurse acknowledges his level of acceptance of dying and death. The patient's acceptance or denial may seem selective at times. In reality, varying levels of acceptance or denial may serve an adaptive function in which only specific aspects of dying are tolerable at a given point in time. The patient is aided when the nurse accepts and supports his coping in this way to deal with the extensive and intensive challenges during the living-dying interval (Kastenbaum, 1997).

Medical science has limitations, and patients often feel dehumanized during some medical procedures. In addition to addressing comfort needs, patients need assurance that their humanity will be respected and valued. The nursing profession has reawakened to the importance of integrating spiritual care within total patient care. Patients have indicated that their spiritual needs are best met through nurses listening to, talking with, supporting religious practices of, and being with them (O'Neill & Kenny, 1998). If a nurse feels inadequate or uncomfortable assisting dying patients in this area in any way, a pastoral care referral may be indicated. In addition, the patient may desire to have clergy closely involved even if the nurse is comfortable meeting the patient's spiritual needs.

Saying good-bye is painful for the patient with a terminal illness, for his significant others, and for the nurse. Discerning when (timing) and how (tone) to say and facilitate others' saying good-bye takes sensitivity (touch, emotional, and/or physical) and skill (training/technique) on the nurse's part. This intervention can be illustrated as follows:
Discernment of readiness to facilitate good-byes = nurse sensitivity (touch) and skill (training/technique) → when (timing) and how (tone)

An important question to ask when caring for the patient who is dying from and living with a terminal illness is "What type of patient has the disease, rather than what type of disease does the patient have?" (Harris, 1991, p. 111). Respecting and affirming the patient as a unique and valuable human being will help promote wholeness during a time of brokenness. As the individual is faced with his imminent death, he must reorient his life to adapt to this realization and the accompanying losses. Minimizing losses due to isolation, rejection, and loss of control can decrease the individual's suffering (Rando, 1984). Optimizing patient strengths is essential in helping the patient achieve the quality of life he would like to pursue in this living-dying interval.

Chronic sorrow is the "periodic recurrence of permanent, pervasive sadness or other grief related feelings associated with a significant loss" (Eakes et al., 1998, p. 179). Chronic sorrow may be triggered if the individual senses a disparity with norms. For example, he may feel he is different from others. Situations, such as hospitalization, accentuate this discrepancy to the individual. Both patients and significant others may experience chronic sorrow.

Counseling can assist individuals with chronic sorrow by helping the individual anticipate trigger events and reinforce effective internal and external management strategies. Internal strategies would be continuing involvement in interests and activities, having a positive attitude, focusing on one day at a time, and emphasizing the positive aspects in the individual's life. External strategies are those provided by health care professionals and view chronic sorrow as a normal experience for individuals dealing with chronic, life-threatening illness. Interventions found to be helpful by patients and their significant others include: listening, being supportive and reassuring, addressing feelings, and affirming the uniqueness of each patient and significant other (Eakes et al., 1998).

The nurse may advocate for a patient with a terminal illness by employing the following interventions: advancement of grief work, encouraging health-promoting strategies despite a compromised health state, making referrals, meeting with significant others, utilizing cognitive reframing of negative patterns, and engaging the patient in individual or group therapy to work through unresolved situations. The nurse may be asked to work with support staff and significant others to help them accept, support, and/or devise strategies to work with a patient or significant other that have a dysfunctional approach to suffering and loss.

Significant Others

The family of a patient dying from and living with a terminal illness experiences great turmoil and disequilibrium. Often, the illness becomes the focal point of family activity and organization. If the patient is a child and has siblings, the family struggles at maintaining life within the household, as well as preparing for the death of one of its members. The child simultaneously may be growing in many ways while dying in others. Treatment programs and appointments may consume much of the family's energy, possibly for extended periods of time. Helping the family maintain a sense of normalcy and balance throughout this period will be important tasks for the nurse. Keeping the family as involved as possible in the patient's care applies to the patient with a terminal illness of any age (Rando, 1984).

The question of where the patient and his/her significant others would like the anticipated death to occur must be answered. With shortened hospital stays, significant others have been forced to assume extended and at times intensive care responsibilities for the dying patient in addition to their usual role expectations and demands. Helping the patient and his/her significant others decide how to care for him/her and where and when this care will take place becomes an important goal in the patient's care and the care of his/her significant others (Lev & McCorkle, 1998). The patient may wish to die at home, in a hospice setting, in a hospital, or another setting. Assisting the patient and his/her significant others to communicate what they each can handle at different stages of the patient's dying will be critical.

A family's response to the patient's death is as unique as the individuals making up the family constellation. A family may seek or need to be referred for counseling if maladaptive symptoms develop. Family bereavement therapy involves assessing the circumstances related to the family member's death, the role of the deceased in the family before and after death, timing of the death in relation to family member's stage of growth and development, previous and current levels of family functioning, the context of the death, and the meaning assigned by the family to the death (Kiser et al., 1998, p. 97).

However, the nurse must now focus her attention on helping the significant others begin the tasks of bereavement: accepting the reality of the loss, experiencing the pain of grief, adjusting to an environment without the deceased, and reinvesting energy into other relationships (Worden, 1991). Backer et al. (1994, p. 165) have identified guidelines for counseling the bereaved as follows:

1. Help actualize the loss by talking about the loss.
2. Identify and express feelings related to the loss.
3. Help the bereaved in decision making.
4. Facilitate emotional withdrawal and development of new relationships.
5. Provide time to grieve and be cognizant of holidays and anniversary dates.
6. Reassure the bereaved that their behavior is normal and that they are not abnormal because of their feelings.
7. Allow for individual differences in the bereavement process.
8. Provide support.
9. Examine individual defenses and coping styles (be aware of problems with alcohol or other substance abuse).
10. Identify pathological behaviors and refer to treatment.

The length of time for intense grief to be resolved varies from individual to individual. As long as the bereaved's grieving behavior does not interfere significantly with their physiological or psychosocial functioning, it is not considered to be abnormal. In general, intense responses to grief generally subside in about 6–12 months (Rando, 1984). Grieving, however, continues throughout the bereaved's life. The loss, in some cases, may be replaced, but in all cases, it is never recovered.

The living-dying interval comes to an end with the death of the patient. How does one know when grieving ends for the bereaved? Parkes and Weiss (1983) identified 10 major areas for assessment of recovery:

1. Functioning has returned to a level equal to or better than before bereavement.
2. Outstanding problems are being solved.
3. Acceptance of the loss has occurred.
4. Socialization is as effective as before the death.
5. The future is viewed positively and realistically.
6. General health is at pre-bereavement level.
7. Anxiety or depression levels are appropriate.
8. Guilt or anger levels are appropriate.
9. Self-esteem levels are appropriate.
10. Coping with future loss is feasible.

Completion of bereavement varies from individual to individual. For some, total resolution may never occur (Rando, 1984). Through appropriate interventions, the nurse can help the bereaved adapt to their loss in a way that will foster their growth and wholeness as well.

CONCLUSION

Living with and dying from a terminal illness results in many losses—for the patient, his significant others, and for the nurse. The nurse is both a facilitator and participant in this process. The nurse adds objectivity while the patient and significant others resolve the many feelings, issues, and decisions necessitated by the living-dying experience.

This period of time frequently involves suffering in multiple dimensions. The nurse can utilize technical skills to alleviate certain attributes of the suffering, such as the patient's physical pain. When these technical skills are accompanied by the nurse's sensitivity, compassion, and empathy, the patient and significant others are better equipped to face the other attributes of suffering as well. Thus, the nurse, as a caring professional, may contribute meaningfully to the wellness of the patient and his/her significant others through one of life's most challenging and difficult transitions.

Education Plan 9.1   Plan for Achieving Competencies: Loss, Suffering, Bereavement, and Grief

Knowledge Needed	Attitude	Skills	Undergraduate Behavioral Outcomes	Graduate Behavioral Outcomes	Teaching/Learning Strategies
Living with and dying from terminal illness: The nurse's role.	*Express comfort and commitment in caring for individuals who are terminally ill and their families. *Acknowledge personal attitudes regarding dying and death.	*Assure the patient and family that their needs will be met.	*Communicate effectively and compassionately with terminally ill patient and family. *Provide holistic care that addresses the basic needs of the terminally ill patient and family.	*Provide comprehensive care for the terminally ill patient and family, recognizing complex needs.	*Ask students in post-conference or seminar to remember a significant loss they had in their lifetime and identify what were their attitudes towards loss and death and what was most helpful and least helpful to them during the experience.

Education Plan 9.1 *(continued)*

Knowledge Needed	Attitude	Skills	Undergraduate Behavioral Outcomes	Graduate Behavioral Outcomes	Teaching/Learning Strategies
					*Complete a death anxiety questionnaire and determine the score. Discuss possible reasons for their score. *Brainstorm as a class euphemisms on death. Discuss their usage and how they reflect their attitudes towards dying and death.

Education Plan 9.1 *(continued)*

Knowledge Needed	Attitude	Skills	Undergraduate Behavioral Outcomes	Graduate Behavioral Outcomes	Teaching/Learning Strategies
Experience of loss and suffering across the life span.	*Appreciate differences in the interpretation of death across the life span. *Accept diverse responses to loss as normal responses.	*Act in accordance with the developmental age of the individual experiencing loss, bereavement, and grief.	*Provide appropriate care to individuals experiencing loss, bereavement, and grief at various developmental stages.	*Educate others as to differences in the needs of individuals experiencing loss, bereavement, and grief at various developmental ages.	*Interview individuals of different age groups who have experienced a loss. Compare their beliefs regarding death and their responses to loss. Present the findings in a written paper, or in a postconference or seminar presentation.
Theories on death and dying.	*Value theories in developing knowledge regarding dying and death.		*Apply theories about death in providing effective and compassionate care to terminally ill patients and families.	*Evaluate theories about death in the care of terminally ill patients and families.	*Ask students to identify a personal loss and evaluate the experience in light of a given theory regarding dying and death.

Education Plan 9.1 *(continued)*

Knowledge Needed	Attitude	Skills	Undergraduate Behavioral Outcomes	Graduate Behavioral Outcomes	Teaching/Learning Strategies
Dimensions of Loss, Suffering, Bereavement, and Grief: —Definitions —Significance and meaning of the relationship.	*Appreciate the value of social, intimate, and therapeutic relationships in supporting individuals experiencing loss, bereavement, and grief.	*Demonstrate competence in establishing therapeutic relationships with individuals experiencing loss, bereavement, and grief.	*Provide effective and compassionate care for individuals experiencing loss, bereavement, and grief.	*Role model effective and compassionate care for individuals experiencing loss, bereavement, and grief.	*Using a case study, identify the significance and meaning of various relationships within the context of end of life. *Role play the development of a therapeutic relationship with individuals experiencing loss, bereavement, and grief.

Education Plan 9.1 *(continued)*

Knowledge Needed	Attitude	Skills	Undergraduate Behavioral Outcomes	Graduate Behavioral Outcomes	Teaching/Learning Strategies
Assessment of the Nurses' Attitudes and Feelings Towards Loss, Bereavement, and Grief.	*Acknowledge students'/nurses' own attitudes and feelings related to loss, bereavement, and grief.	*Demonstrate constructive self-disclosure of feelings in assisting individuals in acknowledging and resolving loss and grief.	*Utilize the insights gained through personal experiences of loss, bereavement, and grief to offer supportive care to others.	*Assist colleagues in identifying and working toward resolving their own feelings of loss, bereavement, and grief in caring for patients and families at the end of life.	*Conduct a self-reflection exercise in which students/nurses prepare a creative presentation to examine how people in various cultures handle loss and grief. *Assist students to work through their own issues of loss and grief by establishing a peer support group.

Education Plan 9.1 *(continued)*

Knowledge Needed	Attitude	Skills	Undergraduate Behavioral Outcomes	Graduate Behavioral Outcomes	Teaching/Learning Strategies
					*Ask students/nurses what unfinished business they would attempt to complete if they knew they would die within a week. Share responses in a small group setting. *Have students/nurses discuss in small groups what they believe would be a good death and bad death. Have two students report to the larger group to consolidate the findings.

Education Plan 9.1 *(continued)*

Knowledge Needed	Attitude	Skills	Undergraduate Behavioral Outcomes	Graduate Behavioral Outcomes	Teaching/Learning Strategies
					*Ask students to imagine their caring for a dying patient and family and answer the following questions: —What do they fear about death?; —How would they offer care that is special or unique? *Ask students to write down what legacy they would like to leave and why this is important to them.

Education Plan 9.1 *(continued)*

Knowledge Needed	Attitude	Skills	Undergraduate Behavioral Outcomes	Graduate Behavioral Outcomes	Teaching/Learning Strategies
Assessment of Patients and Families Experiencing Life-threatening Illness	*Appreciate the diverse feelings, perceptions, and responses of individuals experiencing loss, bereavement, and grief.	*Perform an assessment related to loss and grief for patients, and families, including children.	*Accurately assess patients' and families' immediate and specific needs related to loss, bereavement, and grief. *Assist patients and families in maintaining control over many areas of their lives as death approaches. *Determine individuals who are at high risk for dysfunctional grieving and the need for appropriate referral.	*Accurately assess patients' and families' immediate and specific needs related to loss, bereavement, and grief in complex caregiving situations.	*Conduct an assessment of a patient and family member in the clinical area who have experienced a loss. Based on the assessment, identify their specific and immediate needs, and indications of those at high risk. Present the assessment findings and diagnoses in post-conference or seminar.

Education Plan 9.1 *(continued)*

Knowledge Needed	Attitude	Skills	Undergraduate Behavioral Outcomes	Graduate Behavioral Outcomes	Teaching/Learning Strategies
Normal Grief Reactions and Related Factors	*Consider the various factors that influence normal grief.	*Perform a loss and grief assessment that evaluates the factors influencing the grief reaction.	*Assist patients and families in recognizing normal responses to grief and the factors that influence the grief reaction.	*Educate health professionals regarding normal grief responses and factors that influence the grief reaction.	*Utilizing a case study, identify the physical, emotional, social, and spiritual factors that influence the grief reaction, and the responses to normal grief for individuals of various developmental ages.

Education Plan 9.1 *(continued)*

Knowledge Needed	Attitude	Skills	Undergraduate Behavioral Outcomes	Graduate Behavioral Outcomes	Teaching/Learning Strategies
					*Distribute three-by-five cards and have students/nurses identify one physical, emotional, social, or spiritual response they have experienced related to loss and grief. Gather the cards as to the physical, emotional, social, or spiritual responses and review the responses, noting the frequency of symptoms.

Education Plan 9.1 *(continued)*

Knowledge Needed	Attitude	Skills	Undergraduate Behavioral Outcomes	Graduate Behavioral Outcomes	Teaching/Learning Strategies
Risk Factors for Complicated Grief	*Judge experiences of loss that place individuals at high risk for complicated grief.		*Identify individuals who are experiencing complicated grief and make appropriate referrals.	*Coordinate interdisciplinary initiatives in caring for individuals at risk for or experiencing complicated grief.	*In post-conference or seminar discuss students'/nurses' responses and reactions to the potential or actual death of their patient in the clinical area. Discuss their behaviors and responses in caring for the deceased and their family.

Knowledge Needed	Attitude	Skills	Undergraduate Behavioral Outcomes	Graduate Behavioral Outcomes	Teaching/Learning Strategies
Context of Caregiving and Related Interventions	*Express sensitivity, energy, compassion, and patience in caring for dying patients and their family. *Affirm the need for nurses' self-care within the context of offering end of life care.	*Demonstrate care that is focused more on "being with" the patient and "caring," instead of "doing for" the patient and "curing."	*Establish a therapeutic relationship in which the physical, emotional, social, and spiritual needs of patients and families at the end of life are addressed. *Empower patients and family experiencing life-threatening illness to work through unresolved issues, participate in health-promoting activities despite compromised health, and decide on goals of care and death-related plans. *Assist families in the tasks of bereavement.	*Provide intensive interventions to address the physical, emotional, social, and spiritual needs of patients and families in complex caregiving situations and for those experiencing complicated grief. *Lead a bereavement group or conduct individualized counseling. *Participate in or conduct research related to the experience of loss, bereavement, and grief.	*Ask students/nurses to think about someone who had died within their family, and discuss their relationship to the person, the type and duration of the illness, positive and negative interactions they had with health care providers, and suggestions for improving care. *Invite a guest speaker to class to discuss their loss experience and those interventions that were helpful or not helpful to them in their bereavement. *Develop a plan of care for an individual experiencing bereavement. Critique the plan in class, post-conference, or seminar.

REFERENCES

Backer, B. A., Hannon, N. R., & Gregg, J. Y. (1994). *To listen, to comfort, to care: Reflections on death and dying.* Albany: Delmar Publications Inc.

Bowlby, J. (1980). *Attachment and loss: Loss, sadness and depression (Vol. III).* New York: Basic Books.

Brady, P. F. (1997). The therapeutic relationship. In B. S. Johnson, *Psychiatric-mental health nursing—adaptation and growth* (4th ed.) (pp. 49–57). New York: Lippincott.

Buckman, R. (1993). Communication in palliative care: A practical guide. In D. Doyle, G. W. C. Hanks, & N. Macdonald (Eds.), *Oxford textbook of palliative medicine* (pp. 47–61). Oxford, England: Oxford Medical Publications.

Callanan, M., & Kelley, P. (1992). *Final gifts.* New York: Poseidon Press.

Cassell, E. (1991). *The nature of suffering and the goals of medicine.* New York: Oxford University.

Copp, G. (1997). Patients' and nurses' constructions of death and dying in a hospice setting. *Journal of Cancer Nursing, 1*(1), 2–13.

Copp, G. (1998). A review of current theories of death and dying. *Journal of Advanced Nursing, 28*(2), 382–390.

Corr, C. A. (1992). A task-based approach to coping with dying. *Omega, 24*(2), 81–94.

Danis, M. (1998). Improving end-of-life care in the intensive care unit: What's to be learned from outcome research? *New Horizons, 6*(1), 110–118.

Eakes, G. G., Burke, M. L., & Hainsworth, M. A. (1998). Middle-range theory of chronic sorrow. *Image: Journal of Nursing Scholarship, 30*(2), 179–184.

Engel, G. L. (1964). Grief and grieving. *American Journal of Nursing, 64,* 93–98.

Evans, A. J. (1994) Anticipatory grief: A theoretical challenge. *Palliative Medicine, 8*(2), 159–165.

Ferrell, B. R., Taylor, E. J., Sattler, G. R., Fowler, M., & Cheyney, B. L. (1993). Searching for the meaning of pain. *Cancer Practice, 1*(3), 185–194.

Frank, E., Prigerson, H. G., Shear, M. K., & Reynolds, C. F. (1997). Phenomenology and treatment of bereavement-related distress in the elderly. *International Clinical Psychopharmacology, 12*(supplement 7), S25–S29.

Freud, Sigmund. (1957). The disillusionment of the war. In J. Strachey (Ed.), *The complete psychological works of Sigmund Freud, Vol. XIV (1914–1916).* London: The Hogarth Press and the Institute of Psychoanalysis.

Fulton, R., & Fulton, J. A. (1971). A psychosocial aspect of terminal care: Anticipatory grief. *Omega, 2,* 91–99.

Geis, H. K., Whittlesey, S. W., McDonald, N. B., Smith, K. L., & Pfefferbaum, B. (1998). Bereavement and loss in childhood. *Child and Adolescent Psychiatric Clinics of North America, 7*(1), 73–85.

Georgesen, J., & Dungan, J. M. (1996). Managing spiritual distress in patients with advanced cancer. *Cancer Nursing, 19*(5), 376–383.

Glasser, B. G., & Strauss, A. L. (1965). *Awareness of dying.* Chicago: Aldine.

Goodkin, K., Blaney, N. T., Feaster, D. J., Baldewicz, T., Burkhalter, J. E., & Leeds, B. (1999). A randomized controlled clinical trial of a bereavement support group intervention in human immunodeficiency virus type I-seropositive and -seronegative homosexual men. *Archives of General Psychiatry, 56*(1), 52–59.

Harris, J. M. (1991). Death and bereavement. *Problems in veterinary medicine, 3*(1), 111–117.

Horowitz, M. J., Bonanno, G. A., & Holen, A. (1993). Pathological grief: Diagnosis and explanation. *Psychosomatic Medicine, 55,* 260–273.

Kalish, R. A. (1979). The onset of the dying process. In Kalish, R. A. (Ed.), *Death, dying, transcending* (pp. 5–17). New York: Baywood Publishing Company, Inc.

Kastenbaum, R. A. (1997). *Death, society, and human experience.* Boston: Allyn and Bacon.

Kazanowski, M. (1999). Loss, death, and dying. In D. D. Ignatavicius, M. L. Workman, & M. A. Mishler (Eds.), *Medical-surgical nursing across the health care continuum* (3rd ed.) (pp. 173–184). Philadelphia: W. B. Saunders Company.

Kiser, L. J., Ostoja, E., & Pruitt, D. B. (1998). Dealing with stress and trauma in families. *Child and Adolescent Psychiatric Clinics of North America, 7*(1), 87–103.

Kissane, D. W., Bloch, S., & McKenzie, D. P. (1997). Family coping and bereavement outcome. *Palliative Medicine, 11*(3), 191–201.

Koop, P. M., & Strang, V. (1997). Predictors of bereavement outcomes in families of patients with cancer: A literature review. *Canadian Journal of Nursing Research, 29*(4), 33–5.

Kubler-Ross, E. (1969). *On death and dying*. New York: MacMillan.

Kurtz, M. E., Kurtz, J. C., Given, C. W., & Given, B. (1997). Predictors of post-bereavement depressive symptomatology among family caregivers of cancer patients. *Support Care Cancer, 5*(1), 53–60.

Lev, E. L., & McCorkle, R. (1998). Loss, grief, and bereavement in family members of cancer patients. *Seminars in Oncology Nursing, 14*(2), 145–151.

Lewis, M. L. (1998). Culture and loss: A project of self-reflection. *Journal of Nursing Education, 37*(9), 191–201.

Lindemann, E. (1944). Symptomatology and management of acute grief. *American Journal of Psychiatry, 101,* 141–148.

Mallinson, R. K. (1999). Grief work of HIV-positive persons and their survivors. *Nursing Clinics of North America, 34*(1), 163–177.

McCall, J. B. (1999). *Grief education for caregivers of the elderly.* New York: The Haworth Pastoral Press.

McIntier, T. M. (1995). Nursing the family when a child dies. *RN, 2,* 50–55.

Mitchell, K. R., & Anderson, H. (1983). *All our losses, all our griefs.* Philadelphia: Westminster Press.

O'Neill, D. P., & Kenny, E. K. (1998). Spirituality and chronic illness. *Image: Journal of Nursing Scholarship, 30*(3), 275–280.

Parkes, C. M., & Weiss, R. S. (1983). *Recovery from bereavement.* New York: Basic Books.

Pattison, E. M. (1977). *The experience of dying.* New York: Simon and Schuster.

Pennebaker, J. W., Mayne, T. J., & Francis, M. E. (1997). Linguistic predictors of adaptive bereavement. *Journal of Personality and Social Psychology, 72*(4), 863–871.

Prigerson, H. G., Bierhals, A. J., Kasl, S. V., Reynolds, C. F., Shear, M. K., Day, N., Beery, L. C., Newsom, J. T., & Jacobs, S. (1997). Traumatic grief as a risk factor for mental and physical morbidity. *American Journal of Psychiatry, 154*(5), 616–623.

Pritchett, K. T., & Lucas, P. M. (1997). Grief and loss. In B. S. Johnson, *Psychiatric-mental health nursing—Adaptation and growth* (4th ed.) (pp. 199–218). New York: Lippincott.

Rando, T. A. (1984). *Grief, dying, and death.* Champaign, IL: Research Press Company.

Sherman, D. W. (1998). Reciprocal suffering: The need to improve family caregivers' quality of life through palliative care. *Journal of Palliative Medicine, 1*(4), 357–366.

Siegel, K., Karus, D. G., Raveis, V. H., Christ, G. H., & Mesagno, F. P. (1996). Depressive distress among the spouses of terminally ill patients. *Cancer Practice, 4*(1), 25–30.

Spencer, L. (1994). How do nurses deal with their own grief when a patient dies on an intensive care unit and what help can be given to enable them to overcome their grief effectively? *Journal of Advanced Nursing, 19,* 1141–1150.

Stewart, A. L., Teno, J., Patrick, D. L., & Lynn, J. (1999). The concept of quality of life of dying persons in the context of health care. *Journal of Pain and Symptom Management, 17*(2), 93–108.

Stuart, G. W., & Sundeen, S. J. (1991). *Principles and practices of psychiatric nursing.* Boston: Mosby Year Book, Inc.

Sudnow, D. (1967). *Passing on: The social organization of dying.* Englewood Cliffs, NJ: Prentice-Hall.

The American Heritage Dictionary of the English Language (1992). Boston: Houghton Miflin Company.

Viorst, J. (1987). *Necessary losses.* New York: Ballantine Books.

Warren, B. J. (1999). Cultural competence in psychiatric nursing: An interlocking paradigm approach. In N. L. Keltner, L. H. Schwecke, & C. E. Bostrom (Eds.), *Psychiatric nursing* (3rd ed.). Boston: Mosby.

Worden, J. W. (1991). *Grief counseling and grief therapy: Handbook for the mental health practitioner.* New York: Springer Publishing Company.

PART 4

Physical Aspects of Palliative Care

July 3, 2000

Up until this last week Candy has been relatively independent with her activities of daily living. She was having occasional right-sided chest pain, which she rated as a "3" in intensity, but was relieved by 2 Percocet. In the past week, the pain increased in frequency and intensity, and she had dyspnea at rest. In the past 3 days, Candy became very weak, with no appetite, and she spent most of her time sitting in her "Lazy Boy" chair. Because of her increase in symptoms, I called her daily and visited her every other day. She was extremely lethargic and her husband told me that she became very short of breath on ambulation to the bathroom.

Lethargy and loss of appetite in a person with advanced cancer are common physical symptoms associated with the process of dying. The fact that she was having an increase in symptoms of pain and dyspnea was further evidence that she was nearing death. I called her doctor and asked for a standing order for liquid Morphine and Ativan. I showed Candy and Ron how to administer 5 mg of the morphine in her cheek and recommended repeating the medication dose in 15 minutes if it wasn't effective, and to take the prescribed rescue dose if she experienced heightened pain or shortness of breath.

Today was the first time in the year that I have known Candy that she mentioned dying. I held her hand while she cried and told me how surprised she was that the end was coming so quickly. I suppose these things are surprising when it is clear that the disease will not be cured. Candy asked me to promise her that she would not suffer at the end; it was such a poignant moment. As I hugged her, I told her I would be with her till the end. With the support of members of the Hospice/Palliative Care team, Candy's pain and symptoms were alleviated, and the emotional and spiritual needs of Candy and her family were being addressed.

July 4, 2000

When I arrived at Candy's house today, I saw that her level of conscious-ness had significantly declined. She had not had any oral intake for 2 days, and was only responding occasionally to her name. Her skin was cool and starting to become mottled. Ron said he had given Candy 4 rescue doses of 10 mg of morphine since yesterday. She appeared comfortable and peaceful, with no evidence of grimacing or restlessness, which may indicate pain. Candy did not appear to have difficulty breathing, but her breaths were slow and shallow, and there was a rattle in the back of her throat. I explained that this noise was from secretions in the back of her throat, but that it is usually not distressing to the patient.

I told him that Candy was actively dying and held him as he cried. I suggested to Ron that he get the children if he wanted them to be with her as she died. They came in and crawled into the bed with their mom and lay in her arms for the last time. Ron put his arms around them all, as they prayed together. I was thinking what a good job Candy had done with her kids that they were so comfortable to be with her during this time; I don't know where Ron got his strength to support his family in this way. The love and faith were almost palpable. I stayed at the foot of her bed and did Reike on Candy's feet, something she had always liked me to do during my visits. She opened her eyes, looked at each of us, stopped breathing, and died.

Ron held the children and told them what had happened. Fortunately, there were family and friends in the house to be with the children, as Ron stayed with me to bathe Candy's body. He wanted to do this final act for her because she never liked to leave the house looking "messy." He talked to her as we prepared her to leave her home for the last time.

As I reflect on this nursing experience, I realize the importance of our relationship that we had developed over time. This family allowed me to care for them at one of the most vulnerable times of their lives. I learned so much from Candy about life, living, and ultimately about dying. These are gifts given to us by our patients at the end of life. Palliative care nursing transcends traditional caregiving experiences. In a very intimate way, nurses co-journey with their patients and families who are experiencing life-threat-ening illness and help them to live as fully as possible until death. With the knowledge and skills to alleviate the physical, emotional, social, and spiritual pain and suffering, and by bearing witness to the precious moments of life as patients and their family say their last good-bye and express eternal love, nurses experience the joy and rewards of hospice/palliative care nursing. Through competent and compassionate care at the end of life, nurses can make a difference in the quality of life and quality of dying for their patients and their families.

10

Symptom Management in Palliative Care

Mary K. Kazanowski

AACN Competencies

#7: Use scientifically based standardized tools to assess symptoms (e.g., dyspnea, constipation, anxiety, fatigue, nausea and vomiting, and altered cognition) experienced by patients at the end of life).

#8: Use data from symptom assessment to plan and intervene in symptom management using state-of-the-art traditional approaches.

> People have come both to fear a technologically over-treatment and protracted death and to dread the prospect of abandonment and untreated physical and emotional distress.
> —Institute of Medicine (1997)

Research regarding care at the end of life validates the knowledge that individuals near death often experience physical symptoms of distress. Recognition and treatment of physical and nonphysical symptoms of distress is essential to achieve and maintain comfort and peace until death.

By virtue of their close proximity to those who are sick, and their commitment to patients throughout the life cycle, nurses play a pivotal role in identifying and treating symptoms of patients near death. The provision of quality care near end of life is contingent on nurses receiving adequate education in the treatment of pain and symptoms.

Curriculum content for undergraduates should include signs and symptoms, etiologies and standard treatment for: pain, dyspnea, nausea, vomiting, anxiety, agitation, fatigue, and constipation. Curricula for Advanced Practice nurses should include this content as well as content related to 1) pathophysiology related to advanced disease states; 2) assessment of the emotional, social, and spiritual components of suffering; 3) effective pharmacological and nonpharmacological interventions; 4) measurement issues and assessment tools; and 5) ethical and legal issues related to terminal dehydration, terminal restlessness, refractory symptoms, access to care, barriers to care, and health care policy.

The majority of research on end-of-life symptoms is found in the palliative care literature, with most studies involving clients with terminal cancer (Kazanowski, 1996). Symptoms of distress cited in these studies include but are not limited to pain, anorexia, fatigue, weakness, nausea, vomiting, dyspnea, constipation, anxiety, and delirium (Coyle, Adelhardt, Foley, & Portenoy, 1990). Studies vary somewhat in identifying which symptoms are the most prevalent causes of physical distress near death. However, there is general consensus that pain, dyspnea, delirium, nausea, and vomiting often cause distress in this patient population (Fainsinger, Miller, Bruera, Hanson, & Maceachern, 1991; Kazanowski, 1996).

As death nears, symptoms of distress may escalate, stay the same, or decrease in intensity. To ensure client comfort and family coping, symptoms must be recognized as a threat to client comfort, effectively treated, and monitored, to ensure that they remain controlled.

To decrease suffering, symptoms of distress such as pain, dyspnea, delirium nausea and vomiting generally require the use of medications such as analgesics, sedatives, and/or antiemetics. Once symptoms of distress occur, medications are usually administered around the clock until death to prevent recurrence and attain control. With the appropriate knowledge and resources, medication management of symptoms near death can usually be achieved. In fact, studies show that symptoms of distress, such as pain near death, can be effectively controlled in more than 90% of cases (Management of Cancer Pain Guideline Panel, 1994) when clients have access to health care providers knowledgeable in pain management. Although the research base for the presence of symptoms (other than pain) near death is weaker, problems such as dyspnea, nausea, and vomiting near death have also been shown to be effectively controlled (Gavrin & Chapman, 1995). The problem is that palliative care providers are underutilized, and many individuals lack quality care near death (Fields & Cassell, 1997).

The goals of symptom management for clients near end of life are to control symptoms, promote meaningful interactions between patients and significant others, and facilitate peaceful deaths. To achieve these goals, analgesics and adjunct medications are given at doses titrated for individual patient needs. Certain standard medications are recommended which have been shown to be successful in attaining and maintaining the control of symptoms. Standard medications may at times, however, fail to provide comfort, and complex, multimodal therapy may be required to achieve optimal control. Side effects related to treatment of symptoms also need to be understood and treated. Most health care practitioners outside of palliative care settings lack the knowledge to manage the common as well as the complex symptoms near death, and many lack the knowledge to effectively treat these symptoms. It is essential that health care providers in all settings become prepared to provide quality care at end of life. Given the multiple needs of patients and families, this often requires an interdisciplinary approach to care.

Although studies show that the majority of clients with access to palliative care receive effective symptom management near death, a small percent (< 5 to 10%) of clients experience symptoms of distress which are refractory to treatment (Levy, 1999). This group of people may require such high doses of analgesia, that sedation occurs as a side effect, or they may actually need to be sedated to control symptoms of distress.

Although sedation is not ideal, its occurrence as a side effect of treatment may be acceptable to clients who have no alternative for comfort. It is important that health care providers and the public understand that adequate management of symptoms may at times result in sedation. The sedation that occurs is a side effect of treatment, neither a treatment goal nor an effect meant to hasten death. Administration of medications for symptoms of distress at the end of life is guided by protocols using doses of medications that are considered safe. Use of guides/protocols for management of symptoms is done with the intention of alleviating suffering, not hastening death. The occurrence of an untoward effect of a medication is, however, a risk. According to the Guideline panel for Management of Cancer Pain (1994) "when the patient's death is imminent because of the progression of primary disease, an increased risk of earlier death counts little against the benefit of pain relief and painless death. The ethical duty to benefit the patient through relieving pain is by itself adequate to support increasing doses to alleviate pain, even if there might be life-shortening and expected side effects" (p. 64). This same doctrine of double effect related to other symptoms of distress near the end of life.

ASSESSMENT AT THE END OF LIFE

Clients near the end of life should be conscientiously assessed for any sign or symptom that could potentially cause distress. When first recognized, each symptom should be assessed comprehensively, in terms of intensity, frequency, duration, quality, exacerbating factors, and relieving factors. A method for rating the intensity of that symptom should then be chosen to facilitate ongoing assessments of that symptom, evaluate treatment response, and assess symptom management over time. Family caregivers and health care providers may need to be taught how to interpret some of these tools. Tools that can be easily explained and interpreted with a minimal amount of time and effort should be used. The use of such tools promotes early recognition of symptoms and changes in symptomotology, and facilitates communication of this change to other providers.

Assessment of symptoms should be ideally based on the patient's perception of the symptom with choice of tools based on each patient's understanding. If scales for certain symptoms are not available, a simple flow sheet can be used to prompt health care providers and family caregivers to assess common symptoms of distress. An example of such a flow sheet is found in Table 10.1. Flow sheets such as this are commonly used in palliative care to ensure that priority assessments are consistently performed with each nurse-client encounter.

As one nears the end of life one commonly grows weak and lethargic, sleeping for longer periods of time. This lethargy and sleep may progress to the point that the client has a decreased level of consciousness, rousing only to touch. In most cases, the ability of the client to communicate verbally decreases along with their decreased level of consciousness, making it difficult to assess the client's perception of symptoms. When caring for clients who are unable to communicate their distress or needs, it is essential that health care providers identify alternative ways to assess symptoms of distress. Professional caregivers should teach family caregivers to watch closely for objective signs of discomfort such as restlessness, grimacing, or moaning, and identify when these symptoms occur in relation to positioning, movement, medication, or other external stimuli. For example, grimacing when turning from side to side in the bed is indicative of pain or discomfort with movement. An increase in respiratory rate and effort when the head of the bed is flat is indicative of shortness of breath when lying flat, which is referred to as orthopnea.

Although the client's point of view is likely to be the most valid indicator of comfort or distress, the perception of symptoms that family members have is also important. Family perceptions of symptoms should be obtained as part of each client's symptom assessment. Research has shown that family caregivers, health care providers, and patients may differ in their perceptions of symptoms, in terms of intensity, significance, and meaning (Curtis & Fernsler, 1989; Masters & Shontz, 1989; McMillan, 1996a; McMillan, 1996b; McMillan & Mahon, 1994a; McMillan & Mahon, 1994b; Weitzner, Moody, &

TABLE 10.1 Hospice/Supportive Care Patient Flow Sheet

Date												
Assess respiratory status												
Temperature												
Apical/Radial pulse												
Respiratory rate												
BP												
Breath sounds:												
Left												
Right												
Edema												
Left												
Right												
Sputum: amount/color												
Does patient appear dyspneic?												
Rating of dyspnea with activity?												
(0–5 scale)												
Dyspnea at rest?												
(0–5 scale)												
Is oxygen required?												
Is patient alert?												
Is patient oriented?												
Is patient agitated?												

(continued)

TABLE 10.1 *(continued)*

Date											
Is patient taking medication for dyspnea?											
# times medication taken/24 hrs.											
Other interventions for dyspnea?											
Fan/air conditioner											
Is patient taking medication for anxiety?											
# times medication taken/24 hrs.											
Assessment GI Status											
Is patient nauseated?											
# episodes of nausea/24 hrs.											
# episodes of vomiting/24 hrs.											
# times medication taken for N/V/24 hrs.											
Date of last BM											
Is abdomen distended?											
Are bowel sounds present?											

Adapted with permission from: VNA Transitional Care and Hospice, 1850 Elm Street, Manchester, NH 03104.

McMillan, 1997). Whereas health care providers are often more adept at identifying symptoms of distress, families are often more knowledgeable about client habits and preferences, which often reflects client needs. Health care providers need to incorporate all client-related information into the plan for management of symptoms, working with clients and families toward a common goal.

INTERVENTIONS AT END OF LIFE

The literature indicates that unrelieved pain is one of the most common causes of somatic distress in the months, weeks, and days before death (Paice, 1999). Pain is also the most feared symptom near end of life (Brescia et al., 1990). Assessment and interventions for pain near end of life are discussed comprehensively in chapter 10. Assessment and interventions for common symptoms of distress other than pain (e.g., dyspnea, nausea, vomiting, anxiety, and delirium) will be discussed in this chapter. Control and prevention of recurrent symptoms require administering medication around the clock to maintain or prevent symptoms of distress, which are likely to reoccur. Optimal treatment and control of symptoms near death requires that interventions are planned prior to the occurrence of the symptoms, to facilitate administration of appropriate treatment. Any barrier to obtaining or administering medications for symptoms near death can impact client's suffering at end of life.

The concept of Symptom Relief Kits (or Emergency Kits) addresses the need to have appropriate medications readily available in the home, extended care facility, or hospital. Hospice agencies and pharmacies, with the knowledge that the timing of the dying process cannot consistently be predicted developed the concept of Symptom Relief Kits. The kit generally contains small amounts of various medications that have been found effective in treating common symptoms of distress in clients near death (Appendix 1).

As is the case with analgesics for pain, the oral route is the preferred route for administration of medications for symptoms of distress near the end of life. However, oral administration of medications can become problematic if and when clients have a decrease in their level of consciousness. A decreased level of consciousness, which commonly occurs near the end of life, can make swallowing difficult and/or unsafe. Capsules or sustained-release tablets, which cannot be chewed or crushed, are particularly problematic when a client cannot safely swallow solids. When faced with this situation, the nurse needs to consider alternative routes for medications. The guiding principle for choice of route is to choose the least invasive with the most effective treatment (Coluzzi & Fairbairn, 1998). Identification of appropriate routes and dosages for medications often requires the input of a physician or nurse knowledgeable in palliative care. Access to a pharmacist who is able to advise and/or compound medications for alternative routes are also advantageous.

Sublingual or buccal (cheek or lower lip) administration of certain short-acting medications is often effective using liquefied small crushed tablets. The volume of medication that can be absorbed from the oral cavity, however, limits these routes. Volumes of 1 cc or less are generally well tolerated. Volumes that are not adequately absorbed should be administered by another route (e.g., rectal, intravenous, or subcutaneous).

An alternative route for medications for symptoms near death is the rectal route. Advantages of this route are that dosing requirements of certain oral medications remain the same. Retaining the same dosing requirements thus eliminates the need to calculate equianalgesic doses, and the need to obtain and purchase new prescriptions. Not only does a switch from oral to rectal administration of analgesics save family and health care providers' time and money; it also facilitates ongoing control of symptoms, by avoiding major changes in the treatment plan. Although the rectal route is a good alternative for some dying clients, it is not a good alternative for all clients. Clients with loose stool, constipation, or rectal bleeding may not adequately absorb the medication given rectally. Clients with low platelet counts will be at risk for bleeding from insertion of medication into the rectum. Clients with lesions of the anus or rectum may also experience pain. Rectal administration of analgesics may also pose problems for caregivers assuming the responsibility for administration of medications near death. Problems cited by family caregivers include caregiver aversion to touching the rectum, client aversion to having the rectum touched, and difficulty turning the client and/or inserting the medication in the rectum. It should also be noted that not all oral medications can be administered rectally. Assessment for potential problems related to rectal administration of a medication would be necessary to determine the appropriateness and effectiveness of the rectal route.

Subcutaneous or intravenous routes may need to be utilized for administration of medications if control of symptoms cannot be achieved via the oral or rectal routes or if rapid titration of medication is necessary. Clients with existing central venous access are the preferred candidates for intravenous medications, because they will not require frequency restarts of peripheral catheters that can cause pain. The subcutaneous route is the preferred route for clients without existing venous access, if the medication can be safely administered by that route.

DYSPNEA NEAR THE END OF LIFE

Dyspnea is a subjective experience described as an uncomfortable awareness of breathing, breathlessness, or severe shortness of breath (Hospice and Palliative Nurses Association, 1996) which may be associated with copious secretions, cough, chest pain, fatigue, or air hunger. It is a frequent symptom of distress near the end of life, occurring in 50–70% of dying clients (Bruera, Macmillan, Pither, & MacDonald, 1990) and it is thought to be a marker for the terminal phase of life (Escalante et al., 1996). Dyspnea is considered by many patients, families, and health care providers as the worst symptom of distress because it conveys an image of suffering, invoking fear on the part of the patient and the family. Severe dyspnea is also quite difficult to control, which enhances its negative perception.

Causes of dyspnea can be directly related to the client's primary diagnosis (e.g., lung cancer, breast cancer, or coronary artery disease); secondary to the primary diagnosis (e.g., pleural effusion, metastasis to lung or pleura); related to treatment of the primary disease (e.g., congestive heart failure related to chemotherapy or constrictive pericarditis related to radiation therapy; anemia related to chemotherapy); or to an etiology unrelated to the primary disease (e.g., pneumonia). Depending on the cause, the pathophysiology can involve: a) obstructive, restrictive, or vascular disturbances in the airways with tumor or nodal involvement; b) pulmonary congestion secondary to fluid overload and/or cardiac dysfunction; c) bronchoconstriction and bronchospasm as seen with a respiratory infection, COPD, or airway encroachment by a tumor; d) a decreased hemoglobin carrying capacity as with anemia; or e) hyperventilation secondary to neuromuscular disease with limited movement of the diaphragm.

ASSESSMENT OF DYSPNEA

Research shows that dyspnea near the end of life is inadequately assessed (Escalante et al., 1996). Because of its association with suffering and its resistance to treatment, dyspnea should be routinely assessed in all clients nearing the end of life. The nurse reviews the past medical history of the client for risks of dyspnea related to the primary disease, secondary conditions, and/or the clinical condition of the client. For example, clients with a history of congestive heart failure, or a primary diagnosis of lung cancer or renal failure are at risk for dyspnea because of their primary disease and/or past history. Clients with ascites are at risk for dyspnea related to fluid volume excess.

Symptoms of dyspnea are assessed with particular attention to the client's perception of his/her breathing and the meaning of the dyspnea for the client and/or family. Assessment is performed using the descriptor that most closely reflects the individual experience of each client. Breathlessness may characterize the experience for some whereas discomfort, pain, or difficulty breathing may characterize it for others.

Signs of dyspnea are assessed by inspecting the client's respiratory rate and respiratory effort, and auscultating breath sounds. Respiratory rates greater than the client's norm or greater than 20 per minute (for adults), labored respirations manifested by use of accessory muscles and distended neck veins, diminished breath sounds, and/or auscultation of adventitious lung sounds (e.g., rhonchi or rales) are signs often associated with dyspnea. Absence of these abnormalities does not, however, refute its existence since like pain, dyspnea is a subjective experience, based on primarily the patient's self-report.

Once dyspnea is identified, the nurse obtains information about the frequency, nature, and intensity of the dyspnea, as well as information regarding associated factors that trigger, aggravate, and relieve it. Asking the client or family to describe when the dyspnea occurs and how it relates to activity or positioning is often helpful to clients trying to describe the experience. On initial assessment of dyspnea, the nurse also assesses for prior episodes of this symptom, etiologies of prior episodes, treatment, and effect of treatment at that time.

Assessment of the intensity of dyspnea at end of life is most commonly done by determining the presence or absence of the symptom and the relation of the symptom to activity. Ideally, a tool with a visual analogue scale should be used to track the symptom over time. Visual analogue scales are available with numbers or markers representing "no dyspnea" or "not at all breathless" at the low end of the scale and "dyspnea as bad as it can be" or "severely breathless" at the high end (Harwood, 1999). Although visual analogue scales measure only one aspect (i.e., intensity) of a person's dyspnea, they are useful for evaluating a change in the symptom over time, and response to treatment, and they can be utilized with a minimal time commitment.

More comprehensive assessment tools for dyspnea are available which have been found both reliable and valid in client populations with or without malignant disease. Use of these tools, however, is generally reserved for research activities because they require too much time to use them in the clinical setting. Examples of more comprehensive tools for assessment of dyspnea include the American Thoracic Society Standardized Questionnaire (American Thoracic Society, 1978); the Pulmonary Functional Status and Dyspnea Questionnaire (Lareau, Carrieri-Kohlman, Janson-Bjerklie, & Roos,

1994); the Modified Baseline Dyspnea Index (Stoller, Ferranti, & Feinstein, 1986); the Shortness of Breath Assessment Tool (Lareau, Kohlman-Carrieri, Janson-Bjerklie, & Roos, 1986); and the Transition Dyspnea Index (Mahler, Weinberg, Wells, & Feinstein, 1984). In addition to measuring intensity, these tools often measure functional ability and impairment related to the symptom.

INTERVENTIONS FOR DYSPNEA

The goals for the client with dyspnea near the end of life is to treat the primary cause, relieve the psychological distress and autonomic response that accompany the symptom (Gavrin & Capman, 1995). Because diagnostic testing to identify the cause is usually inappropriate, the etiology is determined by physical assessment and knowledge of the underlying condition. If the etiology of dyspnea cannot be successfully treated, interventions are aimed at alleviating the distress.

Dyspnea is a very difficult symptom to control. Because of this, interventions to decrease its intensity and maintain control should be implemented as soon as possible after its occurrence. Use of standard kits such as Symptom Relief Kits facilitates prompt treatment of dyspnea at end of life (Appendix 1) in a person who cannot safely swallow (Kazanowski, 1999; Petrin, 1998).

MEDICATIONS

OPIODS

Morphine sulfate is highly effective in relieving dyspnea and it is considered the standard treatment for the relief of dyspnea near death (Hospice and Palliative Nurses Association, 1996). Opiods affect dyspnea by altering the individual's perception of breathlessness, reducing respiratory drive, and reducing oxygen consumption (Harwood, 1999). Although morphine may decrease the respiratory rate, lead to an increase in pCO_2, and a decrease in arterial pH, it generally does not severely compromise one's respiratory status. The primary side effect of morphine is somnolence, which may be managed by decreasing the dose.

Morphine for dyspnea can be administered by mouth, sublingually, per rectum, parenterally via intravenous or subcutaneous boluses or drips, or via nebulizer. Although not intended to be given sublingually, morphine concentrates and soluble tablets can be administered under the tongue or in the cheeks in patients who can no longer swallow. Recent studies of morphine administered in this way have found that the majority of the morphine is actually swallowed, thus not absorbed via oral mucosa (Coluzzi, 1998), but is effective.

Nurses need to understand that individuals who are opiod naive (have not been receiving daily opiods) should be initially started on low doses of morphine (e.g., 5 mg–10 mg po or sublingually), which can be repeated if necessary. Individuals taking opiods for pain will need to have their breakthrough dose of morphine increased by 50% their usual dose, for effective treatment of dyspnea.

If intravenous access is available, health care providers may order 1–2 mg of morphine to be given every 5 to 10 minutes until relief is obtained. Given the discomfort associated with needle sticks, health providers should not, however, initiate intravenous access in dying clients unless it is absolutely necessary to achieve comfort. If clients are unable to safely swallow, effective treatment can also be provided by administering morphine subcutaneously.

Morphine via a facial nebulizer is another option for dyspnea near end of life. Although some research suggests that the nebulized route is no more effective than the oral route, anecdotal reports indicate that nebulized morphine is effective, easy to administer, and has no side effects. The suggested dose for nebulized morphine is 4 mg morphine with 2.5 cc normal saline (Wrede-Seaman, 1996).

DIURETICS, BRONCHODILATORS, CORTICOSTEROIDS, AND ANTIBIOTICS

Individuals with signs of fluid volume excess manifested by dyspnea, crackles/rales on auscultation of breath sounds, peripheral edema, and/or signs of heart failure (+ S3) should be given a diuretic such as Furosemide (Lasix) to decrease blood volume, reduce vascular congestion, and reduce the workload of the heart. Furosemide can be administered by mouth, intravenously, subcutaneously, or in the muscle (IM). Intravenous administration, which is effective in the pulmonary vascular within minutes,may be preferred for congestive heart failure and pulmonary edema.

Bronchodilators such as Albuterol via metered dose inhalation or nebulizer may be given for symptoms of bronchospasm (e.g., wheezes on auscultation of breath sounds). Corticosteroids may also be given for bronchospasm and inflammatory problems within and exterior to the lung. Superior vena cava syndrome and lymphangitis carcinomatosis both can cause dyspnea, which may respond to corticosteriods.

Antibiotics may be indicated in clients with dyspnea secondary to a respiratory infection. A thorough work-up for a respiratory infection is not appropriate in clients imminently near death. However, if clients have developed dyspnea along with an elevated temperature, adventitious breath sounds, and a congested cough, it is safe to assume they have an upper respiratory infection. A trial of an appropriate antibiotic should be considered for clients with dyspnea of infectious origin near death, to provide symptom relief and facilitate comfort.

ANTICHOLINERGICS

Secretions in the respiratory tract and oral cavity may contribute to a client's dyspnea near death. Loud wet respirations (referred to as death rattle) are also disturbing to family and caregivers, even when they do not seem to cause dyspnea or respiratory distress. Anticholinergics such as Hyoscyamine (Levsin PO/SL) or Scopolamine transdermal) are used to reduce secretion production (Appendix 1).

Clients with retained sputum or tenacious secretions may benefit from mucolytic agents. However, steam or nebulized saline will probably be as effective (Levy, 1997).

OXYGEN

The use of oxygen for individuals with hypoxemia is recognized as an important part of treatment. However, oxygen for dyspnea has not been established as a standard of care for all individuals (Harwood, 1999). Studies evaluating oxygen therapy in dyspnea patients vary in their findings (Booth, Kely, Cox, Adams, & Guz, 1996; Bruera, de Stoutz, Velasco-Leiva, Schoeller, & Hanson, 1993; Bruera, Schoeller, & MacEachern, 1992; Liss & Grant, 1988).

The need for oxygen for dyspnea at end of life is dependent on the client's perception of the need, and their perception of its effect. Many practitioners believe that oxygen is not necessary near the end of life, that it can actually cause discomfort, and that comfort can be better achieved using morphine. Indeed, many clients with dyspnea near death frequently remove their oxygen, and can be kept comfortable without it. It is imperative, however, that clients with dyspnea who do not promptly respond to morphine (or other medications), be given a trial dose of oxygen to assess its effect, irregardless of whether or not they are hypoxemic.

ANXIOLYTICS (SEDATIVES)

Sedatives are commonly used when morphine does not fully control the client's dyspnea. Either benzodiazepines or phenothiazines can be used for their effect on anxiety, fear, and the autonomic responses that accompany dyspnea.

The benzodiazepine, Lorazepam (0.5 mg PO/SL), is commonly given every 4 hours or around the clock, to prevent/control dyspnea and/or anxiety. Benzodiazepines are more commonly used because phenothiazines have the potential for extrapyramidal side effects. Phenothiazines that have been used for dyspnea include chlorpromazine hydrochloride (Thorazine).

Nonpharmacological Interventions

If dyspnea occurs near death, pharmacological interventions should be initiated early. Nonpharmacological interventions are used in conjunction (not in place) of medications to decrease the impact of the dyspnea on the client. Multi-modal interventions are planned in advance of the actual dying process, particularly when it is known that the client is at high risk for dyspnea.

Nonpharmacological interventions include: altering the environment to facilitate circulation of cool air, cooling of the body, positioning the client to facilitate chest expansion, intervening to conserve client energy, and facilitating the client's rest. An electric fan or air conditioned room helps decrease the impact of dyspnea. Positioning should be such that the individual's head of the bed is elevated and the feet flat or down, with the upper body supported to facilitate diaphragmatic excursion. This can be accomplished with a hospital bed, with pillows, or with the client out of bed in a chair. Clients who suffer from dyspnea when exerting to void are offered a foley catheter, the insertion of which will eliminate the need for exertion to void. This strategy is particularly effective for clients taking diuretics. Research indicates that terminally ill clients are appropriate candidates for urinary catheterization when the goal is comfort, and that the benefit can far outweigh morbidity (e.g., secondary to bacteriuria) (Fainsinger, MacEachern, Hanson, & Bruera, 1992).

Complementary therapies that promote relaxation should also be offered and implemented to reduce the impact of dyspnea. These include imagery, massage, breathing exercises, therapeutic touch, Reiki, music, and aromatherapy.

NAUSEA AND VOMITING NEAR THE END OF LIFE

Although not as common a problem as pain or dyspnea, nausea and vomiting are thought to occur in approximately 40% of terminally ill individuals during the last week of life (Waller & Caroline, 1996). Nausea and vomiting are particularly prevalent in individuals with breast, stomach, and gynecologic cancers, and in individuals with AIDS (Dworkin, 1992).

The mechanisms and mediators of nausea and vomiting are complex and remain incompletely defined (Gavrin & Chapman, 1995). Both central and peripheral factors play a role. The chemoreceptor trigger zone and the nucleus solitarius are located in a highly vascular area of the brain stem which is rich with opiod, dopaminergic, cholinergic, histaminergic, and serotonergic receptors. It is hypothesized that activation of these receptors stimulates an emetic center that produces nausea and/or vomiting. A vestibular component is particularly prevalent with opiod-induced nausea, and it can be stimulated by movement.

Nausea and vomiting at the end of life are commonly seen with: 1) the initiation of opiod therapy (nausea usually limited to a few days); 2) uremia; 3) hypercalcemia; 4) increased intracranial pressure secondary to brain metastasis; 5) vaginal stimulation secondary to oral candidasis; 6) stretching of the hepatic capsule; 7) constipation or impaction; and 8) bowel obstruction.

ASSESSMENT OF NAUSEA AND VOMITING

The client's self-report of nausea is the most reliable way to assess its presence. Clients and family are asked to keep a daily diary noting the time of each episode of nausea and vomiting, along with associated activities such as movement, coughing, eating, and the frequency of bowel movements. Health care providers can assess and monitor nausea and vomiting using a flow sheet such as shown in Table 10.1.

When clients have a decreased level of consciousness, it is very difficult to assess them for nausea. However, retching and gagging can occur even when clients are unresponsive.

INTERVENTIONS FOR NAUSEA AND VOMITING

Any client experiencing nausea and/or vomiting on a daily basis should be given antiemetics around the clock, to control the symptoms, and ideally prevent their reoccurrence. There are a variety of antiemetics that can be used for nausea and vomiting occurring near the end of life. The Phenothiazine, Prochlorperazine (Compazine), is commonly administered as a rectal suppository (25 mg) or intravenously (5–10 mg). The antiemetic and gastrointestinal stimulant Metoclopramide (Reglan) can be given rectally or parenterally, as a single agent or in combination with other antiemetics. Metochlopramide is often the drug of choice with incomplete or high gastrointestinal obstruction or chronic nausea of unknown etiology. This drug, however, should not be used in clients with complete bowel obstruction or clients with colicky abdominal pain.

Clients receiving Metochlopramide (Reglan) need to be monitored for signs and symptoms of dystonic reactions, an infrequent but serious side effect of this drug. Dystonic reactions include akathisia (restlessness), anxiety, agitation, and tardive dyskinesia, manifested as muscle rigidity. Dystonic reactions secondary to Metochlopramide are more common in individuals under 30 years of age, and are more likely to occur when clients are receiving Haloperidol (Haldol) in addition to Metochlopramide (Reglan). If dystonic reactions secondary to Metochlopramide (Reglan) occur, Diphenhydramine (Benadryl) 50 mg is given to reverse the dystonic effect. If Metochlopramide (Reglan) needs to be continued, Diphenhydramine (Benadryl) 50 mg is given with each subsequent dose (Waller & Caroline, 1996).

A compounded antiemetic known by the pneumonic ABHR (Ativan [Lorazepam], Benadryl [Diphenhydramine], Haldol [Haloperidol], and Reglan [Metochlopramide]) is commonly used by palliative care providers for severe cases of nausea and/or vomiting. It can be compounded into suppositories, trochés, or a gel for transdermal use (Petrin, 1998). Although doses of each drug can vary, a common ABHR dose is Ativan 1 mg, Benadryl 25 mg, Haldol 1 mg, and Reglan 10 mg. A limitation to use of ABHR is the need for access to a pharmacist who can compound the medication. ABHR is also associated with significant sedation, which may not be acceptable to clients and/or their families.

Corticosteroids such as Dexamethasone (Decadron) are also used for their antiemetic effects for terminal nausea. Decadron is particularly effective in nausea/vomiting related to increased intracranial pressure, gastrointestinal obstruction, hypercalcemia, and uremia. Daily doses range from 8 to 60 mg daily, which can be given as single agents or in combination with other drugs such as Ativan (Lorazepam), Benadryl (Diphenhydramine), and Reglan (Metochlopramide). ABDR (Ativan, Benadryl, Decadron, and Reglan) is used when clients do not respond to ABHR or ABCR (Ativan, Benadryl, Compazine, and Reglan) compounds.

ANXIETY AND ALTERED COGNITION

Symptoms of anxiety and altered cognition commonly occur together at the end of life, and the presence of one often relates to the development of the other. Anxiety is defined as a feeling of deep unease, without an identifiable cause. Altered cognition is often associated with an acute confessional state or delirium, which represents a disturbance of consciousness with reduced ability to focus or shift attention (March, 1998).

There are multiple causes of anxiety and altered cognition near the end of life. Causes of anxiety include poorly controlled pain, altered physiologic states (e.g., hypoxia, septicemia, hypoglycemia, hypocalcemia), medications (e.g., corticosteriods in high doses, metoclopramide in high doses, neuroleptic medications), withdrawal from alcohol, narcotics, or sedatives), psychologic, emotional, or spiritual distress, or a preexisting anxiety disorder (Hospice and Palliative Nurses Association, 1996).

Etiologies of delirium or altered cognition near the end of life include physiologic impairments (e.g., metabolic encephalopathy due to organ failure, electrolyte imbalance, central nervous system abnormalities such as malignancies or opportunistic infections of the brain, hypoxia, dehydration, septicemia, pain, urinary retention, constipation, fatigue, sensory disturbance, sensory alterations, nausea, extreme temperatures, puritis, or immobilization, alcohol or drug withdrawal); and psychological distress, which is often related to spiritual distress.

Delirium associated with restlessness at end of life is often referred to as terminal restlessness or terminal agitation. Terminal restlessness is defined as an observable syndrome characterized by the inability to rest, occurring in clients with varying diagnoses during the last days of life (March, 1998). Observable manifestations of terminal restlessness include frequent, nonpurposeful motor activity, the inability to concentrate or relax, disturbances in sleep/rest patterns, fluctuating levels of consciousness, and cognitive failure and/or anxiety (Hospice and Palliative Nurses Association, 1997).

Anxiety and altered cognition are disturbing to clients and families, but terminal restlessness often causes tremendous distress and can put the client and family at risk for injury. Because anxiety and altered cognition often precede terminal restlessness, symptoms should be identified and treated early to obtain and maintain symptom control and facilitate client comfort.

ASSESSMENT OF ANXIETY AND ALTERED COGNITION

Assessment of anxiety and altered cognition is initially focused on identifying a physical cause, which may be reversible. The nurse initially assesses for pain, urinary retention, and/or constipation as the cause. Anxiety that continues in the absence of these problems prompts the nurse to review medications, to identify new additions and recent changes, and consider their anxiety-provoking potential. Withdrawal of benzodiazepines in clients near death is a common cause of delirium near death. Delirium, however, can also occur secondary to an increase in benzodiazepines (Levy, 1999).

If delirium continues despite treatment of reversible causes (e.g., pain, urinary retention, and changes in medications), consideration should be given to the possibility that hypoxemia, hypercalcemia, kidney, and/or liver failure are contributing causes. However, it is inappropriate to investigate metabolic causes by invasive means (e.g., laboratory analysis). Invasive procedures often inflict pain and they are usually unsuccessful in establishing the cause of delirium (Burke, 1997).

In the absence of a physiologic impairment, clients with anxiety and delirium are assessed for their familiarity with the environment, their perceived readiness to die, and their perception of spiritual concerns. Clients in an unfamiliar environment (e.g., hospital), with unfinished business and spiritual concerns are more likely to be anxious than clients without these stresses (March, 1998).

The Mini Mental Status Exam (Folstein, 1983) is considered the gold standard for evaluating delirium. Spiritual and psychosocial assessment tools are also available for use in clients with social and/or spiritual concerns. However, clients near death are often unable to respond to questions on these assessment tools because they are obtunded, moribund, or agitated. A systematic assessment for sources of delirium and agitation in clients near death is often unobtainable. If the client is verbal, the nurse and family should listen for statements reflecting client concerns. Clients may want to discuss spiritual matters, beliefs about death, God, and/or a search for meaning in life. Every effort should be made to discuss areas of concern.

When caring for a client near death, it is imperative that anxiety, delirium, and terminal restlessness be distinguished from movement disorders such as myoclonus and extrapyramidal symptoms. Myoclonus is defined as a sudden, brief, shock-like, involuntary movement caused by active muscular contractions of symmetrical muscle groups (Sjogren, Jonsson, Jensen, Drenck, & Jensen, 1993). A major concern with myoclonic spasms is that the jerking or twitching may progress to recurrent convulsions. Myoclonus is often related to rapid increases and high doses of opiods such as morphine and its accumulated metabolites. Myoclonus may also result from a lowered seizure threshold related to medications (metoclopramide, phenothiazines, antihistamines, Haloperidol, tricycle antidepressants, anticholinergics), organ failure, brain lesions, hypoxia, dehydration, withdrawal syndromes, and electrolyte or glucose abnormalities (Back, 1992; deStoutz, Bruera, & Suarez-Almazor, 1995).

The assessment should also differentiate between extrapyramidal symptoms and other movement abnormalities. Extrapyramidal symptoms occur as side effects of neuroleptic medications such as the phenothiazines (Chlorpromazine, Prochlorperazine, Butyrophenones, and Metoclopramide). Examples of extrapyramidal symptoms include muscle rigidity, acute dystonia, akathisia (restlessness), cogwheeling, and akinesia.

INTERVENTIONS FOR ANXIETY AND ALTERED COGNITION

Given that pain is a common cause of anxiety at end of life, initial treatment often involves administration of a fast-acting analgesic such as morphine (liquid) PO/SL or PR. If the anxiety is relieved in response to the analgesic, around-the-clock doses should be continued or increased. Clients near death may also experience anxiety secondary to urinary retention, which may occur as a side effect of anticholinergics agents or smooth muscle relaxants. Anxiety in the presence of a distended bladder may resolve with intermittent or indwelling urinary catherization.

Benzodiazepines

Benzodiazepines are often considered the drugs of choice for anxiety, restlessness, or myoclonus near death. Lorazepam (Ativan) 1–2 mg is often crushed and given sublingually with a few drops of water, and continued at 0.5–2 mg every 6 to 8 hours around the clock. If paradoxical agitation occurs, Lorazepam is changed to another benzodiazepines. Alprazolam (Xanax) is another short-acting benzodiazepine that can be used for agitation.

Until recently, long-acting benzodiazepines such as Diazepam (Valium) were not recommended for agitation near death. The long-acting effect of these medications is now considered helpful in the control of anxiety near death, and Diazepam (Valium) and Clonazepam (Klonopin) are now being used more commonly. Valium has the added benefit of having a rapid onset. Recommended doses of these long-acting benzodiazepines are Diazepam (Valium) 10–20 mg PR at first sign of restlessness, followed by 5–10 mg every 8 to 12 hours around the clock, and Clonazepam (Klonopin) 0.3–0.5 mg SC every 12 hours.

Midazolam (Versed) is another benzodiazepine that has a rapid onset. Its use, however, is generally reserved for terminal agitation that does not respond to more commonly used benzodiazepines and barbiturates (described in next section). Use of Midazolam (Versed) is described further on in this chapter under "Sedation for Refractory Symptoms."

Barbiturates

When benzodiazepines fail to control anxiety, delirium, or restlessness near death, barbiturates are administered. Phenobarbital 60 mg PR every 4 to

12 hours as needed, is rapidly effective, although quite sedating (March, 1998). Phenobarbital also serves a dual purpose of treating myoclonus or preventing seizures. Alternative barbiturates include Pentobarbital, Secobarbital, Thiopental, and Propofol. Thiopental and Propofol are reserved for use in extraordinary cases of agitation, where sedation is needed for comfort. Sedation for comfort is discussed in further detail under "Sedation for Refractory Symptoms."

Neuroleptics

With the occurrence of hallucinations or paranoia, the neuroleptic Haloperidol (Haldol) is given at a starting dose of 1–2 mg PO or SC every 1 hour as necessary. Haloperidol may be increased but should not exceed 5 mg every 4 hours, because of the risk of myoclonus (Levy, 1999).

Chlorpromazine (Thorazine) is another neuroleptic that is routinely used for terminal anxiety. It can be used in individuals who responded to Haloperidol, but need more sedation, are considered safe at high doses, and can be given PO, PR, or IV. Common doses of Chlorpromazine (Thorazine) are 25–50 mg PR every 4–12 hours, or 12.5 mg IV every 4–8 hours. For terminal restlessness, a suggested starting dose of Thorazine is 100 mg PO or PR, followed by maintenance of 25–50 mg every 4–12 hours.

SEDATION FOR REFRACTORY SYMPTOMS

Refractory symptoms at end of life are defined as symptoms of distress that cannot be adequately controlled, despite aggressive effort to identify therapy that does not compromise consciousness (Levy, 1999). Delirium and myoclonus are at times refractory to aggressive interventions as well as pain, dyspnea, and emesis. The decision to utilize sedation for refractory agitation should be made on a case-by-case basis, by experts in palliative care. Sedation may be employed when providers are confident that appropriate medications have failed; standard interventions risk excessive and intolerable morbidity, and/or standard interventions are incapable of providing adequate relief in a tolerable time frame.

An increase in doses of opiods, benzodiazepines, and neuroleptics to the point of sedation is one method of sedation for refractory symptoms. This method is the most routine, and it generally involves increasing analgesia, Lorazepam, Alprazolam, Haloperidol, or Chlorpromazine (Levy, 1999). Infrequently, clients may need sedation for refractory symptoms using Diazepam, Pentobarbital, Secobarbital, Amobarbital, or Phenobarbital. In rare cases of refractory symptoms of distress, clients may need extraordinary medications to relieve distress. Medications recommended for extraordinary situations of refractory distress include the Midazolam (Versed), Thiopental, or Propofol.

Midazolam (Versed) is a rapid-acting benzodiazepine that is administered by subcutaneous or intravenous route. The initial dose of Midazolam is 0.4–0.8 mg/hour, with a range of 0.2–8.3 mg/hour. The onset of Midazolam is 1–5 minutes, with a duration of 60–120 minutes, and a half-life of 1–4 hours. Clients on Midazolam drips should have their blood pressure, pulse, respiratory rate, and level of comfort monitored, with upward and downward titration to maintain comfort and anticipated drug accumulation. If clients become obtunded and the family wants them more awake, the Midazolam can safely decreased by as much as 25% of their total dose.

NONPHARMACOLOGICAL INTERVENTIONS

Pharmacological interventions are generally initiated at the early onset of anxiety or agitation near death, because of the risk that these symptoms will accelerate. There are, however, several nonpharmacological therapies that could be tried in conjunction with pharmacological therapy, in an attempt to decrease anxiety and agitation in the client near death (see Chapter 2).

Fanslow (1984) reported using therapeutic touch to elicit a sense of peace and calm in dying patients. Reiki therapy could also be tried. Aromatherapy using combinations of essential oils such as lavender, marjoram, or geranium could be applied to hands and feet of clients or vaporized (only in the absence of oxygen administration) to promote relaxation (James, 1998). A trial of Therapeutic Touch or Reiki would require a practitioner who has had training in these therapies. Aromatherapy would require consultation with a professional aromatherapist (Snyder & Lindquist, 1998).

CONSTIPATION

Clients near death usually demonstrate a gradual decline in their physical condition, often manifested by a decrease in oral intake and decrease in mobility. Although these are potential risk factors for constipation in this client population, the fact is that many of these people have actually been dealing with constipation for some time. Recognition of factors that increase the risk for constipation of clients with terminal disease is addressed throughout the course of the illness. These factors include inadequate dietary bulk or fiber), decreased mobility, metabolic disturbances (e.g., hypercalcemia and hyperkalemia), decreased muscular or neurologic function, and side effects related to medications. The usual pattern of bowel elimination should also be assessed.

Constipation in clients with cancer is primarily due to the colonic effects of opiods which are taken for cancer-related pain (Robinson et al., 2000). Constipation occurs when opiods decrease peristalsis that inhibits intestinal contents from being propelled forward (Cameron, 1992). Although it is not a universal problem, constipation secondary to opiods is so common and so potentially distressing, that it warrants prophylactic treatment when opiods are initiated, and ongoing monitoring for the remainder of the person's life.

INTERVENTIONS FOR CONSTIPATION

Bowel protocols or algorithms are often used to prevent and treat constipation. Prophylactic treatment with a stool softener (e.g., docusate sodium) and stimulant laxative such as senna is commonly prescribed because of its direct effect on the colon, and demonstrated effect in these patients (Nursing Drug Handbook, 2000). Patients are commonly instructed to take 1–2 tablets orally at bedtime. Dosage of the laxative with the stool softener (i.e., Senokot-S) or without the stool softener (Senokot) can be increased gradually up to 4 tablets TID as needed to maintain a comfortable elimination pattern for the patient (Robinson et al., 2000).

The nurse at admission to the health care agency should assess the usual bowel elimination pattern for each individual. Although there are variations in elimination patterns, absence of bowel elimination for 3 or more days should prompt the nurse to assess for other signs and symptoms of constipation (e.g., abdominal distention, nausea, vomiting, or rectal impaction). If the patient is relatively comfortable, without nausea, vomiting or impaction, 30 ml of Milk of Magnesia can be given to stimulate the bowel, with a follow-up assessment within 24 hours. Evidence of symptoms of discomfort from constipation mandates that a digital rectal exam be performed to rule out impaction, and an aggressive bowel protocol with rapid-acting laxatives be implemented.

Constipation in a client without nausea or vomiting can be treated with oral laxatives such as Lactulose 45–60 ml po, magnesium citrate 8-oz po, or Fleet Phospho-Soda po. Palpation of stool in the rectum calls for Ducolax suppositories or a Fleet enema by rectum. Disimpaction is required if stool is hard and cannot be evacuated via these methods, and the client is in distress. Ideally, disimpaction is preceded by administration of an oil retention enema (120 cc) several hours or the night before the procedure (Waller & Caroline, 1996). Ten minutes prior to the procedure, the rectum is instilled with 10 ml of 1% Lidocaine jelly, and the patient is premedicated with intravenous morphine and/or Midazolam. The nurse should begin the procedure by lubricating the surface of the anus and her/his index finger with Lidocaine jelly.

As death nears, appetite and oral intake commonly decreases. Constipation in the immediate period near death is generally not problematic if clients have been monitored. However, clients with abdominal pain, escalation of their usual pain, anxiety, agitation, nausea, or vomiting, need to be assessed for possible constipation and impaction as a cause. Administration of enemas and/or manual disimpaction is indicated in the period near death only if constipation is contributing to client discomfort.

INTESTINAL OBSTRUCTION

A potential complication of a fecal impaction is a bowel obstruction. Bowel or intestinal obstructions can also occur in individuals near end of life as a result of a primary or secondary malignant tumor or a nonmalignant cause such as adhesions (Waller & Caroline, 1996).

Distinction of a fecal impaction from a bowel obstruction is important to determining treatment. Bowel obstructions are particularly common in clients with primary colon, ovarian, stomach, pancreatic, and renal cancers, and retroperitoneal sarcoma. Obstructions can also occur with metastasis to the abdomen from lung, breast, esophageal, or cervical cancers or malignant melanoma (Waller & Caroline, 1996).

Depending on the etiology of an obstruction and the goals for the patient, clients may be admitted to a hospital for nasogastric suction, and in some instances, surgery to release the obstruction. However, the majority of terminally ill patients with intestinal obstruction can be managed medically without nasogastric suction or intravenous fluids (Waller & Caroline, 1996).

Bowel obstructions in clients with advanced cancer are characterized by abdominal distention and tenderness, which occurs in a slow, progressive fashion. Colicky abdominal pain occurs in approximately 75% of patients (Waller & Caroline, 1996), and is characterized as "crampy" pain that comes and goes with relatively pain-free intervals. Episodes of colicky pain may be associated with audible borborygmi.

Continuous or steady abdominal pain occurs in more than 90% of patients with cancer and bowel obstruction (Waller & Caroline, 1996). Unlike colicky pain which comes and goes, steady pain is produced by stretching of the liver capsule or abdominal distention, and it responds well to opioids such as morphine. Other symptoms suggestive of obstruction include intermittent borborygmi, absence of bowel sounds, and intermittent or continuous vomiting. A flat plate x-ray of the abdomen can be ordered to rule out bowel obstruction versus constipation.

INTERVENTIONS FOR INTESTINAL OBSTRUCTION

In the presence of colicky abdominal pain and abdominal distention, all laxatives should be discontinued. Clients taking Metoclopramide (Reglan) may need to discontinue this medication in the presence of colicky pain, although this is controversial and client specific. Metoclopramide (Reglan) may be the drug of choice for incomplete obstructions, and it is often an effective antiemetic. Metoclopramide, however, should probably be discontinued for complete obstruction.

Colicky pain is poorly relieved by opiods, and responds better to antispasmodics such as Loperamide (Imodium) or Hyoscyamine (Levsin). Loperamide (Imodium) is available in oral or sublingual form. Hyoscyamine (Levsin) 0.125 mg can be given sublingually every 4 hours as needed. Another alternative is a transdermal Scopolamine patch (1.5 mg) which can be applied every 4 days behind the ear.

Steady abdominal pain is treated with a continuous subcutaneous infusion of opiods by pump. Pain that is specifically localized suggests a perforation or an ileal or colonic strangulation. Pain increasing with palpation indicates probable peritoneal irritation possibly due to early perforation.

Nausea and vomiting are commonly seen with individuals with intestinal obstruction. The goals for individuals near death are to eliminate the nausea, and reduce the vomiting to once or twice daily. Waller and Caroline (1996) recommend a combination of Haloperidol (Haldol) 1.5 mg, Hydroxyzine (Vistaril) 25 mg, and Octreotide 0.3 mg in a continuous subcutaneous infusion over 24 hours. Dexamethasone (Decadron) 1–8 mg may also be given orally, intravenously, or intramuscular every AM.

Clients with intestinal obstructions at end of life may be allowed to eat and drink as tolerated, as the goal is patient comfort. Intractable vomiting (> 2 episodes/8 hours) that does not respond to pharmacological measures may indicate the need for nasogastric intubation to provide comfort (Waller & Caroline, 1996).

FATIGUE

When clients and family are asked to identify symptoms they experience near end of life, fatigue and sleepiness are among the most commonly cited

(Kazanowski, 1996). Health care providers give inadequate attention to fatigue and sleepiness, and it is generally not considered a symptom of distress. From the perspective of clients and families, however, fatigue is the source of a tremendous amount of distress. Because of its prevalence and its negative impact on quality of life, fatigue cannot be ignored. Fatigue should be assessed with other symptoms of distress in all clients at the end of life.

Treatment of fatigue at the end of life differs from that provided for other symptoms of distress with regard to use of medications. Administration of medications to prevent and suppress symptoms such as pain, dyspnea, nausea, vomiting, and anxiety are usually the interventions of choice. Administration of medications to suppress fatigue is not, however, the primary intervention for this symptom.

Theories on fatigue suggest that passive strategies such as rest compound the fatigue experience (Ream & Richardson, 1999). Theorists recommend active and innovative measures for its management, including light exercise, diversional activities,relaxation and visualization, and attempts to balance activity with rest.

Although individuals near death are often extremely weak, lethargic, and bedbound, they can be assessed for their interest in participating in diversional activities. They should be asked what activities they enjoy most, and given permission to rest or sleep during less enjoyable activities to conserve energy. This may involve limiting or excluding certain visitors, and prioritizing others. Music and imagery could also be used to stimulate and or relax the client at various times of choice, providing sounds and sights that are pleasant for the patient. A video describing a favorite pastime like golf or football may be an excellent source of diversion and enjoyment.

TERMINAL DEHYDRATION

Dehydration in a healthy individual is generally associated with discomfort related to fluid and electrolyte imbalance, often manifested as fatigue, weakness, muscle cramps, nausea, vomiting, and headaches (Musgrave, 1990). The goal for dehydration in the healthy individual is to reverse the condition through means of hydration, and achieve fluid and electrolyte balance, with consequential revitalization and comfort.

Unlike dehydration in healthy individuals, dehydration in individuals at the end of life is considered a normal physiologic process that occurs to prepare the body for death. Reduced desire and intake of food and fluids is also a normal physiologic process near death. Although decrease intake and consequent dehydration may be associated with weakness, fatigue and thirst, it is not considered an uncomfortable condition for the patient that merits reversal. Furthermore, dehydration may actually have some beneficial effects in terms of symptom palliation (Zerwekh, 1983; Musgrave, 1990). Zerwekh (1983) contended that intake cessation leads to a reduced fluid load which serves to reduce urinary output, nausea and vomiting, pulmonary congestion, and edema. Printz (1992) described a possible endogenous benefit of intake cessation citing the effects of ketosis and increased levels of endorphins on the central nervous system in rats. Increased endorphins in humans may lead to a heightened state of well-being.

Many palliative care authors contend that with skilled nursing care, patients with terminal disease can die comfortably without artificial hydration (Morita, Tsunoda, Inoue, & Chihara, 1999). Research also indicates that palliative care providers believe that dehydration near the end of life is not only unnecessary and futile, but also potentially harmful and capable of causing discomfort (Meares, 1994). Forcing fluids or food on a person who has no or little appetite risks causing nausea, vomiting, and aspiration. Insertion and maintenance of intravenous catheters or nasogastric/feeding tubes is often painful for patients. Fluids from intravenous infusions or nasogastric tube feedings can increase respiratory secretions, which in turn increases pulmonary congestion, cough, and sensations of dyspnea. Administration of intravenous fluids will also increase urine output, increasing the occurrence of incontinence or need for Foley catheters. Intravenous fluids will also increase total body water, which could result in an increase in fluid retention in the form of edema, ascites, or pleural effusions. Intravenous and nasogastric fluids would also increase gastric secretions, which could contribute to nausea and vomiting.

In the last days of life individuals rarely feel hunger and thirst. Comfort can be achieved by such interventions as moistening mouth and lips. Salivart, which is artificial saliva, can be given as 1–2 sprays in the mouth every hour as needed for comfort.

A major problem that terminal dehydration presents for patients, families, and palliative care providers are the emotional impact that withholding fluids and food has on the family. In most cultures, food and eating is equated with love; withholding food and fluids is considered abandonment. Research has shown that the point in time when patients can no longer eat represents a major life transition and loss for family caregivers (Meares, 1995).

It is essential that nurses assess patients' and families' perceptions about terminal dehydration, and discuss the advantages and disadvantages of each, maintaining an open dialogue about the topic. Nurses should provide families with reading materials which explain the normal physiologic process at end of life, and allow families time to absorb the information. If, despite explanations, families continue to be uncomfortable with a decision to withhold food and fluids, the option of intravenous or subcutaneous therapy may be offered. Intravenous or subcutaneous fluid could be given at a rate not to exceed 1–1.5 liters per day, using Furosemide as needed to control symptoms of over-hydration (Waller & Caroline, 1996).

CONCLUSION

To prevent suffering near death, clients need to be consistently assessed for signs and symptoms of distress such as pain, dyspnea, anxiety, agitation, nausea and vomiting, fatigue, and constipation. Systematic assessment of these symptoms and evaluation of the effect of treatment can be accomplished using a symptom-specific tool measuring level of intensity or a flow sheet as found in Table 10.1. Table 10.2 outlines interventions to relieve distressing symptoms that people approaching the end of their life may experience. The occurrence of dyspnea, nausea and vomiting, agitation, and altered cognition requires ongoing treatment to prevent escalation of symptoms and to maintain client comfort near death.

Treatment of symptoms near death should ideally be directed at the cause of the symptom. When the cause cannot be identified or eliminated, the goal is changed to treating the symptom itself. Successful interventions reduce or eliminate the symptom. Algorithms or protocols developed by palliative care providers are used to guide pharmacological treatment of symptoms near death. Protocols should be used in conjunction with input from the palliative care interdisciplinary teams, to ensure that assessments are comprehensive, and that all factors contributing to the symptom of distress has been considered.

Inadequate control of symptoms of distress using standard interventions mandates a consult with a palliative care provider to identify other options for symptom management. Changes in medication management should be made as soon as medications are deemed ineffective. Delays in changing medication regimens can cause unnecessary suffering for clients and families. Client and family suffering at the end of life should be perceived by all as unacceptable.

More research is needed regarding the occurrence of symptoms in clients with nonmalignant causes of death. More research is also needed on treatments for dyspnea, anxiety, agitation, and terminal restlessness in the client near death considering the impact of the environment on the symptom, availability of resources, access to care, and family caregiver experiences treating and experiencing symptoms of distress near death.

TABLE 10.2 Symptom Management

Medications	Indications
Dyspnea	
Step 1	
Opiods—	Sensation of breathlessness
Morphine sulfate—	Pulmonary congestion
PO/SL/SC/IV	
Starting dose 5 mg–10 mg PO/SL if patient opiod naïve. Repeat q 2 hours prn.	
For patients taking opiods for pain, increase MS04 by 50% their usual breakthrough dose	
Step 2 as indicated by clinical findings:	
Diuretics	Pulmonary congestion (seen with cardiac dysfunction and/or fluid volume overload)
Furosemide (Lasix)	
IM/IV (20–40 mg +)	
Bronchodilators	Bronchoconstriction/spasm
Albuterol	
or Ipratropium bromide	
Inhalation	
Corticoster oids IV/SC	For inflammation within and exterior to lung (e.g., Superior vena cava syndrome; lymphagitis carcinomatosis)
Dexamethasone	
(Decadron)	
Antibiotics	Respiratory distress likely due to infection, manifested by copious secretions
Erythromycin PO	
Anticholinergics Hyoscyamine	Secretions
(Levsin) 0.125–.25 mg q 6 hr	
PO/SL prn	
Scopolamine	
(transdermal)	
Atropine 1–2 mg IM/SC/or	
Inhalation	
Anxiolytics	Sense of breathlessness, anxiety, fear
(Sedatives)	
Benzodiazepines—Sedatives of choice	
Lorazepam 0.5 mg	
PO/SL q 4 hours PRN or ATC	
or	
Phenothiazines	
Chlorpromazine hydrochloride	
(Thorazine) Or haloperidol (Haldol)	
Mucolytic agents	Thick secretions
Nebulized saline	

TABLE 10.2   *(continued)*

Medications	Indications
Nausea/Vomiting	
Phenothia zines	Nausea/vomiting of any etiology
Prochlorperazine (Compazine) PR/IV/ PO	
GI Stimulant	Incomplete or high GI obstruction or
Metoclopramide (Reglan) PR/IV/PO/Trouche	Chronic nausea of unknown etiology
Compounds	Severe nausea or vomiting
ABHR (Ativan [Lorazepam], Benadryl [Diphenhydramine], Haldol [Haloperidol], and Reglan [Metochlopramide]	
Corticosteroids	Nausea/vomiting r/t increased intra-
Dexamethasone (Decadron) PO/PR/IV	cranial pressure, gastrointestinal obstruction, hypercalcemia, and uremia.
Anxiety	
Opiods	Signs and symptoms of discomfort
Morphine sulfate (liquid) PO/SL or PR.	
Benzodiazepines	Anxiety, restlessness, or myoclonus
Lorazepam (Ativan) SL or Alprazolam (Xanax)	
Diazepam (Valium) PR	Anxiety, restlessness, or myoclonus
Clonazepam (Klonopin) SC	Myoclonus
Midazolam (Versed) IV/SC	Reserved for terminal agitation that does not respond to more commonly used Benzodiazepines and barbiturates
Barbiturates	When Benzodiazepines fail to control
Phenobarbital PR	anxiety.
or Pentobarbital	Myoclonus.
or Secobarbital	Seizures prevention.
Thiopental and Propofol	Reserved for use in extraordinary cases of agitation, where sedation is needed for comfort.
Neuroleptics	Hallucinations or paranoia
Haloperidol (Haldol) PO/SC	
Chlorpromazine (Thorazine) PO/PR	Terminal restlessness

(continued)

TABLE 10.2   *(continued)*

Medications	Indications
Constipation	
Oral Laxative	In patient taking opiods
Senna with stool softener PO	
Milk of Magnesia (MOM)	If senna not effective
Lactulose, Magnesium Citrate, or Fleet Phospho-Soda PO	If MOM not effective
Ducolax suppositories or Fleet enema	Stool in rectum, or if constipation with nausea/vomiting
Oil retention enema	Stool impaction

Education Plan 10.1 Plan for Achieving Competencies: Symptom Management in Palliative Care

Knowledge Needed	Attitude	Skills	Undergraduate Behavioral Outcomes	Graduate Behavioral Outcomes	Teaching/Learning Strategies
The need for symptom management at the end of life.	*Accept the pivotal role of nurses in symptom management at the end of life.		*Address symptom management in patients' plan of care.	*Advocate for aggressive symptom management for patients and family at the end of life.	*Evaluate case studies for evidence of effective or ineffective symptom management.
Symptom Assessment: —Dyspnea —Nausea and Vomiting —Anxiety —Altered Cognition —Constipation —Intestinal Obstruction —Fatigue —Terminal Dehydration	*Accept that symptoms are what the patient says they are.	*Perform a comprehensive assessment to determine symptoms at the end of life, utilizing various measurement instruments.	*Accurately identifies symptoms and related suffering of patients and family at the end of life.	*Utilize advanced knowledge to diagnose complex symptoms and related suffering of patients and family at the end of life.	*Utilize case studies to identify symptoms and suffering issues at the end of life for patients and family. *Assess patients in clinical setting, and utilize measurement instruments to identify symptoms and suffering experienced at the end of life. Present findings during post-conference or interdisciplinary team meetings.

357

Education Plan 10.1 *(continued)*

Knowledge Needed	Attitude	Skills	Undergraduate Behavioral Outcomes	Graduate Behavioral Outcomes	Teaching/Learning Strategies
Pharmacological and Nonpharmacological Management of Symptoms and Suffering: —Dyspnea —Nausea and Vomiting —Anxiety —Altered Cognition —Constipation —Intestinal Obstruction —Fatigue —Terminal Dehydration	*Recognize and suspend practitioner bias related to pharmacological and non-pharmacological interventions. *Value the role of the interdisciplinary team and the potential need for consultation with other experts.	*Administer optimal treatment for the management of symptoms and suffering. *Guide pharmacological treatment of symptoms utilizing established protocols and algorithms developed by palliative care providers.	*Provide optimal symptom management and relief of suffering based on prescribed plan of care or through consultation with members of other disciplines.	*Prescribe a plan of care, utilizing pharmacological and non-pharmacological modalities to alleviate symptoms and suffering of patients and family at the end of life. *Collaborate with other disciplines when needed for optimal symptom management.	*Present a clinical experience to peers in post-conference or seminar, for critique of the plan of care as related to symptom management. *Evaluate case studies for the effectiveness of interventions. *Using case studies, identify appropriate pharmacological and non-pharmacological interventions.

REFERENCES

American Thoracic Society (1978). Recommended respiratory disease questionnaires for use with adults and children in epidemiological research. *American Review of Respiratory Disease, 14*(7), 53.

Back, I. N. (1992). Terminal restlessness in patients with advanced malignant disease. *Palliative Medicine, 6,* 293–298.

Booth, S., Kely, M. J., Cox, N. P., Adams, L., & Guz, A. (1996). Does oxygen therapy help dyspnea in patients with cancer? *American Journal of Respiratory Critical Cared Medicine, 153,* 1515–1518.

Brescia, F. J., Adler, D., Gray, G., Ryan, M. A., Cimino, J., & Mamtini, R. (1990). Hospitalized advanced cancer patients: A profile. *Journal of Pain and Symptom Management, 5*(4), 221–227.

Bruera, E., de Stoutz, N., Velasco-Leiva, A., Schoeller, T., & Hanson, J. (1993). Effects of oxygen on dyspnea in hypoxemic terminal-cancer patients. *Lancet, 342,* 13–14.

Bruera, E., Macmillan, T., Pither, J., & MacDonald, N. (1990). Effects of morphine on the dyspnea of terminal cancer patients. *Journal of Pain and Symptom Management, 5,* 341–344.

Bruera, E., Schoeller, T., & MacEachern, T. (1992). Symptomatic benefit of Supplemental oxygen in hypoxemic patients with terminal cancer: The use of the N of 1 randomized controlled trial. *Journal of Pain and Symptom Management, 7,* 365–368.

Burke, A. (1997). Palliative care: An update in "terminal restlessness." *Medical Journal of Australia, 166*(1), 39–42.

Coluzzi, P. H. (1998). Sublingual morphine: Efficacy reviewed. *Journal of Pain and Symptom Management, 16,* 187–192.

Coluzzi, P. H., & Fairbairn, B. S. (1999). The management of pain in terminally ill cancer patients with difficulty swallowing. *American Journal of Hospice & Palliative Care, 16,* 731–737.

Coyle, N., Adelhardt, J., Foley, K., & Portenoy, R. K. (1990). Character of terminal illness in the advanced cancer patient: Pain and other symptoms during the last four weeks of life. *Journal of Pain and Symptom Management, 5,* 83–93.

Curtis, A. E., & Fernsler, J. I. (1989). Quality of life of oncology hospice patients: A comparison of patient and primary caregiver reports. *Oncology Nursing Forum, 16,* 49–53.

deStoutz, N. D., Bruera, E., & Suarez-Almazor (1995). Opiod rotation for toxicity reduction in terminal cancer patients. *Journal of Pain and Symptom Management, 10,* 378–384.

Dworkin, B. M. (1992). Gastrointestinal manifestations of AIDS. In G. P. Wormser (Ed.), *AIDS and other manifestations of HIV infection* (2nd ed.) (pp. 419–432). New York: Raven Press.

Escalante, C. P., Martin, C. G., Eltin, L. S., Cantor, S. B., Harle, T. S., Price, K. J., Kish, S. K., Manzullo, E. F., & Rubenstein, E. B. (1996). Dyspnea in cancer patients: Etiology,resource utilization, and survival-implications in a managed care world. *Cancer, 78,* 1314–1319.

Fainsinger, R. L., MacEachern, T., Hanson, J., & Bruera, E. (1992). The use of urinary catheters in terminally ill cancer patients. *Journal of Pain and Symptom Management, 7,* 333–338.

Fainsinger, R., Miller, M. J., Bruera, E., Hanson, J., & Maceachern, T. (1991). Symptom control during the last week of life on a palliative care unit. *Journal of Palliative Care, 7*(1), 5–11.

Fanslow, C. A. (1984). Touch and the elderly. In C. C. Brown (Ed.), *The many facets of touch* (pp. 183–189). Skillman, NJ: Johnson & Johnson.

Fields, M., & Cassell, C. (1997). *Approaching death: Improving care at the end of life.* Washington, DC: National Academy Press.

Folstein, M. F. (1983). The mini-mental state examination. In T. Crooke, S. Rerris, & R. Bartus (Eds.), *Assessment in geriatric psychopathology* (pp. 47–51). New Canaan, CT.

Gavrin, J., & Chapman, C. R. (1995). Clinical management of dying patients. In Caring for patients at the end of life [Special Issue]. *Western Journal of Medicine, 163,* 268–277.

Harwood, K. V. (1999). Dyspnea. In C. H. Yarbro, M. H. Frogge, & M. Goodman (Eds.), *Cancer symptom management* (2nd ed.) (pp. 45–57). Boston: Jones and Bartlett.

Hospice and Palliative Nurses Association (1996). *Clinical practice protocol: Dyspnea.* Pittsburgh, PA: Hospice and Palliative Nurses Association.

Hospice and Palliative Nurses Association (1997). *Clinical practice protocol: Terminal restlessness.* Pittsburgh, PA: Hospice and Palliative Nurses Association.

James, K. (1998). In M. Snyder & R. Lindquist (Eds.), *Complementary/alternative therapies in nursing,* (3rd ed.) (pp. 139–147). New York: Springer.

Kazanowski, M. (1996, June). *Review of the literature on symptoms near death in patients with terminal cancer.* Paper presented at conference on research-based clinical practice. Dartmouth-Hitchcock Medical Center and Saint Anselm College, Nashua, NH.

Kazanowski, M. (1999). Loss, death, and dying. In D. Ignatavicius, M. L. Workman, & M. A. Mishler, *Medical-Surgical nursing across the health care continuum* (3rd ed.) (pp. 173–184). Philadelphia: W. B. Saunders.

Lareau, S. C., Carrieri-Kohlman, V., Janson-Bjerklie, S., & Roos, P. J. (1994). Development and testing of the Pulmonary Functional Status and Dyspnea Questionnaire (PFSDQ). *Heart and Lung, 23,* 242–250.

Lareau, S., Kohlman-Carrieri, V., Janson-Bjerklie, S., & Roos, P. J. (1986). Functional levels and dyspnea in patients with COPD. *American Review of Respiratory Disease, 133,* 163A.

Levy, M. (1997). *Symptom control in advanced cancer.* Australia: Pharmacia & Upjohn.

Levy, M. (1999, October 28). *Sedation in palliative care: Walking an ever-fine line.* 1999 Annual Conference New Hampshire Cancer Pain Initiative and New Hampshire Hospice Organization, Portsmouth, NH.

Liss, H. P., & Grant, B. J. B. (1988). The effect of nasal flow on breathlessness in patients with chronic obstructive pulmonary disease. *American Review of Respiratory Disease, 137,* 1285–1288.

Mahler, D. A., Weinberg, D. H., Wells, C. R., & Feinstein, A. R. (1984). The measurement of dyspnea: Contents, interobserver agreement, and physiologic correlates of two new clinical indexes. *Chest, 85,* 751–758.

Management of Cancer Pain Guideline Panel (1994). *Management of cancer pain: Clinical practice guidelines,* AHCPR Pub. No. 94-0592, Rockville, MD: Agency for Health Care Policy and Research, Public Health Service, U.S. Department of Health and Human Services.

March, P. A. (1998). Terminal restlessness. *American Journal of Hospice & Palliative Care, 15*(1), 51–53.

Masters, M., & Shontz, F. C. (1989). Identification of problems and strengths of the hospice client by clients, caregivers, and nurses. *Cancer Nursing, 12,* 226–235.

McMillan, S. C. (1996a). Quality of life of primary caregivers of hospice patients with cancer. *Cancer Practice, 4,* 191–198.

McMillan, S. C. (1996b). The quality of life of patients with cancer receiving hospice care. *Oncology Nursing Forum, 23,* 1221–1228.

McMillan, S. C., & Mahon, M. (1994a). Measuring quality of life in hospice patients using a newly developed Hospice Quality of Life Index. *Quality of Life Research, 3,* 437–447.

McMillan, S. C., & Mahon, M. (1994b). The impact of hospice services on the quality of life of primary caregivers. *Oncology Nursing Forum, 21,* 1189–1195.

Meares, C. J. (1994, May/June). Terminal dehydration: A review. *American Journal of Hospice & Palliative Care,* 10–14.

Meares, C. J. (1995). The Dinnerhour and other losses: Caring for a hospice patient who ceased nutrition. (Doctoral dissertation, Boston College, Chestnut Hill, MA, 1995). *Dissertation Abstracts International, 56*(10), 5420.

Morita, T., Tsunoda, J., Inoue, S., & Chihara, S. (1999). Perceptions and decision-making on rehydration of terminally ill cancer patients and family members. *American Journal of Hospice & Palliative Care, 16,* 509–516.

Musgrave, C. F. (1990). Terminal dehydration: To give or not to give intravenous fluids. *Cancer Nursing, 13*(1), 62–66.

Nursing Drug Handbook (2000). Philadelphia: Saunders.

Paice, J. (1999). Pain. In C. H. Yarbro, M. H. Frogge, & M. Goodman (Eds.), *Cancer symptom management* (2nd ed.) (pp. 118–147). Boston: Jones and Bartlett.

Petrin, R. (1998). The symptom relief kit for hospice patients. *International Journal of Pharmaceutical Compounding*, *2*(2), 116–117.

Printz (1992). Terminal dehydration, a compassionate treatment. *Archives of Internal Medicine*, *152*(4), 697–700.

Ream, E., & Richardson, A. (1999). From theory to practice: Designing interventions to reduce fatigue in patients with cancer. *Oncology Nursing Forum*, *26*, 1295–1303.

Robinson, C. B., Fritch, M., Hullett, L., Petersen, M. A., Sikkema, S., Theuninck, L., & Timmer, K. (2000). Development of a protocol to prevent opiod-induced constipation in patients with cancer: A research utilization project. *Clinical Journal of Oncology Nursing*, *4*, 79–84.

Sjogren, P., Jonsson, T., Jensen, N., Drenck, N., & Jensen, T. (1993). Hyperalgesia and myoclonus in terminal cancer patients treated with continuous intravenous morphine. *Pain*, *55*, 93–97.

Snyder, M., & Lindquist, R. (1998). *Complementary/Alternative therapies in nursing* (3rd ed.). New York: Springer.

Stoller, J., Ferranti, R., & Feinstein, A. (1986). Further specification and evaluation of a new index for dyspnea. *American Review of Respiratory Disease*, *134*, 129–134.

Waller, A., & Caroline, N. L. (1996). *Handbook of palliative care in cancer*. Newton, MA: Butterworth-Heinemann.

Weitzner, M. A., Moody, L. N., & McMillan, S. C. (1997). Symptom management issues in hospice care. *American Journal of Hospice & Palliative Care*, *14*, 190–195.

Wrede-Seaman, L. (1996). *Symptom management algorithms for palliative care*. Yakima, WA: Intellicard.

Zerwekh, J. V. (1983, January). The dehydration question. *Nursing*, 47–51.

11

Pain Assessment and Management in Palliative Care

Nessa Coyle and Mary Layman-Goldstein

AACN Competencies

 # 2: Promote the provision of comfort care to the dying as an active, desirable, and important skill, and an integral component of nursing care.

 # 9: Evaluate the impact of traditional, complementary, and technological therapies on patient-centered outcomes.

In a recent survey to evaluate end of life content in a sample of nursing textbooks, virtually no information was found regarding pain at the end of life (Ferrell, Virani, & Grant, 1999). The intent of this chapter is to provide nurses with up-to-date information on pain assessment and management at end of life. The chapter is divided into three sections. Section One addresses pain assessment and a pharmacologic approach to management. Section Two addresses integration of nondrug interventions into a comprehensive pain management plan. Section Three highlights the needs of special populations including the elderly, the communication impaired, those with a history of substance abuse, and pediatrics. The norm in working with patients in pain at the end of life is to combine the pharmacologic with the nondrug approaches.

SECTION 1: PAIN ASSESSMENT AND PHARMACOLOGIC INTERVENTIONS

Few things are of more concern to patients at end of life and to their families than that pain will be well controlled. In the words of one patient, "It is not dying that I'm afraid of—but how to get from A to D (alive to dead)—I don't want to suffer." Unrelieved pain can consume the attention and energy of those who are dying, and create an atmosphere of impotency and despair in their families and caretakers.

The fear of unrelieved pain, expressed by patients and their families, is sadly often reflective of what they have or will experience (Lynn, Teno, Phillips, Wu, & Desbiens, 1997; SUPPORT, 1995; VonRoenn, Cleeland, Gonin, Hatfield, & Pandya, 1993). This fear has been one of the driving forces for the national movement to legalize physician-assisted suicide in the terminally ill (Foley, 1991). And yet, with the knowledge and art that is now available, we have the ability to relieve the majority of pain including pain at the end of life (Jacox et al., 1994). In few areas has the emerging role of the advanced practice nurse had a greater impact on quality of life for the dying and their family than in pain management.

Cancer is a useful model in which to review pain assessment and management at the end of life. Cancer is the second leading cause of death in the United States (American Cancer Society, 1999), and is frequently associated with significant pain (Lynn et al., 1997; Morris, Mor, Goldberg, Sherwood, Greer, 1986; SUPPORT, 1995). The assessment and management of cancer pain will be used as the framework for this chapter.

BARRIERS

Physicians, patients, and the general public, through a series of surveys have defined the numerous barriers that interfere with adequate pain management (Cherny & Catane, 1995; Cleeland et al., 1994; Foley, 1998; Gonzales & Coyle, 1992; Grossman et al., 1991; Jacox et al., 1994; Levin, Cleeland, & Dar, 1985; Von Roenn, Cleeland, Gonin, Hatfield, & Pandya, 1993). These barriers have been broadly characterized as patient related, physician related, and institution related. The patient-related barriers include: (1) reluctance to report pain; (2) reluctance to follow treatment recommendations; (3) fears of tolerance and addiction; (4) concern about treatment related side-effects; (5) fears regarding disease progression; and (6) belief that pain is an inevitable part of cancer and must be accepted. In a study by Ward et al. (1993), which evaluated these patient-related barriers, a higher level of concern was associated with the elderly, the less educated, and those with lower incomes and was correlated with under-medication of pain.

Closely related to patient-related barriers are clinician-related issues. Surveys have demonstrated the failure of clinicians to evaluate or appreciate the severity of the pain problem (Grossman et al., 1991; Von Roenn et al., 1993; Wallace, Reade, Pasero, & Olsson, 1995). It is suggested that inaccurate assessment of the severity of a patient's pain is a major predictor of inadequacy of relief. Unless it is acknowledged that the expert on determination of the severity of the pain and adequacy of pain relief is the person who is experiencing it, then inadequate pain control is likely to continue.

Institutional-related barriers to adequate control of pain include: lack of visibility of pain, lack of a common language to describe pain, lack of commitment to pain management as a priority, and failure to use validated pain measurement tools in clinical practice (Bookbinder et al., 1995; Foley, 1998; Max et al., 1995). Economic factors and legal restrictions to drug prescribing and drug availability are further impediments to adequate pain treatment (Foley, 1998; Joranson, Cleeland, & Weisman, 1992; Max et al., 1995).

To address these various barriers, specific programs have been developed that focus on making pain visible within an institution. For example, incorporating a pain measurement tool into institutional daily clinical practice thereby making pain the fifth vital sign (Figure 11.1), and introducing broad educational efforts to change attitudes, behaviors, and knowledge deficits in patients, clinicians, and institutions (Bookbinder et al., 1995). The use of continuous quality improvement (CQI) programs have been demonstrated to be effective in providing the framework for initiatives for change (Bookbinder et al., 1995).

BASIC PRINCIPLES OF PAIN ASSESSMENT AT THE END OF LIFE

Pain is defined as "an unpleasant sensory and emotional experience associated with actual or potential tissue damage or described in terms of such damage. Pain is always subjective . . . " (International Association for the Study of Pain, 1979). The patient is the expert on the severity of his or her pain and the adequacy of relief obtained. The interdisciplinary team's expertise is in identifying the different etiologies of the pain and arriving at effective management strategies. Although verbal report of pain and adequacy of pain relief is considered the gold standard, some individuals at end of life are unable to communicate verbally (American Pain Society, 1999; Twycross & Lichter, 1998). Other behavioral measures for assessing pain are therefore required. For example, patients who are semiconscious

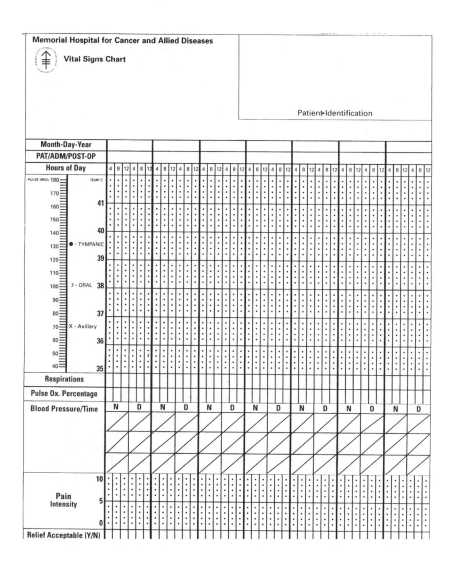

FIGURE 11.1 Pain as the fifth vital sign.

From Bookbinder, M., et al. (1995). Improving pain management practices. In D. B. McGuire, C. H. Yarbro, & B. R. Ferrell (Eds.), *Cancer pain management* (2nd ed., p. 347). Boston: Jones and Bartlett. (Reprinted with permission.)

or in a coma may moan or cry out or exhibit other signs of distress when moved. Although these behaviors are not necessarily associated with pain, the likelihood of pain should be strongly considered. If the decision is made to medicate the patient for pain, subsequent signs of diminished distress on movement would indicate that pain had been present. If such a patient had been on an analgesic regimen prior to diminution of consciousness, analgesics should be continued or increased until the patient shows signs of comfort.

Assessment of pain at end of life is often complicated by the presence of multiple other symptoms including cognitive impairment, common in the last few days of life (Coyle, Adelhardt, Foley, & Portenoy, 1990; Curtis, Krech, & Walsh, 1991; Portenoy et al., 1994). In addition, the suffering that patients experience at the end of life is not necessarily related to the severity of the symptom. Mild symptoms may cause considerable distress especially in the individual who has not yet come to terms with dying (Twycross & Lichter, 1998). Unrelieved pain, however, can deprive a patient and their family of interaction at the end of life around anything other than pain. A time of potential growth, communication, and reconciliation can be lost. Nurses have an extraordinary responsibility to be patient advocates in the assessment and management of pain throughout the course of a disease process, but especially at the end of life (American Nurses' Association, 1990).

Because of its complexity, the assessment of pain requires a multidimensional and interdisciplinary approach (Ingham & Coyle, 1997). The tissue damage response leading to the complaint of pain, the suffering component of the pain, and the meaning of the pain to the individual and their family all need to be addressed. Although this comprehensive pain assessment is usually interdisciplinary, it is the nurse who brings that assessment and plan to the bedside. The assessment of pain is carried out within the framework of goals of care, knowledge of the disease process, and nearness of the individual to death.

TYPES OF PAIN—NEUROPHYSIOLOGICAL MECHANISMS OF PAIN

Three types of pain, *somatic*, *visceral*, and *neuropathic*, are described based on their neurophysiological mechanisms (Foley, 1996, 1998; Portenoy, 1992). Understanding these basic mechanisms is a necessary background for the nurse to arrive at a reasoned analgesic management approach.

Somatic or *nociceptive* pain occurs as a result of activating pain sensitive structures or nociceptors in the cutaneous and deep musculoskeletal tissues. This pain is typically well localized and may be felt in the superficial cutaneous or deeper musculoskeletal structures. Examples of somatic pain include bone metastases, postsurgical incisional pain, and pain accompanying myofascial or musculoskeletal inflammation or spasm (Payne & Gonzales, 1998). Somatic pain is responsive to the nonsteroidal anti-inflammatory drugs and to the opioid drugs.

Visceral pain results from infiltration, compression, distension, or stretching of thoracic or abdominal viscera (e.g., liver metastases or pancreatic cancer). This type of pain is poorly localized, often described as deep, squeezing, pressure, and may be associated with nausea, vomiting, and diaphoresis (especially when acute). Visceral pain is often referred to cutaneous sites which may be remote from the site of the lesion, for example, shoulder pain associated with diaphragmatic irritation. Tenderness and pain on touching the referral cutaneous site may occur. Visceral pain is responsive to the nonsteroidal anti-inflammatory drugs and to the opioid drugs (Payne & Gonzales, 1998).

Neuropathic pain results from injury to the peripheral and/or central nervous systems. In the cancer patient, neuropathic pain most commonly occurs as a consequence of tumor compressing or infiltrating peripheral nerves, nerve roots or the spinal cord. In addition, surgical trauma, chemical or radiation-induced injury to peripheral nerves or the spinal cord from cancer therapies may result in this type of pain. Examples of common neuropathic pain include metastatic or radiation-induced brachial or lumbosacral plexopathies, epidural spinal cord and/or cauda-equina compression, postherpetic neuralgia and painful chemotherapy-induced neuropathy. Neuropathic pain is often described as having sharp, shooting, electric shocklike qualities which are unfamiliar to the patient. It can also be described as a constant dull ache, sometimes with a pressure or viselike quality with episodic paroxysms of burning and/or electric shocklike sensations. Neuropathic pain is often severe, very distressing to the patient, and sometimes difficult to control. Although partially responsive to the nonsteroidal anti-inflammatory drugs and to the opioid drugs, neuropathic pain is also responsive to adjuvant drugs such as antidepressants, anticonvulsants, and local anesthetics (Elliot & Foley, 1988; Payne & Gonzales, 1998).

TEMPORAL PATTERN OF PAIN

Pain can also be defined on a temporal basis, for example, acute pain and chronic pain. Patients at the end of life can have a combination of both acute and chronic pain (Cherny & Portenoy, 1994; Foley, 1998; Merskey, 1986).

Acute pain is characterized by a well-defined pattern of onset. Generally the cause of the pain can be identified and frequently the pain is accompanied by physiological signs of hyperactivity of the central nervous system such as a rapid pulse and elevated blood pressure. Acute pain usually has a precipitating cause, for example, small bowel obstruction, a painful dressing change, or a pathological fracture. The pain tends to be time limited and responds to analgesic drug therapy, and where possible, treatment of the precipitating cause. Acute pain can be further subdivided into subacute pain and intermittent or episodic types (Foley, 1998). Subacute pain describes pain that comes on over several days, often with increasing intensity, and may be associated with a variety of causes such as a progressive pathological process or an analgesic regimen that has not been titrated upward to accommodate for a progressive painful disease process. Episodic pain refers to pain that occurs during defined periods of time, on a regular or irregular basis (Foley, 1998). Intermittent pain is an alternative way to describe episodic pain. Such pain may be associated with movement, dressing changes, or other activities. Because the trigger for intermittent pain can often be identified, the nurse, through appropriate use of analgesics prior to the pain-provoking event, can have a significant impact on decreasing these painful episodes for the patient. The fear of pain associated with these activities is therefore lessened for the patient.

Chronic pain differs from acute pain in its representation. These differences are essential for the nurse to assess as patients with chronic pain are at risk to have their pain unrecognized, untreated, or undertreated. Chronic pain is defined as pain that persists for more than three months (Foley, 1998). Adaptation of the autonomic system occurs and the patient does not exhibit the objective signs of pain found so frequently in those with acute pain (e.g., there is no rapid pulse or elevated blood pressure). Poorly relieved chronic pain at the end of life can contribute to fatigue, depression, insomnia, general despair, withdrawal from interaction with others, and desire for death (Ferrell, Rhiner, Cohen, & Grant, 1991; Coyle, 1992, 1995).

Breakthrough pain is a more recent classification within the various types of pain. Breakthrough pain is defined as a transient increase in pain to greater than moderate intensity, occurring on a baseline pain of moderate intensity or less (Portenoy & Hagen, 1990). Breakthrough pain has a diversity of characteristics. In some patients, for example, it is characterized by marked worsening of pain at the end of the dosing interval of regularly scheduled analgesics. In other patients it occurs by the action of the patient or the nurse, for example, when turning or having a dressing change, and is referred to as incident pain. Patients frequently have a combination of these different types of pain; noting the patterns of pain in a particular individual is an essential component of pain assessment. Attention to such details is the essence of symptom control at the end of life. A pain diary or log, kept by the patient or family, can help identify the pattern of pain. The log can indicate, over the course of the day, the patient's rating of pain, medication taken, activity level, and any other pain relief measures tried (McCaffery & Beebe, 1989). Additional information on this intervention is included in Section Two.

CLINICAL ASSESSMENT OF PAIN

The previously described mechanisms of pain, and types of pain that can be experienced by patients towards the end of life, are a useful background from which to start a clinical pain assessment. The clinical assessment is based on a process of both observation and interview. The basic principles of a pain assessment are outlined in Table 11.1. Taking a history of the pain complaint involves the following parameters:

Onset

When did the pain begin? Was it associated with a particular activity or known medical event? Did other symptoms accompany the onset of pain such as nausea or vomiting?

Site(s)

Ask the patient to point to the site or sites of pain. Frequently individuals with cancer have multiple sites of pain. Each site needs to be assessed as the management approach may differ depending on the etiology of the pain (Grond, Zech, Diefenbach, Radbruch, & Lehmann, 1996; Twycross & Lack, 1983).

Quality of the Pain

Have the patient describe the quality of the pain. Word descriptors used by patients to describe their pain help the clinician to arrive at an inferred pain mechanism. This in turn influences the choice of pharmacotherapy. For example, sharp, shooting, electric shock description of pain, often described by the patient as being "unfamiliar," suggests a neuropathic component to the pain (Elliot & Foley, 1988). Such pain may be responsive to the adjuvant drugs as well as to opioid analgesics.

Severity of the Pain

Have the patient describe the severity of the pain. It is particularly important that the nurse recognizes the significance of escalating pain within the

TABLE 11.1   Clinical Assessment of Pain: Basic Principles

- Believe the patient's complaint of pain. The patient is the expert on the pain being experienced. The multidisciplinary staff are the experts in determining the etiology of the pain.
- Take a careful history of the pain complaint and place it within the context of the patient's medical history and goals of care. If the patient is unable to communicate verbally, obtain a history from those most involved in the patient's care, both family and formal health care providers.
- Observe the patient for nonverbal communication regarding pain, for example, guarding, wincing, and moaning, or crying out when turned or moved.
- Recognize that the patient near the end of life may have multiple symptoms complicating pain assessment.
- Assess the characteristics of each pain, including the site, pattern of referral, what makes it better and what makes it worse, and the impact of the pain on the individual's activity of daily living and quality of life; for example, mood, sleep, movement, and interaction with others.
- Clarify the temporal aspects and pattern of the patient's pain; for example, acute, chronic, baseline, intermittent, breakthrough, or incident.
- Assess the psychological state of the patient and the meaning of the pain to the patient and their family.
- Examine the site of the pain.
- Facilitate an appropriate diagnostic work-up making sure that the patient's pain is adequately managed during the work-up.
- Provide continuity of care for the patient and family during ongoing pain assessment and management.
- Assess and reassess the effectiveness of the pain management regimen both for baseline pain and breakthrough pain.
- Give a time frame where you would expect to see evidence of patient comfort after the start or adjustment of a pain management approach. If this is not evident, reassess the patient. Ongoing reassessment is essential in the setting of a complex patient with multiple symptoms.
- Assess and reassess for the presence of adverse side effects from the pain management regimen.

construct of that particular patient's disease process, value system, goals of care, and nearness to death. Treatment decisions take all of these factors into account. For measuring severity of the pain a variety of tools are available for use in clinical practice (DeConno et al., 1994; Fishman et al., 1986; Jacox et al., 1994). These include numerical estimates, for example, 0 indicating no pain and 10 indicating the worst pain imaginable; word descriptors such as none, mild, moderate, and severe (Wallenstein, Rogers, Kaiko, & Houde, 1986); visual analogue scales where a 10 centimeter line is anchored at one end by no pain and the other end by the worst possible pain (Ahles, Ruckdeschel, & Blanchard, 1984); and happy/sad faces (McGrath, 1990).

Numerical estimates are the most frequently used method of assessing severity of pain and adequacy of pain relief (Bookbinder et al., 1995). Some patients, however, cannot use a numerical estimate and one of the other tools may be more appropriate. It is important that the staff be consistent in using a particular assessment tool with an individual patient so that communication regarding that patient's pain management is enhanced.

Assess Pain Severity at Times of Different Activity

Pain intensity should be assessed at rest, on movement, and in relation to daily activity and the patient's analgesic schedule. Asking questions such as: "How much pain is relieved when you take the pain medication?" "How long does the relief last?" and "Are side effects present?" helps establish if the appropriate drug has been selected, dose efficacy, and if the time interval between doses for this patient is correct. A more global 24-hour assessment of the adequacy of pain management in general includes asking the patient their pain scores—"right now," "at its best," "at its worst," and "on average" (Daut, Cleeland, & Flanery, 1983).

Exacerbating and Relieving Factors

Identifying factors that increase or relieve the patient's pain can be helpful both in arriving at a pain diagnosis and in giving the nurse the opportunity to reinforce techniques that the patient has found useful in the past to relieve pain. A patient with cancer who reports rapidly escalating back pain, with a bandlike quality, which is worse when lying in bed and better when standing, is considered to have cord compression until proved otherwise (Posner, 1995). Early recognition of cord compression and treatment, frequently by steroids and/or radiation therapy, may prevent paraplegia in the last few weeks or months of a patient's life. Escalating back pain may be the only sign of the impending cord compression. To reiterate, it is imperative that the nurse caring for a patient at the end of life recognizes the significance of escalating pain within the construct of that particular patient's disease process and goals of care.

Impact of the Pain on the Patient's Psychological State

The interface between pain and suffering has been well defined (Cherny & Coyle, 1994; Cherny & Portenoy, 1994; Fishman, 1991; Foley, 1991). In clinical situations, when patients are asked, "What does this pain mean to you?", What do you think is causing the pain?", a flood of suffering and fear is often expressed. Patients are fearful of what their dying will be like, of uncontrolled and agonizing pain, of being a burden on their family, and of being "drugged out" on morphine. The same questions are asked by the patient and family time and time again, and need to be responded to in a sensitive, accurate, and reassuring manner. Some clinicians, when meeting a patient in severe pain for the first time, ask if the pain has ever been so bad that the individual has thought of harming him or herself. Again, the response may indicate that suicide has been considered as an option if the pain is not controlled or if things get "too bad." These are important questions for an experienced clinician to ask, so that the patient's vulnerabilities and anxieties are verbalized, suicide vulnerability factors identified, and education and support from other members of the interdisciplinary pain team including psychiatrists and social workers mobilized (Cherny & Coyle, 1994; Cherney & Portenoy, 1994; Foley, 1991).

Pain Treatment History and Responses to Previous and Current Analgesic Regimens

The patient needs to be asked very specifically about what approaches have been used to manage pain in the past, both pharmacological (including over-the-counter medication), and nonpharmacological, and how effective those approaches have been. Included should be analgesics that have been previously prescribed, dosages, time intervals, routes of administration, effects, side effects, and the reasons why a particular approach was discontinued. Fear of recurrence of previously experienced side effects (e.g., sedation, nausea, mental haziness, and constipation) may make a patient reluctant to start a new analgesic regimen. Focusing attention on their concerns and a clear explanation of how side effects will be managed if they do occur, can do much to allay these fears. This is a commitment that will require close monitoring of the patient's response to therapy and a rapid response to the management of any adverse side effects should they occur.

Examine the Patient and the Site of the Pain

Examining the site of the pain and possible referral sites may help identify the source of the pain (Foley, 1998). This is always done within knowledge of the patient's disease process, extent of disease, possible referral sites of pain, and goals of care. The source of the pain may be obvious, for example, a distended abdomen associated with bowel obstruction or liver distention, a prior skin eruption with postherpetic neuralgia, a bony deformity or inability to use a limb due to a pathological fracture, or an open fungating infected wound. In other instances, pain may be reproduced when palpating or moving an extremity or when manipulating or palpating the spine. Figure 11.2 gives an example of an initial pain assessment tool.

In the advanced cancer patient, the cause of pain is frequently multifactorial requiring a multimodal approach (Jacox et al., 1994; McGuire, 1995). Whenever possible, within the constraints of nearness to death and goals of care, an attempt is made to treat the cause of the pain as well as the pain itself. The extent of the diagnostic work-up depends on the goals of care, and the likely impact of the results of the diagnostic work-up on the patient's treatment plan and overall quality of life. The benefit to burden ratio to the patient is of uppermost concern and needs to be discussed fully with the patient and family or the patient's health care proxy (Latimer, 1991).

COMPONENTS OF PAIN MANAGEMENT

Pain is a multidimensional experience that involves sensory, affective, cognitive, behavioral, and sociocultural components (McGuire, 1995). Although pharmacotherapy is the foundation of pain management, pharmacotherapy alone will not be an effective approach to pain management at the end of life. A multimodal approach is usually required including attention to the suffering and spiritual or existential component to the patient's pain (Byock, 1997; Cherny & Coyle, 1994; Coyle, 1995; Twycross & Lichter, 1998). In addition, the needs of the family must be addressed. Figures 11.3 and 11.4 illustrate two models which demonstrate the multidimensional nature of pain at the end of life and the multimodal approach to its management.

PHARMACOLOGIC THERAPY

Inadequate knowledge of analgesic pharmacotherapy is one of the most commonly cited reasons for undertreatment of pain (Ferrell et al., 1991; Jacox et al., 1994). Developing expertise in the use of analgesic drugs is an integral part of nursing care at the end of life.

Over a decade ago, an expert committee, convened by the cancer unit of the World Health Organization (WHO), developed a three-step analgesic ladder approach to the selection of drugs for the treatment of cancer pain (WHO, 1990, 1996) (Figure 11.5). The basic principles of analgesic selection developed by this committee apply to pain management at the end of life. Three categories of analgesic drugs are included in the three-step analgesic ladder: nonsteroidal anti-inflammatory drugs (NSAIDs), opioids, and adjuvant analgesics. With a focus on end-of-life care, discussion around these

---

FORM 3.1 Initial Pain Assessment Tool

Date _____

Patient's Name _____ Age _____ Room _____

Diagnosis _____ Physician _____

Nurse _____

1. LOCATION: Patient or nurse mark drawing.

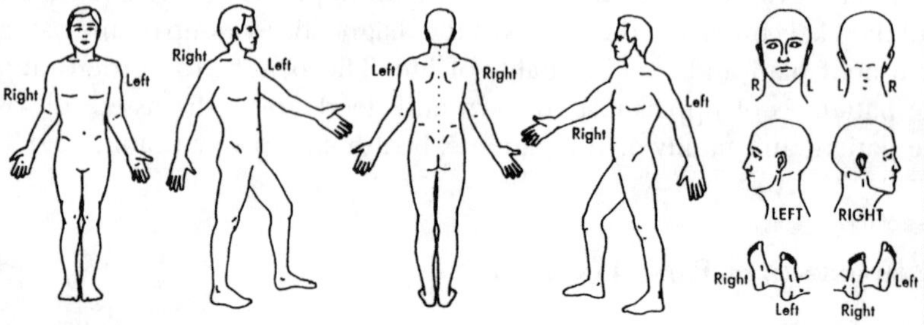

2. INTENSITY: Patient rates the pain. Scale used _____

   Present: _____
   Worst pain gets: _____
   Best pain gets: _____
   Acceptable level of pain: _____

3. QUALITY: (Use patient's own words, e.g., prick, ache, burn, throb, pull, sharp) _____

4. ONSET, DURATION, VARIATIONS, RHYTHMS: _____

5. MANNER OF EXPRESSING PAIN: _____

6. WHAT RELIEVES THE PAIN? _____

7. WHAT CAUSES OR INCREASES THE PAIN? _____

8. EFFECTS OF PAIN: (Note decreased function, decreased quality of life.)
   Accompanying symptoms (e.g., nausea) _____
   Sleep _____
   Appetite _____
   Physical activity _____
   Relationship with others (e.g., irritability) _____
   Emotions (e.g., anger, suicidal, crying) _____
   Concentration _____
   Other _____

9. OTHER COMMENTS: _____

10. PLAN: _____

FIGURE 11.2   Example of an initial pain assessment tool.

From McCaffery, M., & Pasero, C. (1999). *Pain: Clinical Manual* (2nd ed., p. 60). St. Louis: Mosby. (Reprinted with permission.)

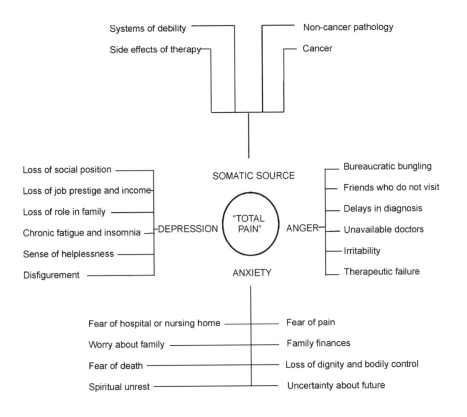

Systems of debility ——————

Side effects of therapy—

Non-cancer pathology

Cancer

Loss of social position ——————

Loss of job prestige and income—

Loss of role in family ——————

Chronic fatigue and insomnia —

Sense of helplessness ——————

Disfigurement ——————

SOMATIC SOURCE

DEPRESSION

"TOTAL PAIN"

ANGER—

ANXIETY

Bureaucratic bungling

Friends who do not visit

Delays in diagnosis

Unavailable doctors

Irritability

Therapeutic failure

Fear of hospital or nursing home ——————

Worry about family ——————

Fear of death ——————

Spiritual unrest ——————

Fear of pain

Family finances

Loss of dignity and bodily control

Uncertainty about future

FIGURE 11.3 Multidimensional nature of pain.

From Twycross, R., & Lack, S. A. (1983). *Symptom Control in Far Advanced Cancer: Pain Relief.* London: Pitman Books, p. 46. (Reprinted with permission.)

groups of drugs will include rationale for selection, dose titration, routes of administration, and side-effect management.

Nonsteroidal Anti-inflammatory Drugs

The NSAIDs include many subclasses, are frequently used in all steps of the "analgesic ladder" and are analgesic, antipyretic, and anti-inflammatory (American Pain Society, 1999; Rawlins, 1998) (Table 11.2). Aspirin is the prototype of the NSAIDs. Acetaminophen, although lacking in significant anti-inflammatory effects, and with a different side-effect profile, is often classified within this group. Nonsteroidal anti-inflammatory drugs are most effective in treating mild to moderate pain when there is an inflammatory

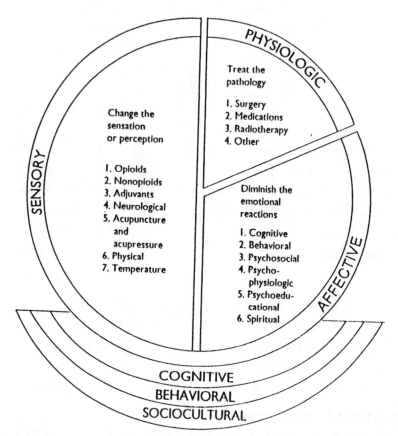

FIGURE 11.4 Multidimensional approach to pain management.

From McGuire, D. B. (1995). The multiple dimensions of cancer pain: A framework for assessment and management. In McGuire, D. B., Yarbro, C. H., & Ferrell, B. R. (Eds.), *Cancer pain management* (2nd ed., p. 12). Boston: Jones and Bartlett. (Reprinted with permission.)

component present and are used in Step 1 of the Analgesic Ladder. When greater relief is needed they are continued along with the opioid drugs in Steps 2 and 3 of the Analgesic Ladder. The NSAIDs can be extremely effective when combined with an opioid drug in treating bone pain in cancer patients (Prostaglandins, which are rich in the periosteum of the bone, are implicated in pain modulation [Paice, 1999]). Unlike the opioid drugs, the NSAIDs have a ceiling effect (a dose beyond which added analge-

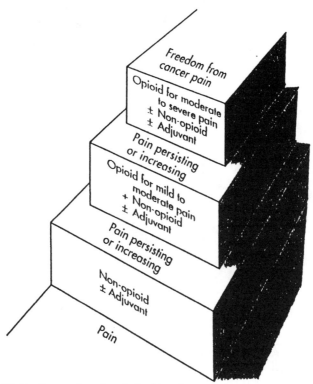

FIGURE 11.5   3-step "analgesic ladder."

World Health Organization. (1990). *Cancer pain relief and palliative care*. Geneva: World Health Organization. (Reprinted with permission from World Health Organization.)

sia is not obtained) (American Pain Society, 1999). These drugs do not produce tolerance or physical dependence, and are not associated with psychological dependence (addiction) (American Pain Society, 1999). This class of drugs may also have an opioid sparing effect in some patients.

Mechanism of Action

The nonsteroidal anti-inflammatory drugs impact pain perception in three ways. First, they inhibit the conversion of arachinidonic acid to prostaglandin G2 by inhibiting the enzyme cyclo-oxygensase (American Pain Society, 1999; Jenkins & Bruera, 1999). There are two known types of cyclo-oxygenase enzymes: COX-1 which is part of normal cells and COX-2 which is induced

TABLE 11.2 Nonsteroidal Anti-inflammatory Drugs and Acetaminophen Commonly Used at End of Life
(Please refer to the PDR for current information as dosing recommendations change. This Table is to be used as a guide only and does not replace a more comprehensive review.)

Chemical class	Generic name	Half-life (H)	Dosing schedule	Recommended starting dose** (MG)	Maximum dose recommended (MG/Day)	Comments
p-aminophenol derivatives	acetaminophen	2–4	q 4–6 h	650	6,000	-Overdosage produces hepatic toxicity. No GI or platelet toxicity.
COX-2 Inhibitors	celecoxib		q 12 h	200	400	-No effect on platelets.
	rofecoxib		q 24 h	12.5	25	-No effect on platelets.
Salicylates	aspirin	3–12	q 4–6 h	650	6,000	-Standard for comparison. May not be as well-tolerated as some of the newer NSAIDs.
	diflunisal	8–12	q 12 h	500	1,500	-Less GI toxicity than aspirin.
	choline magnesium trisalicylate	8–12	q 12 h	500–1,000	4,000	-Minimal GI toxicity. No effect on platelet aggregation.
	salsalate	8–12	q 12 h	500–1,000	4,000	

TABLE 11.2 (*continued*)

Chemical class	Generic name	Half-life (H)	Dosing schedule	Recommended starting dose** (MG)	Maximum dose recommended (MG/Day)	Comments
Proprionic acids	ibuprofen	3–4	q 4–8 h	400	4,200	Available as a suspension.
	naproxen	1–3	q 12 h	250	1,500	
	fenoprofen	2–3	q 6 h	200	3,200	
	ketoprofen	2–3	q 6–8 h	100	300	
	flurbiprofen	5–6	q 8–12 h	100	300	
	oxaprozin	40	q 24 h	600	1,800	
Acetic acids	indomethacin	4–5	q 8–12 h	25	200	Higher incidence of GI and CNS side effects than proprionic acid. Available in slow-release preparations.
	tolmetin	1	q 6–8 h	200	2,000	
	sulindac	14	q 12 h	150	400	
	diclofenac	2	q 6 h	25	200	
	ketorolac	4–7	q 4–6 h	***	Refer to PDR for age-related dosing guidelines.	Use not recommended for > 5 days. Parenteral and oral preparations.

(continued)

379

TABLE 11.2 *(continued)*

Chemical class	Generic name	Half-life (H)	Dosing schedule	Recommended starting dose** (MG)	Maximum dose recommended (MG/Day)	Comments
Oxicams	piroxicam	45	q 24 h	20	20	Administration of 40 mg for > 3 weeks is associated with high incidence of peptic ulcer disease particularly in the elderly.
Pyranocarboxylic acids	etodolac	7	q 8 h	200	1,200	
Naphtyl alka-	nabumetone	22–30	q 12 h	500	2,000	

*Table based on clinical experience of the authors and a variety of published sources.
**Starting dose should be one half to two thirds recommended dose in the elderly, those on multiple drug or those with renal insufficiency.
***30–60 load, then 15–30 q 6 h (parenteral), 10 q 6 h (oral).
q = ever; h = hour.

From Coyle, N., Cherny, N. I., & Portenoy, R. K. (1995). Pharmacologic management of cancer pain. In D. B. McGuire, C. H. Yarbro, & B. R. Ferrell (Eds.), *Cancer pain management* (2nd ed.) (pp. 91–92). ©1995 Boston: Jones & Bartlett Publishers. (Reprinted with permission.)

in the inflammatory process. Inhibition of COX-2 is responsible for the anti-inflammatory processes of the NSAIDs, whereas COX-1 inhibition is responsible for many of the side effects of the NSAIDs (American Pain Society, 1999; Jenkins & Bruera, 1999; Rawlins, 1998). A new group of NSAIDs drugs have been developed which selectively inhibit COX-2 cyclo-oxygenase, while leaving the more protective COX-1 cyclo-oxygenase intact.

The second way in which NSAIDs affect pain perception is through their action on the cell membranes of neutrophils to inhibit the release of inflammatory mediators. These two mechanisms reduce inflammation in tissues and thus decrease the release of substance P and pain-producing cytokines, thereby reducing nociception (Jenkins & Bruera, 1999). A third way by which the NSAIDs may have impact on pain perception is through mechanisms at the brain and spinal cord level (Yaksh, Dirig, & Malmberg, 1998).

Acetaminophen, although lacking in significant anti-inflammatory effects, is often classified with the NSAIDs. Its mechanism of action is not known (American Pain Society, 1999). Acetaminophen has fewer adverse effects than the NSAIDs. Gastrointestinal toxicity is rare, and there are no adverse effects on platelet function or cross-reactivity in patients with aspirin hypersensitivity (American Pain Society, 1999). Hepatic toxicity can occur, however, and patients with chronic alcoholism and liver disease can develop severe hepatotoxicity even when the drug is taken in usual therapeutic doses (Whitcomb & Block, 1994).

Adverse Effects and Their Management

Patients at the end of life are very susceptible to adverse side effects of pharmacotherapy. A careful balance is needed between achieving the desired effect of the selected drug for the patient, and the potential for adverse effects. This is particularly important in this group of drugs. Unlike the opioids where the adverse effects are usually dose dependent and controllable, NSAIDs have a largely "hidden" side effects profile (Jenkins & Bruera, 1999). These adverse effects, although they occur in a minority of patients, are often "silent," not producing symptoms until a major event occurs such as gastrointestinal bleeding without prior warning. The nurse is an active participant in assessing this risk/benefit ratio for the patient and needs to become familiar with the relative side-effect profile for each of the drugs within this category. The potential adverse effects of the NSAIDs (excluding acetaminophen, which have been described earlier) include those affecting the hematologic, gastrointestinal, renal, and central nervous systems. As noted earlier, the COX-2 inhibitors differ in their side-effect profile from other NSAIDs in relation to potential for gastric irritation and interference with platelet aggregation.

Hematologic Effects.   Nonsteroidal anti-inflammatory drugs (with the exception of COX-2 inhibitors) inhibit platelet aggregation resulting from inhibition of prostaglandin synthetase. This results in prolonged bleeding time. Single doses of aspirin above 40 mg irreversibly inhibit platelet aggregation (normal platelet function is expressed only by those platelets produced after cessation of aspirin therapy) (Sunshine & Olsen, 1993). Consequently, aspirin may prolong bleeding for many days after administration ceases. In contrast, other NSAIDs produce reversible platelet aggregation inhibition. These drugs render the patient more susceptible to bleeding only for the period during which drug circulates in the plasma (American Pain Society, 1999).

   A bleeding diathesis of any cause is a strong relative contraindication to the use of these drugs. The COX-2 inhibitors, however, do not interfere with platelet aggregation, and should be considered for patients at risk for hematologic adverse effects. Similar to the nonacetylated salicylates, such as choline magnesium trisalicylate, they do not change bleeding time, and also may be a safer NSAID to choose in patients at risk for bleeding (Sunshine & Olson, 1993).

Gastrointestinal Effects.   Nonsteroidal anti-inflammatory drugs can cause ulceration throughout the gastrointestinal tract, most commonly in the stomach, but also in the small and large bowel (Hawkey, 1990; Jenkins & Bruera, 1999). Overall the risk of ulceration is threefold in patients using NSAIDs (excluding the COX-2 inhibitors) over the general population (Jenkins & Bruera, 1999). This ulceration occurs by two mechanisms. The first is through direct irritation of the gastric mucosa. This is felt to play a minor role in gastric ulceration, and can be overcome by using enteric-coated products or a route other than the oral for administration.

   The second, and more important mechanism is through NSAID-induced decrease in the production of cytoprotective prostaglandins. People with previous ulcer disease and older adults appear to be most at risk (Roth, 1988). Those patients with a relatively high risk for developing ulceration should be considered for the prophylactic use of gastroprotective therapy (e.g., misoprostol) (American Pain Society, 1999; Hawkey & Yeomans, 1998). The NSAIDs should not be used concomitantly with other drugs that have the potential to cause gastric erosion (e.g., corticosteroids).

Renal Effects.   In the palliative care population, the renal adverse effect of most concern is NSAID-induced renal failure. Patients at increased risk include older adults and those with congestive heart failure, chronic renal insufficiency, and cirrhosis with ascites. In addition, patients who have a decreased effective circulating volume and are dependent on prostaglandin-mediated renal vasodilation to maintain their renal blood flow are at risk (American Pain Society, 1999; Jenkins & Bruera, 1999).

Central Nervous System Effects. Tinnitus, deafness, headache, and dizziness, well-known manifestations of salicylate toxicity, can also be side effects of other NSAIDs (Goodwin & Regan, 1982). The direct impact of NSAIDs on cognition at end of life has not been studied. Terminally ill patients have a high incidence of delirium, which is multifactoral (Breitbart, Bruera, Chochinov, & Lynch, 1995; Pereira, Hanson, & Bruera, 1997). The adverse effects of NSAIDs on renal function may contribute to end-of-life delirium through the mechanisms previously described.

Hypersensitivy Reactions. Two subgroups of aspirin-sensitive patients have been reported. One subgroup develops a respiratory reaction with rhinitis, asthma, or nasal polyps. The second develops urticaria, wheals, angiodema, and hypotension (Clissold, 1986; Szczeklik, 1986). Bronchospasm with NSAIDs occurs in 8 to 20% of the population with asthma, nasal polyps, and chronic urticaria (Jenkins & Bruera, 1999). These hypersensitivities usually develop within minutes of ingestion, and almost always within an hour. Patients who are sensitive to aspirin may also develop sensitivities to the other NSAIDs. A history of aspirin intolerance is therefore a contraindication to use drugs within this category.

Principles of Administration of the NSAIDs

Drug Selection. A careful medical and pain history provides the nurse with information about potential benefits and risks for a patient about to receive a NSAID. An analgesic history should illuminate the patient's prior exposure to the NSAIDs, including frequency of administration and both analgesic effects and side effects. Information regarding the timing interval of other analgesics is important so that a prescribed NSAID regimen fits in with the patient's total analgesic plan. For example, if a patient is on an 8- or 12-hour dosing regimen of a controlled release morphine preparation, a NSAID with a similar dosing profile would be appropriate (refer to Table 11.2). This may aid patient compliance and cut down on the feeling of having to constantly take medication.

Choice of a Starting Dose and Dose Titration. A NSAID is combined with an opioid drug in Step 2 and Step 3 of the analgesic ladder. Doses are often started at the lower end of the recommended scale in these medically fragile individuals who are coming to the end of their lives and are increased as needed (Table 11.2). Although several weeks are needed to evaluate the efficacy of a dose when NSAIDs are used in the treatment of grossly inflammatory conditions such as arthritis, clinical observation suggests that a shorter time period, usually a week, is adequate for pain relief in a patient with cancer pain. Pain and other symptoms should be monitored before and after starting the NSAIDs to document any improvement or adverse effects. If no benefit is seen or if adverse effects are noted, consideration should be given to discontinuing the drug or switching to an alternate NSAID, as marked variability has been noted in patients' response to different NSAIDs. Indicators of an effective response would be either a significant improvement in pain, or a significant decrease in the opioid use with a subsequent reduction in opioid-related side effects. The degree of monitoring for adverse effects from the NSAIDs should be individualized to the patient. Table 11.3 provides guidelines to the nurse for the selection and use of NSAIDs in the management of pain.

The Opioid Drugs

Opioid analgesics are the mainstay of pain treatment at the end of life (WHO, 1996). These drugs are used for moderate to severe pain in Step 2

TABLE 11.3   Guidelines for Selection and Use of NSAIDs in the Management of Pain

- Avoid NSAIDs if possible in patients with gastroduodenopathy, bleeding diathesis, renal insufficiency, hypertension, severe encepalopathy, and cardiac failure; avoid acetaminophen in patients with severe liver disease.
- If NSAIDs strongly indicated in patients with relative contraindications (except severe liver disease) consider acetomenophen; if anti-inflammatory effects are wanted consider gastroprotective therapy, a COX-2 inhibitor or choline magnesium trisalicylate.
- Consider individual differences (note prior treatment outcomes) and patient preferences.
- Be aware of available routes of administration (e.g., oral, rectal, intravenous).
- Begin with a low dose and adjust weekly if dose escalation is needed.
- Increase dose until adequate analgesia achieved, adverse effects occur, or maximum recommended dose reached.

From Coyle, N., Cherny, N. I., Portenoy, R. K. (1995). Pharmacologic management of cancer pain. In D. B. McGuire, C. H. Yarbro, & B. R. Ferrell (Eds.), *Cancer pain management* (2nd ed.) (p. 95). Boston: Jones & Bartlett Publishers. (Reprinted with permission.)

and Step 3 of the analgesic ladder. They are frequently used in combination with a NSAID (American Pain Society, 1999). When combined with a NSAID drug, dose escalation is limited by reaching the maximum recommended daily dose of the NSAID. When used as a single agent, however, there appears to be no ceiling effect (Hanks & Cherny, 1998). Dose escalation may be limited by adverse effects such as sedation, confusion, nausea and vomiting, myoclonus, and (rarely) respiratory depression (Hanks & Cherny, 1998). Dose escalation is governed by the balance between pain relief and intolerable and unmanageable side effects (Hanks & Cherny, 1998). This balance can only be determined by ongoing assessment and documentation of the effects and side effects produced by the opioid.

Mechanism of Action

Opioids produce their effects through binding to receptors in the brain and spinal cord to prevent the release of neurotransmitters involved in pain transmission (Paice, 1999). Opioids can also have a peripheral site of action in the presence of inflammation (Stein, 1995). In addition, opioid receptors are present in immunocompetent cells that migrate to inflamed tissue (American Pain Society, 1999; Sibinga & Goldstein, 1988). The opioids can be divided into agonists, agonist-antagonists, and antagonists classes based on their interactions with the receptor types. Pure opioid agonists, for example, morphine, hydromorphone, oxycontin, fentanyl, and methadone bind primarily to the mu receptors.

Partial agonists and mixed agonist-antagonists either block or remain neutral at the mu opioid receptors while activating kappa opioid receptors (Jaffe & Martin, 1990). Partial agonists, for example, butorphanol, dezocine, and pentazocine, have limited use in palliative care. Their pharmacology is characterized by a ceiling effect to analgesia and the ability to precipitate withdrawal symptoms in patients who are physically dependent on pure agonist drugs (e.g., morphine) (Hanks & Cherny, 1998). The incidence of psychotomimetic effects (agitation, dysphoria, confusion) from the mixed agonist-antagonist is greater than that of pure agonists (morphinelike drugs) (Hanks & Cherny, 1998). The opioid antagonist drugs include nalaxone and naltrexone. These drugs bind to opioid receptors and block the effect of morphine-like agonists. The most commonly used opioids in end-of-life care are briefly reviewed below.

Morphine is the prototype opioid agonist. The WHO placed morphine on the essential drug list and requested that it be made available throughout the world for cancer pain relief (World Health Organization, 1986). Morphine is available in tablet, elixir, suppository, and parenteral form (Hanks, 1996). Various oral-controlled relief preparations provide analgesia with a duration of from 8 to 12 to 24 hours. Alternate routes of drug administration are available for patients who are unable to use the oral or rectal route.

Patients with severe pain are initially titrated with immediate-release morphine tablets, and once stabilized converted to a controlled-release preparation (Hanks, 1996). To manage breakthrough pain or incident pain, immediate-release morphine should be made available to all patients receiving controlled-release preparations. Absorption of morphine after oral administration occurs mostly in the upper small bowel. The average bioavailabilty for oral morphine is 20 to 30% (Gourlay, Plummer, Cherry, & Purser, 1991). This explains why there is a need to increase the patient's opioid dose when changing from the parenteral to the oral route of drug administration (Table 11.4). In patients with normal renal function, the average plasma half life is 2 to 3 hours while the average duration of analgesia is about 4 hours (Hanks & Cherny, 1998). Morphine-6-glucoronide (M-6-G), an active metabolite of morphine and a powerful analgesic, may accumulate in patients with impaired renal function. This accumulation may lead to signs of opioid toxicity (Portenoy, 1991; Portenoy et al., 1992; Tiseo et al., 1995), which will be described later in the chapter. The nurse should be aware of the patient's renal status when administering morphine and monitor accordingly for signs of opioid toxicity.

Hydromorphone and oxycodone are short half-life opioids that are a useful alternative to patients who tolerate morphine poorly. Hydromorphone is more potent than morphine and can be administered by the oral, rectal, parenteral, and intraspinal routes. The half life of hydromorphone of 1.5 to 3 hours is slightly shorter than that of morphine, and it has an oral bioavailability of 30 to 40% (Houde, 1986). The comparative potency of the opioid drugs and bioavailabilty dependent on route of administration underscores the need for nurses to be competent in the use of the equianalgesic table (Table 11.4).

Oxycodone has a high oral bioavailability of 60 to 90% and an oral analgesic potency similar to that of morphine (Loew, Smith, Williams, & Cramond, 1992). It has a half life of 2 to 4 hours and is mainly excreted by the kidneys. Oxycodone is available in combination with aspirin (Percodan) or acetaminophen (Percocet) or as a single immediate-release or controlled-release tablet. The controlled-release tablet (Oxycontin) provides the patient with analgesia for 8 to 12 hours. Both hydromorphone and oxycodone are used in Steps 2 and 3 of the analgesic ladder.

Fentanyl is a potent short half-life opioid that is being used with increasing frequency in palliative care. Fentanyl comes in a transdermal, transmucosal, and parenteral form. In the transmucosal and parenteral form it has a rapid onset of action and personal clinical experience suggests a lower profile of cognitive toxicity. The transdermal fentanyl delivery system consists of a

TABLE 11.4 Equianalgesic Dose Table: Relative Potencies, Half-lives, and Duration of Action of Commonly Used Opioids at End of Life*

Drug	Half-life (H)	Equianalgesic intramuscular dose (mg)**	Intramuscular: oral potency (mg)	Starting oral dose	Comment
Morphine-like agonists					
Morphine	2–3	10	1:3 (after repeat dosing) (in the opioid tolerant patient)	15–30	Standard of comparison for opioid analgesics. Multiple routes of administration. Controlled-release available. M6G accumulation in patients with renal failure. Lower doses for the elderly.
Oxymorphone		1	—	1	Available in suppository form as Numorphan.
Hydromorphone	2–3	1.5	1:5	4–8	Useful alternative to morphine. No known active metabolite. Multiple routes available.
Methadone	15–190	10***	1:2	5–10	Long half-life; low cost. May accumulate with repetitive dosing.
Levorphanol	12–15	2	1:2	2–4	Long half-life.
Meperidine	2–3	75	1:4	Not recommended	CNS excitatory toxic metabolite, normeperidine. Relatively contraindicated for long-term dosing, for patients with renal failure, and for others receiving MAO inhibitors.

(continued)

387

TABLE 11.4 (*continued*)

Drug	Half-life (H)	Equianalgesic intramuscular dose (mg)**	Intramuscular: oral potency (mg)	Starting oral dose	Comment
Fentanyl	4–7	—	—		Short half-life when used acutely. Parenteral use via infusion. Clinical experience suggests 4 mg IV morphine sulfate/hr = 100 ug transdermal patch. Patches available to deliver 25, 50, 75, 100 ug/hr. Oral transmucosal delivery system also available for breakthrough pain.
Oxycodone	2–3	2		5–10	Available in liquid or tablet preparation. Also in combination with a nonopioid. Controlled-release available.
Codeine	2–3	130	1.5	30–60	Used orally for less severe pain. Usually combined with a nonopioid.
Hydrocodone	4	—	—	5–10	Usually combined with nonopioid.

*Table based on clinical experience of the authors and a variety of published sources.

**Dose that provides analgesia equivalent to 10 mg i.m. morphine. These ratios are useful guides when switching drugs or routes of administration (see text). In clinical practice, the potency of the i.m. route is considered to be identical to the IV and subcutaneous routes.

***When switching from another opioid to methadone, the potency of methadone is much greater than indicated on this table (see text). Frequently 5–10% of the equianalgesic dose is used.

Adapted from Coyle, N., Cherny, N. I., & Portenoy, R. K. (1995). Pharmacologic management of cancer pain. In D. B. McGuire, C. H. Yarbro, & B. R. Ferrell (Eds.), *Cancer Pain Management* (2nd ed.) (pp. 101–102). ©1995 Boston: Jones and Bartlett Publishers.

drug reservoir in the form of a patch that is separated from the skin by a copolymer membrane that controls the rate of drug delivery to the skin surface. This approach provides the means to continuously infuse an opioid drug without the need for needles and pumps (Payne, Chandler, & Einhaus, 1995). Clinical experience with cancer patients suggest that a 100 mcg fentanyl patch is equianalgesic to 4 mg of parenteral morphine per hour (Hanks & Cherny, 1998). Transdermal fentanyl has only been approved for chronic cancer pain. Although most patients maintain satisfactory pain control with a patch change every 72 hours, some patients require the patch to be changed after 48 hours. Careful monitoring of adequacy of pain relief and evidence of end-of-dose failure will guide the nurse in the needs of the particular patient. It is important that the nurse also realize that there is a lag in absorbing fentanyl through the skin. It takes 12 to 16 hours for the patient to see a substantial therapeutic effect and 48 hours to reach steady-state blood concentrations (Hanks & Cherny, 1998; Payne et al., 1995). Availability of a different route of drug administration is therefore necessary during the 12 to 16 hours following the initial patch placement. An alternate route of drug administration is also required for breakthrough pain medication. Significant concentrations of fentanyl remain in the plasma for about 24 hours after removal of the patch because of delayed release from the tissues and subcutaneous depots. Drug side effects (if present) may persist for that length of time.

Oral transmucosal fentanyl (OTFC) is the one FDA-approved drug specifically for breakthrough pain (American Pain Society, 1999; Christie et al., 1998), although many other short half-life opioids are used for this purpose. Oral transmucosal fentanyl citrate is recommended only to be used in patients who are opioid tolerant, and who are receiving the equivalent of no less than 60 mg of oral morphine a day or transdermal fentanyl 50 mcg every 3 days. Oral transmucosal fentanyl differs from other breakthrough pain medication in that there is no relationship between the baseline dose of the patient's pain medication, and the microgram dose of OTFC required to relieve breakthrough pain (American Pain Society, 1999; Streisand et al., 1998). In all other opioid drugs there is a relation between the two. With OTFC (Actiq), the smallest available dose is initially chosen (200 mcg) and titrated up depending on the patient's response (available strengths range from 200 to 1,600 mcg per unit). Table 11.5 outlines a suggested dose titration approach to OTFC. Personal clinical experience with the use of OTFC has indicated its benefit for patients with acute predictable breakthrough pain such as a fungating chest wall dressing change.

Methadone is another useful opioid for the management of pain at the end of life (De Conno, Groff, & Brunelli, 1996; Manfredi, Borsook, Chandler, & Payne, 1997). Clinical experience suggests, however, that it is more difficult

TABLE 11.5   Guidelines for Oral Transmucosal Fentanyl Citrate (Actiq®) Use for Breakthrough Pain

Titration

1. Patients' ATC opioid should be at least 60 mg P.O. morphine equivalents or 50 mcg/h fentanyl patch. There is no correlation between patients' ATC opioid or previous PRN rescue dose and the effective Actiq® dose.
2. Start with 200 mcg units.
3. Dispense 6 units for each titration phase until an effective dose is determined.
4. Have previous PRN rescue dose available for patients.
5. If no relief from 1st unit, patients may suck another unit 15 minutes after completing the 1st unit. If no relief with the 2nd unit, patients should take their regular PRN rescue dose.
6. Use a single dosage strength of Actiq for at least 2–3 episodes of breakthrough pain before titrating to the next higher dose, i.e. 400 mcg.
7. Follow steps 3–6 until an effective dose is found. The goal of titration is to find the dosage strength that controls the majority of breakthrough pain episodes with only one unit.
8. Have patients contact their nurse or physician during the titration phase to monitor effectiveness and assess for side effects.

Patient Teaching

a. Actively suck the whole unit over 15 minutes.
b. Move the unit around in the mouth, especially over the cheek area.
c. Do not bite or chew the unit.
d. Do not drink fluids during administration of the unit.
e. Do not eat anything citrus, acidic, or caffeinated immediately before Actiq® use.
f. Reassure patients that an effective dose will be found for their breakthrough pain.

Table complied by Diane B. Loseth, RN, MSN, OCN, Pain and Palliative Care Service, Memorial Sloan-Kettering Cancer Center.

to administer than other morphinelike opioids because of its variable long half life (range 13 hours to over 100 hours) (Hanks & Cherny, 1998) and a discrepancy between drug half life and the duration of analgesic effect (4 to 8 hours). Patients are at increased risk for drug accumulation and subsequent toxicity when treatment is initiated, the dose is increased, or multiple organ failure develops (Inturrisi, Colburn, Kaiko, Houde, & Foley, 1987; Inturris, Portenoy, Colburn, & Foley, 1990). Patients may become confused, increasingly sedated and progress to a respiratory arrest if not closely monitored especially during the titration period (Fainsinger, Schoeller, & Bruera, 1993; Hunt & Bruera, 1995). Because of this risk, methadone is considered a "second line" drug in the treatment of pain at end of life. The risk of delayed toxicity from methadone accumulation can be reduced if the initial period of dosing is accomplished with "as needed" administration (Ettinger, Vitale, & Trump, 1979). When a steady state has been approached, a fixed dosing schedule of every 4 to 8 hours can be substituted. An opioid with a short half life such as morphine or hydromorphone is frequently used for supplementary or "rescue" dosing although methadone can also be used.

Knowledge of the long half life of methadone has a special relevance for the nurse if severe respiratory depression associated with drug accumulation occurs, and the use of naloxone is felt to be appropriate. Because of the short half life of naloxone in comparison with methadone, either repeated doses or an infusion of naloxone may be required to prevent recurrence of respiratory depression as the effects of the naloxone decline and the methadone rebinds to the opioid binding sites. Table 11.6 illustrates a careful approach to the administration of naloxone which will reverse the respiratory depressant effects of an opioid drug but will not place the patient at risk for the symptoms of withdrawal. The need to reverse the respiratory effects of an opioid drug is unusual in end of life care (Manfredi, Ribeiro, & Payne, 1996). Most patients have been exposed to the opioid drugs over time, and have become tolerant to the respiratory depressant effects of these drugs. Occasionally staff unfamiliar with the dying process and the altered breathing pattern that so frequently occurs at this time, become concerned that continued use of opioids, especially in the higher doses sometimes required to control pain at the end of life, will hasten death. The input and mentoring by a nurse knowledgeable in pain and palliative care, will help refocus the more inexperienced staff on appropriate dosing strategies in the symptomatic dying patient, goals of care, and the normal dying process.

Levorphanol, like methadone, has a long half life of 12 to 16 hours (Dixon, Crews, Inturrisi, & Foley, 1983). It is five times more potent than morphine and has an oral/parenteral ration of 1:2 (Wallenstein, Rogers, Kaiko, & Houde, 1984). Like methadone, the discrepancy between plasma half-life (12 to 16 hours) and duration of analgesic effect (4 to 6 hours) may lead to drug accumulation during the drug titration phase. In clinical practice, however, this appears to be less of a problem than with methadone.

Meperidine is not a drug of choice for the management of chronic pain either at the end of life or earlier on in the disease process. Meperidine has an active metabolite, normeperidine, that is twice as potent as a convulsant and one-half as potent as an analgesic as its parent compound (Kaiko, 1983). The half life of normeperidine is three to four times that of meperidine, and accumulation of the metabolite with repetitive dosing can result in central nervous system excitability characterized by tremor, myoclonus,

TABLE 11.6   Guidelines for Administration of Naloxone in an Opioid Dependent Patient
(Onset of action in 1–2 minutes. Duration of effect approximately 45 minutes, varies).

- Patients receiving opioids for pain are exquisitely sensitive to Naloxone.
- Inappropriate use of this drug can precipitate severe pain and withdrawal symptoms in these patients.
- Patients at the end of life rarely require the use of naloxone.
- Assess the patient. Remember that in the terminally ill, increasing somnolence is frequently part of the dying process.
- If the assessment indicates that the use of Naloxone may be appropriate, stimulate the patient both verbally and nonverbally, and assess responsiveness.
- If appropriate, obtain pulse oximetry and compare to baseline evaluation.
- Review the medication record for administration of other sedative type drugs.

If the patient responds to stimulation and the pulse oximetry is > 90%:
- Hold the opioid until the patient is more responsive.
- When the patient is more responsive and complains of pain, restart the opioid regimen at 50% of the previous dose.

If the patient does not respond to stimulation, respirations are below 8 per minute, or the pulse oximetry is below 90%, and use of Naloxone is appropriate, administer Naloxone as follows:
- Dilute one Naloxone ampoule (0.4 mg/ml) in 9 mls of N/S and give 1–2 ccs IV push over 15 seconds.
- Evaluate responsiveness, i.e., level of consciousness (LOC), respiratory rate, and pulse oximetry.
- If the patient is responsive, with improvement in respiratory rate and pulse oximetry, do not administer further Naloxone. Continue to monitor the patient closely.
- If there is none to minimal improvement in LOC, respiratory rate, and pulse oximetry, repeat the same dose of Naloxone (1–2 ccs) every 2–3 minutes until the patient is more responsive with improvement in respiratory rate and pulse oximetry.
- Continue to monitor for presence of pain.

If the patient responds initially to a single or repeated doses of Naloxone, but then becomes sedated, with respirations below 8/minute and or oximetry < 90%, a continuous infusion of Naloxone may be indicated. Patients who are receiving long half-life drugs such as Methadone or Levorphanol are most at risk. (continued on next page)

TABLE 11.6   *(continued)*

1. Dilute 2 mg (5 × 0.4/mg ampoules) in 500 ml NS or D5W to yield 0.004 mg/ ml (4 mcg/ml).
2. Administer using an infusion device at an hourly rate equal to the amount needed to produce an improvement in LOC, respiratory rate and pulse oximetry (e.g., if 2 ccs of diluted naloxone = .08 mg was the effective dose, administer this dose on an hourly basis = 20 mls/hour).
3. Evaluate the patient hourly for maintenance of acceptable LOC, respiratory status, and pulse oximetry.
4. If the above parameters are not maintained, titrate the dose upwards by increasing the hourly rate by 50–100%.
5. If the above parameters are maintained satisfactorily, wean the patient off the Naloxone infusion by titrating down 50% Q1H × 2 hours and then discontinuing the infusion.
6. Monitor the patient closely for 4 hours.
7. If the pain returns, restart the opioid at a 50% dose reduction and continue to monitor closely.

Guidelines developed based on clinical experience and developed in collaboration with Susan Derby, RN, MA, GNP, Pain and Palliative Care Service, Memorial Sloan-Kettering Cancer Center. It is emphasized that these are merely guidelines and do not substitute for good clinical judgment.

agitated delirium, and seizures (Szeto et al., 1977). Naloxone does not reverse meperidine-induced seizures and potentially could precipitate seizures by blocking the depressant effects of meperidine and allowing the convulsant effects of normeperidine to become manifest (Kaiko et al., 1983; Umans & Inturrisi, 1982).

Principles of Opioid Administration

Numerous factors, both patient related and drug related must be considered in the selection of an appropriate opioid for a patient (Cherny & Portenoy, 1994). The opioid should be compatible with the patient's pain severity, age, dosing and route requirements, underlying illness, and metabolic state. Selection of an opioid that is available as a controlled-release formulation such as morphine or oxycodone, may be an important consideration for some patients. For the older adult or those who have major organ dysfunction, an opioid with a short half life, such as morphine, hydromorphone, or oxycodone is preferable. Patients with marked renal impairment may do better with an opioid other than morphine because of the potential to accumulate the active metabolite M-6-G and to develop toxicity. However, renal impairment is not an absolute contraindication for the use of morphine at the end of life, and would not be a reason to switch drugs if the patient had good pain control and no adverse effects on the current regimen.

The potential for additive side effects and serious toxicities from drug combinations must be recognized by the nurse each time a new drug is added to a patient's regimen (Portenoy, 1994). Patients frequently have many distressing symptoms and are receiving multiple drugs. For example, it is not unusual for a patient toward the end of life to be receiving an opioid, a nonsteroidal anti-inflammatory drug, a tricyclic antidepressant, an anxiolytic, a steroid, an H2 blocker, and a neuroleptic. In these circumstances additive side effects, especially those of sedation, are frequent and yet the opioid drug tends to get blamed in isolation.

Sequential trials of opioid drugs may be needed to find the most favorable balance for the patient between pain relief and adverse effects (Galer, Coyle, & Pasternak, 1992). The patient and family should be warned that this is a possibility so that they do not become discouraged during the process. The sequential trial of opioid drugs requires knowledge by the nurse of equianalgesic potencies among opioid drugs (Table 11.4). When converting from one opioid drug to another in patients with good pain control but significant side effects, reduce the dose to 50 to 75% of the equianalgesic dose (Hanks & Cherny, 1998). When converting from one opioid to another in patients with poor pain control and significant side effects, use 75 to 100% of the equianalgesic dose. When converting to methadone, the equianalgesic dose can usually be decreased by 80 to 90% (Ripamonti et al., 1998). In all instances when an opioid dose is decreased or the drug changed, because of large interpatient variability, the patient must be closely monitored for adequacy of pain relief or presence of adverse side effects (Hanks & Cherny, 1998).

Selecting a Route and Dosing Intervals

Opioids should be administered by the least invasive and safest route capable of producing adequate analgesia. Clinical experience indicates that the majority of patients can use the oral route of drug administration throughout the course of most of their disease. However, at times some patients become unable to use this route and require an alternate approach (Coyle et al., 1990). Nurses must be skilled in selecting among the alternate routes to meet the needs of a particular patient. The most commonly used alternate routes include rectal, sublingual, transmucosal, transdermal, subcutaneous, intravenous, epidural, and intrathecal. Table 11.7 reviews the most commonly used alternate routes of drug administration, patient selection criteria, and advantages and disadvantages of each.

TABLE 11.7 Commonly Used Routes of Drug Administration at End-of-Life

Route	Patient selection criteria	Advantages	Disadvantages	Comments
Oral (PO)	Route of choice. Mild to severe pain. Most common reasons for oral route failure: Amount given not sufficient for severity of pain; Equianalgesic ratios not adhered to when switching from parenteral to oral route; Parenteral to oral change made too quickly; Drug administered at intervals too long for time action curve of the drug.	Most acceptable to patients. Simple. Noninvasive. Longer duration of effect than parenteral route. Controlled-release preparations of morphine available and can be given at 8- to 12-hr intervals. Preparations available in liquid form.	Onset of action slower than parenteral route. Absorption affected by stomach emptying time, presence of food, gastrointestional mobility.	Patients with gastrointestinal disease may not absorb the analgesic and may need an alternate route.

(continued)

TABLE 11.7 *(continued)*

Route	Patient selection criteria	Advantages	Disadvantages	Comments
Sublingual, Buccal, Rectal	Unable to tolerate oral route (e.g., nausea, vomiting). Unable to swallow (e.g., head & neck cancer, esophageal disease).	Avoids need for repeated injections. Easy to administer.	Unpalatable taste (sublingual and buccal). Limited drugs available for sublingual and buccal routes. Rectal route unacceptable to some patients. Tissue irritation (rectal). Onset of action similar to oral (rectal).	Hypodermic, tablets and oral solutions have been used as sublingual and buccal preparations with varying effect. Opioids available in suppository form are morphine, hydromorphone (Dilaudid), and oxymorphone (Numorphan). Suppositories contraindicated in patients with a platelet count of 50 or below.
Transdermal	Inability to use the oral route. Stable pain. Occasionally need to improve patient compliance with opioid therapy.	No need for SC or IV access. Long duration of action, 48–72 hrs, provides continuous administration of an opioid.	Need to alternate route for rescue medication. Relatively slow onset of action. Adverse effects continue after patch removed. Fentanyl only opioid available by this route.	Short half-life opioid recommended for "breakthrough." Difficult to titrate rapidly. Serum fentanyl concentration falls 50% in about 24 hrs. If narcan indicated may need an infusion.

TABLE 11.7 *(continued)*

Route	Patient selection criteria	Advantages	Disadvantages	Comments
Transmucosal	Need for rapid onset of action, short duration.	Rapid onset of action. Short duration of effect.	No relationship between ATC dose of an opioid and the effective transmucosal dose.	Fentanyl the only opioid available by this route. Not for use in opioid naive patients.
Subcutaneous (SC) intermittent or infusion	Moderate to severe pain. Unable to tolerate the oral route. Variable or uncertain PO absorption.	Intravenous access not required. Subcutaneous route can be continuous or intermittent. Onset of action more rapid than oral route. Family can learn administration techniques, both continuous infusion and intermittent injections.	Absorption variable depending on muscle, fat, and blood supply. Peaks and troughs unless continuous SC infusion. Duration of action shorter than oral route (intermittent SC). Patient may be dependent on others to administer the analgesic on time (intermittent SC). Volume restriction.	Intermittent injection contraindicated in patients with a platelet count of 50 or below. Methadone should not be used for continuous SC infusions as it is a tissue irritant. Continuous SC infusion is the method of choice in an obstructed patient being cared at home. A variety of portable pumps are available for continuous SC infusion use.

(continued)

TABLE 11.7 *(continued)*

Route	Patient selection criteria	Advantages	Disadvantages	Comments
Intravenous (IV) bolus infusion	Severe pain (rapid control needed). Dying patient with rapidly escalating pain. Postoperative period. Children unable to take oral medications. Alternative routes ineffective.	Bioavailability 100%. Rapid onset of action (10–15 min). Can be given bolus or continuous. Variety of access ports available. Milligram dose of drug administered not limited by volume requirement.	Need for IV access. Short duration of effect with bolus. Bolus effect with intermittent injections. Hospital constraints (e.g., nurses not permitted to administer IV opioid bolus).	IV opioids do not guarantee adequate pain relief.

TABLE 11.7 *(continued)*

Route	Patient selection criteria	Advantages	Disadvantages	Comments
Epidural (ED) and intrathecal (IT)	–Pain mid-chest or below. –Unable to tolerate side effects of opioids by other routes. –No contraindications: • coagulopathy • altered spinal anatomy • infection	–Selective activation of spinal opioid receptors so that analgesia may be achieved with fewer side effects. –Smaller dose of opioid required than when given by alternate route. –May use local anesthetic and/or clonidine as adjunct to further minimize opioid dose and treat neuropathic pain.	–Adverse effects can be similar to those after systemic administration. –Onset of analgesia may occur later than IV route (30–60 min with morphine). –Respiratory depression from morphine can occur both early (after 1–2 hr) and later (after 6–25 hr). –Adverse effects include facial pruritus and urinary retention (15%). –Mild hypotension may occur with local anesthetic or clonidine.	–Epidural meds are administered as an intermittent bolus and continuous infusion using an external pump. –Intrathecal meds are usually administered via an implanted catheter and subcutaneous reservoir by continuous infusion. –A patient who is tolerant to opioids by the oral or parenteral route will also be tolerant to opioids by the IT or ED route, but not to local anesthetics or clonidine.

Adapted from Coyle, N., Cherny, N. I., & Portenoy, R. K. (1995). Pharmacologic management of cancer pain. In D. B. McGuire, C. H. Yarbro, & B. R. Ferrell (Eds.), *Cancer Pain Management* (2nd ed., pp. 101–102). ©1995 Jones & Bartlett Publishers, Boston.

Patient-controlled analgesia (PCA) in the palliative care arena is a method that refers to parenteral drug administration in which the patient controls a pump that delivers analgesics according to parameters set by the nurse and/or physician. These parameters include concentration of the drug, basal infusion rate, and bolus dose with permitted intervals between doses for "breakthrough" pain. Use of a PCA device is fairly common in palliative care patients requiring a parenteral route of drug administration. This technique can be managed safely at home for most patients, providing a system of education, monitoring, and support is in place (Coyle, Cherny, & Portenoy, 1994).

A switch in route of opioid administration requires that the nurse have knowledge of relative potencies, to avoid overdosing or underdosing (Table 11.4). These times of transition from one drug or route to another, place patients at risk for pain escalation, or the development of adverse effects. Frequent assessment is therefore required during the transition period. The equianalgesic dose table provides a guide to dose selection when these changes are made. The calculated equianalgesic dose is usually reduced 25 to 50% when switching drugs to account for incomplete cross tolerance. As noted previously, a much larger reduction (sometimes as much as 80 to 90%) is necessary when switching to methadone to prevent oversedation.

Patients with continuous or frequently occurring pain generally benefit from scheduled around-the-clock (ATC) dosing. This provides a more stable plasma level of the drug and helps prevent pain from recurring. A "rescue" dose is offered on a "prn" basis and provides a means to treat pain that breaks through the fixed analgesic schedule. The drug used for breakthrough pain is usually the same as that administered on a regular basis. An alternative short half-life drug is recommended when using methadone or transdermal fentanyl (Hanks & Cherny, 1998). Clinical experience suggests that the rescue dose should be calculated as about 25 to 50% of the hourly dose, or 5 to 15% of the 24-hour baseline dose (Hanks & Cherny, 1998; Jacox et al., 1994). For example, a patient receiving 60 mg of a controlled-release oral morphine preparation every 12 hours should have a rescue or supplemental dose of 10 to 15 mg of immediate-release morphine available on a 1- to-2-hour basis.

Choice of a Starting Dose and Dose Titration

A patient who is relatively opioid-naïve should generally begin treatment at an opioid dose equivalent to 5 to 10 mg of parenteral morphine every 4 hours (Cherny & Portenoy, 1994). Titration of the opioid dose is usually necessary at the start of pain therapy and at different points during the disease course. At all times, inadequate relief should be addressed with dose escalation until relief is reported or until intolerable and unmanageable side effects occur. Integration of "around-the-clock" (ATC) dosing with supplemental rescue doses provides a rational stepwise approach to dose escalation and is appropriate to all routes of drug administration. Patients who require more than four to six rescue doses per day should generally undergo escalation of the baseline dose. In all cases, escalation of the baseline dose should be accompanied by a proportional increase in the rescue dose so that the size of the supplemental dose remains a constant percentage of the fixed dose. Nursing assessment of the patient's pattern of pain, rescue use, and level of pain relief is essential for appropriate dose titration. Table 11.8 summarizes the basic principles in the use of opioid drugs to manage pain.

Managing a Pain Crisis

A pain crisis can be defined as pain which is severe, uncontrolled, and distressing to the patient. It may be acute in onset or may have gradually progressed in severity. A pain crisis is considered a medical and nursing care emergency for those at the end of life. At the same time as the pain is being managed the probable etiology of the pain is assessed within the framework of the previous pattern of pain, probable cause of present pain crisis, goals of care, and the most effective long-term management approaches. Refer to Table 11.9 for the pharmacological management of a pain crisis.

In patients who do not respond to opioid titration, or who develop intolerable side effects, the following adjuvants should be considered: (1) A parenteral NSAID, for example, ketorolac, 30 mg times one, and then 15 mg every 6 hours for no longer than 5 days. During this period other more long-term approaches for pain relief should be considered; (2) Parenteral steroids, for example, dexamethasone, 16 mg to 100 mg for the first dose, followed by a dose every 6 hours, the dose being gradually tapered down to the lowest effective dose for the patient. Anecdotal experience has shown the use of parenteral NSAIDs or steroids to be effective in a pain crisis associated with bone pain and neuropathic pain; (3) If the pain is predominantly neuropathic, intravenous lidocaine or intravenous phenytoin can be helpful for some patients (Portenoy, 1998). The efficacy of a nerve block or spinal delivery system of drug administration for this particular clinical situation should be considered (Swarm & Cousins, 1998). The reader is referred to Section Two, invasive interventions, for further informaton. An important consideration in end-of-life care is the option of sedation for the patient if the symptom is refractory (Cherny & Portenoy, 1994).

Sedation at the End of Life

A proportion of patients at the end of life will experience refractory symptoms, including pain, that is not possible to control in the absence of

TABLE 11.8   Principles of Opioid Use in the Management of Pain

- Select a drug from step 2 or step 3 of the analgesic ladder appropriate to the patient's level of pain and analgesic history.
- Take into consideration patient's age, metabolic state, presence of major organ failure (renal, hepatic, or respiratory), and presence of coexisting disease.
- Consider pharmacologic issues (e.g., potential accumulation of active metabolites, effects of concurrent drugs, and possible drug interactions).
- Know the drug class (e.g., agonist, agonist/antagonist), duration of analgesic effects, and pharmacokinetic properties.
- Be knowledgeable about the various drug formulations (e.g., controlled release, immediate release, liquid, transmucosal).
- Be aware of the available routes of administration (e.g., oral, rectal, transdermal, transmucosal, subcutaneous, intravenous, epidural) and equianalgesic dosages among drugs and between routes.
- Select the least invasive route appropriate to the patient's needs.
- Consider issues in patient compliance (e.g., convenience, ease for home management, and cost).
- Administer the analgesic on a regular basis. Make sure that supplemental or "rescue" doses are available.
- Use drug combinations, if appropriate to provide added analgesia (e.g., NSAIDs and adjuvants).
- Avoid drug combinations that increase sedation without enhancing analgesia.
- Anticipate and treat side effects.
- Prevent precipitating an acute withdrawal syndrome in the patient who is physically dependent on an opioid drug (e.g., taper opioids if a patient has a neuroablative procedure and is pain free; do not abruptly stop the opioid).
- Systematically evaluate effectiveness of analgesic regimen (e.g., amount of relief, duration of relief, frequency of breakthrough pain, frequency and pattern of "rescue" use, presence of adverse effects, and satisfaction with mode of therapy.
- Teach the patient and family the principles of analgesic therapy. Address their fears about addiction and tolerance.

From Coyle, N., Cherny, N. I., & Portenoy, R. K. (1995). Pharmacologic management of cancer pain. In D. B. McGuire, C. H. Yarbro, & B. R. Ferrell (Eds.), *Cancer pain management* (2nd ed.) (p. 99). Boston: Jones & Bartlett Publishers. (Reprinted with permission.)

sedation. The number of patients involved is not clear. Ventafridda et al. (1990) reported that approximately 50% of patients followed in an Italian-based home-care program required sedation at the end of life to control intractable symptoms. Other authors have quoted figures in the 5 to 25% range. Recent controversy has arisen in the role of sedation in the care of the dying with some authors suggesting that it is a form of "slow euthanasia" (Billings & Block, 1996). However, the Supreme Court decision on physician-

TABLE 11.9   Guidelines to Managing a Pain Crisis—Pharmacological Approach

These are merely guidelines and do not substitute for good clinical judgment. Dose selection is influenced by the patient's age; pulmonary, renal, and cardiac status; and potential for drug interactions.

A.   In the opioid naïve patient:
- Administer 5–10 mg. of morphine intravenously.
- Repeat same dose in 20 minutes if pain not adequately controlled.
- If pain persists > 5–6/10 or relief is unsatisfactory to the patient and there are no dose limiting side effects such as excessive sedation, increase the dose by 50%.
- Repeat this dose every 20 minutes until there is satisfactory pain relief or unacceptable side effects.
- Remain with the patient during management of the pain crisis.
- The loading dose is the sum of the repeated opioid doses that were needed to make the patient comfortable.
- The loading dose is used as a framework to decide the appropriate around-the-clock (ATC) dose requirements to control the patient's ongoing pain.
- Patients who are comfortable at rest but have pain on movement may be best managed by "as needed" parenteral dosing for the first 12–24 hours. A patient-controlled analgesia device (PCA) may be used to give the patient control over their PRN dosing.

B.   If the patient is to be placed on a parenteral infusion route of administration once the pain has been brought under control, determine the hourly parenteral dose as follows:

1. Divide the loading dose by two times the drug half-life, for example: the half-life of morphine is 4 hours. If the loading dose required to make the patient comfortable was 30 mg. of morphine, then divide the 30 mg. of morphine by 4 times 2 = 8. The hourly parenteral dose of morphine would therefore be 4 mg./hour (refer to Table 11.4 for drug half-life).
2. Set the patient-controlled analgesia pump (PCA) infusion rate to deliver that dose as the hourly or basal rate.
3. Provide the patient with access to a PRN "rescue" dose every 20 minutes.
4. The PRN "rescue" dose should equal 50% of the patient's hourly dose.
5. Monitor the patient for adequacy of pain relief and development of adverse side effects hourly for the first 12 hours. If signs of sedation occur, decrease the infusion rate by 50%. Leave the PRN "rescue" doses unchanged. If sedation persists, discontinue the basal infusion rate but leave the PRN "rescue" doses available to the patient. Patients who are comfortable at rest, but have pain on movement are at risk for over-sedation when initially started on a continuous opioid infusion and must be monitored closely.
6. Assess the etiology of the pain crisis.

(continued)

TABLE 11.9   *(continued)*

C. If the patient is to be placed on an oral route of drug administration after the pain has been brought under control via the parenteral route:

   1. Take the hourly milligram dose the patient is receiving via the parenteral route which is providing adequate pain relief (see dose calculation in section B # 1).
   2. Multiply that hourly dose by the parenteral to oral equianalgesic dose ratio (refer to Table 11.4). For example, intravenous morphine 5 mg. per hour = oral morphine 15 mg. per hour (ration 1:3).
   3. Then multiply that dose by 4 if the patient is to be on an every 4 hourly around-the-clock regimen. For example: morphine 5 mg. per hour intravenously = 15 mg. per hour orally = 60 mg. every 4 hours by mouth.
   4. After 24–48 hours of stable pain relief consider conversion to an 8-, 12-, or 24-hour controlled release preparation. For example, if the patient was receiving 60 mg. of morphine every 4 hours, that dose should be converted to 120 mg. every 8 hours, or 180 mg. every 12 hours of a controlled release morphine preparation.
   5. Continue to provide the patient with a PRN "rescue" doses every 1–2 hours.
   6. The PRN "rescue" dose should be equal to 5 to 15% of the 24-hour baseline dose. The percentage selected depends on the severity of the breakthrough pain and the likelihood that the patient will develop adverse side effects.
   7. Monitor the patient for adequacy of pain relief and development of adverse side effects.

D. In the opioid-tolerant patient presenting in a pain crisis

If on oral opioids:
   • Determine the total oral milligram dose the patient has received in the past 24 hours including the use of PRN "rescue" doses.
   • Convert to an equianalgesic parenteral dose. For example, MS Contin 60 mg. every 12 hours = MS Contin 120 mg. every 24 hours. The oral to parenteral morphine conversion ration is 1:3 (refer to Table 11.4). Oral morphine 120 mg. morphine per 24 hours = intravenous morphine 40 mg. in 24 hours = 1.6 mg. per hour.
   • Administer an intravenous dose equivalent to double the hourly intravenous dose (e.g., 3.2 mg.).
   • Repeat same dose in 20 minutes if pain not adequately controlled.
   • If pain persists > 5–6/10 or relief is unsatisfactory to the patient and there are no dose limiting side effects such as excessive sedation, increase the dose by 50%.
   • Repeat same dose every 20 minutes until there is satisfactory pain relief or unacceptable side effects.
   • Remain with the patient during management of the pain crisis.
   • Once the pain is controlled, determine whether the patient will continue on the parenteral route of drug administration or be converted to the oral route.

TABLE 11.9 *(continued)*

- If the parenteral route is to be continued, determine the loading dose and proceed as described in section B.
- If conversion to the oral route is appropriate, determine the loading dose and proceed as described in section C.

E. If the patient is at home in a pain crisis and does not have access to parenteral drugs:
  - Instruct the patient to take two times their standard oral PRN "rescue" dose stat.
  - Repeat in 1 hour if pain persists > 5–6/10 or relief is unsatisfactory for the patient and there are no limiting side effects such as excessive sedation.
  - Monitor the patient closely via telephone for adequacy of pain relief and presence of side effects.
  - Once the patient has achieved adequate pain relief, adjust the ATC dose and PRN "rescues" dose to their new requirements.
  - If the patient's pain is not controlled despite escalating doses of opioids, the patient must be evaluated that day by the home care nurse. In anticipation of intractable pain, parenteral opioids should be brought to the home as well as clonazepam and haloperidol so that they are available if required.
  - Prepare to admit the patient if that is their choice.

F. If the patient does not respond to the above consider:
  - A parenteral NSAID (e.g., Ketorolac).
  - A parenteral steroid (e.g., dextramethasone).
  - Intravenous lidocaine or phenytoin.
  - Anesthesia procedure (e.g., epidural administration of opioids/local anesthetics; nerve blocks).
  - A ketamine infusion.
  - Sedation.

These guidelines were developed with input from advanced practice nurses and physicians in the Pain and Palliative Care Service, Memorial Sloan-Kettering Cancer Center. It is emphasized that they are merely guidelines and do not substitute for good clinical judgment.

---

assisted suicide strongly endorsed sedation in the imminently dying as appropriate palliative care, distinguishing it from physician-assisted suicide and euthanasia (Burt, 1997).

Numerous surveys of nurses and physicians suggest that clinicians are confused about the application of ethical principles in the care of the dying (Solomon et al., 1993). For example, in a recent survey of neurologists, 40% reported that administering intravenous morphine to a dyspneic amyotrophic lateral sclerosis (ALS) patient could be considered a form of euthanasia (Carver, 1999) and yet this is standard palliative treatment for the management of dyspnea. The American Nurses Association, in their position paper on promotion of comfort and relief of pain in dying patients state unambiguously: "Nurses should not hesitate to use full and effective doses of pain medication for the proper management of pain in the dying patient. The increasing titration of pain medication to achieve adequate symptom control, even at the expense of life, thus hastening death secondarily, is ethically justified" (American Nurses Association, 1990). The principle evoked here is the Principle of "Double Effect." The Principle of Double Effect distinguishes between the compelling primary therapeutic intent—to relieve suffering—and the unavoidable untoward consequences—likely diminution of consciousness and potential for accelerated death (Cherny & Coyle, 1999; Latimer, 1991). Of note, however, in a comparison of patients who were sedated for symptom control versus those who were not, in both hospital and home-based palliative care settings, there was no significant difference in patients time to death (Charter, Vickrey, & Bernat, 1998). In a study of opioid doses in patients cared for in an inpatient palliative care unit, there was no correlation between the opioid doses and the timing of deaths (Brescia, Portenoy, Ryan, Drasnoff, & Gray, 1992).

Palliative care teams need to develop guidelines for the use of sedation in dying patients with intractable symptoms. Such guidelines must include the parameters for the choice of drug and dosage and a titration method correlated to symptom assessment and individualized to the patient. Clear documentation and communication among the team members and with the family is essential. It should reflect: the goals of care clearly stated in unambiguous terms with resuscitation status established; discussion with the patient and/or health care proxy with informed consent; symptom being treated and management approach selected; and end point to be achieved and monitoring parameters. Dose escalation without clear indications should not occur. In this way the integrity of the process is maintained.

Tolerance, Physical Dependence, and Psychological Dependence (Addiction): Clinical Significance in End-of-Life Care

Tolerance is the phenomenon characterized by the need for increasing dose to maintain the same drug effect (American Pain Society, 1999). Usually the reason for dose escalation at the end of life occurs in the setting of increasing pain associated with progressive disease (Coyle et al., 1990; Foley, 1993). Patients with stable disease do not usually require increasing opioid doses (Foley, 1993; Levy, 1989). This observation, integrated with the knowledge that there is no "ceiling" effect to the opioid drugs, implies the following: (1) concern about tolerance to analgesic effects should not impede the use of opioids early in the course of the disease, and (2) worsening pain in a patient on a stable dose of opioids is assumed to be evidence of disease progression until proven otherwise (Coyle & Portenoy, 1995).

Physical dependence is an altered physiologic state that occurs in patients who use opioids on a long-term basis. If the drug is stopped abruptly or an antagonist is given, the patient exhibits signs of withdrawal. Signs of opioid withdrawal include anxiety, alternating hot flashes and cold chills, salivation, rhinorrhea, diaphoresis, piloerection, nausea, vomiting, abdominal cramping, and insomnia (American Pain Society, 1999). The timeframe of the withdrawal syndrome depends on the half life of the drug. For example, abstinence from drugs with a short half life such as morphine and hydromorphone, may occur within 6 to 12 hours of stopping the drug, and be most severe after 24 to 72 hours. After withdrawal of drugs with a long half life such as methadone or levorphanol, the symptoms may not occur for a day or longer (Hanks & Cherny, 1998). Gradual reduction of the opioid dose in the physically dependent patient who no longer has pain will prevent the withdrawal syndrome (American Pain Society, 1999). Clinical experience suggests that administering 25% of the previous analgesic dose will prevent the withdrawal syndrome. Patients must be closely monitored during the tapering process to be sure they are not experiencing symptoms of withdrawal as their needs are variable.

The use of an antagonist such as naloxone in the physically dependent patient will precipitate acute withdrawal symptoms unless carefully titrated. If a drug overdose is suspected in a patient who has received opioids for more than a few days, a dilute solution of naloxone can be used (0.4 mg in 10 ml of normal saline solution) (American Pain Society, 1999). This may be administered in 1 ml bolus injections every one to three minutes until the patient becomes responsive. As the half-life of naloxone is considerably shorter than the majority of opioid drugs, an intravenous infusion of naloxone, carefully titrated to respirations and level of pain, may be the safest approach once the patient has become stable (Table 11.6). It is reiterated that the need to use naloxone to reverse opioid induced respiratory depression at end of life is exceedingly rare (Fins, 1999).

Psychological dependence (addiction) is defined as a pattern of compulsive drug use characterized by a continued craving for an opioid, loss of control, and continued use despite harm. Addiction is rare in patients without a history of drug abuse who are receiving opioids for cancer pain (Porter & Jick, 1980). Concerns about this outcome, however, continue to be a reason for undertreatment of pain (Cleeland, 1989; Foley, 1989b). In the setting of poorly relieved pain, "aberrant" drug-seeking behavior such as "clock watching" requires careful nursing assessment. The term "pseudoaddiction" has been used to describe drug-seeking behavior, reminiscent of addiction, that occurs in the setting of inadequate pain relief and is eliminated by improved analgesia (Weissman, Bunchman, Dinndorf, & Dahl, 1990). For the most part, this behavior signifies inadequate pain relief. Patients and their families need to be reassured that use of opioid drugs in the amount that is needed to control pain, regardless of what that amount is, will not result in addiction. The patient will not die an "addict." The management of pain in patients with a history of drug abuse will be discussed in the section on special populations.

Opioid Side-Effects and Their Management

Constipation. Constipation in the palliative care setting is common and usually multifactorial (Bruera et al., 1994; Portenoy, 1994). It is the most frequently encountered side effect experienced during opioid therapy and the one to which patients' rarely develop tolerance. Opioid binding to peripheral receptors in the gut prolongs colon transit time by increasing or decreasing segmental contractions and decreasing propulsive peristalsis (Sykes, 1998). Because the likelihood of constipation is so great in palliative care patients who are receiving opioid therapy, laxative medications should be prescribed in a preemptive manner (Walsh, 1990). Table 11.10 outlines a nursing approach to the assessment and management of constipation for patients receiving chronic opioid therapy.

Sedation. Some level of sedation is experienced by many patients at the initiation of opioid therapy and during significant dose escalation. Patients usually develop tolerance to this effect in days to weeks (Bruera, Macmillan, & MacDonald, 1989; Portenoy, 1994). Should sedation persist, at a level that is unacceptable to the patient, a careful assessment by the nurse is needed. Confounding factors such as other sedating drugs, metabolic disturbances, sleep deprivation, and the somnolence that may occur at end of life must be identified. Nursing evaluation and management of persistent unwanted sedation in patients receiving opioid therapy is outlined in Table 11.11. Management steps include elimination of nonessential drugs with central nervous system depressant effects, reduction of the opioid dose if feasible, changing to an alternate opioid drug, and if necessary adding a psychostimulent such as dextroamphetamine, methylphenidate, or pemoline (Portenoy, 1994).

Confusion. Like sedation, mild cognitive impairment is common after initiation of opioid therapy (Bruera et al., 1989, 1992; Portenoy, 1994). Patients may express this as feeling "mentally hazy" or "not as sharp as before." Patients should be reassured that these effects are transient in most individuals and last from a few days to a week or two. Persistent confusion attributable

TABLE 11.10   Guidelines in Assessment and Management of Constipation in the Patient Receiving Chronic Opioid Therapy

- Identify "normal" bowel pattern for individual patient.
- Identify present bowel pattern and how it varies from the patient's norm.
- Identify factors that may be contributing to the patient's constipation and address those that are treatable:

  —Drugs in addition to the opioids (e.g., antidepressants).
  —Inactivity.
  —Generalized weakness (e.g., unable to get to the toilet, has to use a bedpan).
  —Lack of privacy when toileting.
  —Dehydration, fever.
  —Lack of bulk and fiber in diet.
  —Metabolic (e.g., hypercalcium, hypokalemia).

- Disimpact patient if necessary (give rescue dose beforehand).
- Establish a bowel-management program appropriate to the patient and level of debility.

  —Anticipate daily bowel regimen will be needed in patients' receiving ATC opioids.
  —Consider combination of stool softener with drug that increases peristalsis as a first-line management approach (e.g., ducusate plus senna).
  —Use bulk agent to supplement fiber in the diet if appropriate; avoid in severely debilitated patients and those with partial bowel obstruction. May increase flactulance, distention, bloating, and abdominal pain in patients with intraabdominal disease.
  —Have "backup" agents available for episodes of refractory constipation (e.g., lactulose, magnesium citrate, rectal suppositories, enema).

- In patients with persistent refractory constipation consider use of:

  —A prokinetic agent to improve colonic transit (e.g., metaclopramide).
  —Oral administration of Naloxone to produce "bowel withdrawal" without concurrent systemic withdrawal. Treatment with oral Naloxone should always incorporate dose escalation (e.g., starting at a dose of 0.8 mg daily [0.4 mg BID], and doubling the dose every 2 to 3 days until a favorable response or any signs of systemic withdrawal occur).

From Coyle, N., Cherny, N. I., & Portenoy, R. K. (1995). Pharmacologic management of cancer pain. In D. B. McGuire, C. H. Yarbro, & B. R. Ferrell (Eds.), *Cancer pain management* (2nd ed.) (p. 112). Boston: Jones & Bartlett Publishers. (Reprinted with permission.)

TABLE 11.11 **Guidelines in Assessment and Management of Persistent Sedation in the Patient Receiving Chronic Opioid Therapy**

- Evaluate potential disease or treatment-related causes for the patient's persistent sedation, including metabolic, sleep deprivation, and closeness to death.
- Evaluate the level of sedation within goals of care for patient, and whether sedation is troublesome to the patient.
- If level of sedation is unacceptable to the patient:
  —Eliminate nonessential CNS depressant medication.
  —If analgesia is satisfactory, reduce opioid dose by 25%.
  —If analgesia is unsatisfactory, or dose reduction is not viable, consider switching to an alternate opioid, especially if current opioid is one with a long half-life such as Methadone.
  —Consider addition of a NSAID or adjuvant analgesic that may allow reduction in opioid use with compromise to analgesia.
- If sedation persists:
  —Consider addition of a psychostimulant (e.g., methylphenidate, caffeine, dextroamphetamine).
  —Consider change to an epidural route to allow dose reduction.
  —Consider use of an anesthetic approach.

From Coyle, N., Cherny, N. I., & Portenoy, R. K. (1995). Pharmacologic management of cancer pain. In D. B. McGuire, C. H. Yarbro, & B. R. Ferrell (Eds.), *Cancer pain management* (2nd ed.) (p. 110). Boston: Jones & Bartlett Publishers. (Reprinted with permission.)

to opioids alone is uncommon. More commonly confusion in patients at the end of life is multifactorial including electrolyte disorders, neoplastic involvement of the CNS, sepsis, vital organ failure, and hypoxia (Portenoy, 1994; de Stoutz, Bruera, & Suarez-Almazor, 1995). Table 11.12 guides the nurse in the evaluation and management of persistent confusion in palliative care patients receiving opioid therapy.

Nausea and Vomiting. Nausea and vomiting are not uncommon at the start of opioid therapy (Portenoy, 1994; Hanks & Cherny, 1998). Tolerance to this effect typically develops within weeks. Both peripheral and central mechanisms are thought to be involved. Opioids stimulate the medullary chemoreceptor trigger zone and increase vestibular sensitivity. Direct effects on the gastrointestinal tract include increased gastric antral tone, diminished motility, and delayed gastric emptying (Portenoy, 1994; Hanks & Cherny, 1998). Constipation may also be a contributing factor. Establishing the pattern of nausea may clarify the etiology of the symptom and guide management approaches (Table 11.13). Frequently a combination of cognitive and pharmacologic approaches are used, depending on the pattern of the nausea

TABLE 11.12   Guidelines in Assessment and Management of Confusion in the Patient Receiving Chronic Opioid Therapy

- Establish whether the patient's confusion is long-standing or new. Identify the pattern.
- Evaluate potential disease or treatment-related causes for the patient's confusion. Treat underlying cause whenever possible.
- Recognize the prevalence of end of life delirium.
- Remember that opioids alone rarely cause persistent confusion.
- Review patient's drug therapy. Eliminate nonessential centrally acting medication.
- If analgesia is satisfactory, reduce opioids by 25%; reassess.
- If analgesia is unsatisfactory or confusion persists, consider switching to an alternate opioid. Select an opioid with a short half-life.
- Consider a trial of a neuroleptic (e.g., haloperidol).
- Consider use of an anesthetic approach to allow for opioid reduction.

From Coyle, N., Cherny, N. I., & Portenoy, R. K. (1995). Pharmacologic management of cancer pain. In D. B. McGuire, C. H. Yarbro, & B. R. Ferrell (Eds.), *Cancer pain management* (2nd ed.) (p. 111). Boston: Jones & Bartlett Publishers. (Reprinted with permission.)

and assumed underlying mechanism. Cognitive techniques might include relaxation training with focused breathing, guided imagery, and distraction (Fishman, 1991). For nausea associated with early satiation and bloating, metoclopramide is often the initial pharmacologic approach. If vertigo or movement-induced nausea are the predominant features, the patient may benefit from an antivertiginous drug such as scopolamine (transdermal) or meclazine. Other options include trials of alternative opioids, treatment with an antihistamine (e.g., hydroxyzine or diphenhydramine), neuroleptic (e.g., haloperidol or chlorpromazine), benzodiazepine (e.g., lorazepam), or a steroid (e.g., dexamethasone). The role of seratonin antagonists (e.g., odansetron) has not been established in opioid-induced nausea and vomiting (Hanks & Cherny, 1998; Portenoy, 1994).

Multifocal Myoclonus.   Mild and infrequent multifocal myoclonus can occur with all opioids (Hanks & Cherny, 1998). The effect is dose-related and the mechanism is unclear. Pronounced myoclonus is extremely distressing to the patient. The uncontrolled, abrupt, jerking movements of the patient's limbs and/or torso can increase already existing pain. Myoclonus can be a sign of opioid toxicity and is a reason to switch to an alternate opioid. In addition, a benzodiazepine, for example, clonazepam, can be used to treat the symptom (Twycross & Lichter, 1998).

TABLE 11.13 Guidelines in Assessment and Management of Nausea and Vomiting Based on Inferred Mechanism in the Patient Receiving Chronic Opioid Therapy

Inferred mechanism	Clinical features	Antiemetic drugs of choice
Stimulation of the medullary chemoreceptor trigger zone	Nausea and vomiting or both shortly after opioid administration	Metoclopramide, prochlorperazine, chlorpromazine, haloperidol, corticosteroids, or lorazepam
Enhanced vestibular sensitivity	Prominent movement-induced nausea and vomiting or vertigo	Scopolamine, meclazine, or lorazepam
Increased gastric antral tone	Early satiation, postprandial bloating or vomiting	Metoclopramide
Constipation	Passage of small, hard, infrequent stool, with difficulty	Proactive bowel regimen

From Coyle, N., Cherny, N. I., & Portenoy, R. K. (1995). Pharmacologic management of cancer pain. In D. B. McGuire, C. H. Yarbro, & B. R. Ferrell (Eds.), *Cancer pain management* (2nd ed.) (p. 114). Boston: Jones & Bartlett Publishers. (Reprinted with permission.)

Urinary Retention.   Urinary retention can occur in patients receiving opioid drugs especially in those who require rapid escalation of the drug, are receiving other drugs with anticholinergic effects such as the tricyclic antidepressants or have compromised bladder function. Older men with an enlarged prostate are particularly at risk. Opioids increase smooth muscle tone and infrequently cause bladder spasm or an increase in spincter tone which may lead to urinary retention (Hanks & Cherny, 1998).

Respiratory Depression.   Fear of respiratory depression is a frequently cited concern among medical and nursing staff when initiating opioid therapy or when rapidly increasing opioid drugs to control pain in a debilitated patient at the end of life. This fear may be accentuated by the current climate and discussion regarding physician-assisted suicide and euthanasia. Clinicians may not want to be seen as hastening death, and confuse good palliative care with appearing to hasten death. *The principle of double effect* is an essential ethical construct for nurses to understand if they are going to adequately control complex symptoms at the end of life. This principle distinguishes between the compelling primary therapeutic intent (to relieve suffering) and unavoidable untoward consequences (such as the likely diminution of interactional function and the potential for hastening death) (Latimer, 1991). The principle of double effect is most commonly evoked in the use of high-dose opioid analgesics or induced sedation in the management of otherwise refractory pain or shortness of breath (Cavanaugh, 1996; Cherny & Portneoy, 1994). It is predicated on the axion that *intent* is a critical ethical concern, and that the distinction between foreseeing and intending an unavoidable maleficent outcome is ethically significant (Latimer, 1991). When caring for patients at the end of life with intractable symptoms invocation of this principle allows suffering to be relieved and symptoms to be controlled. Giving a patient who is dying, hypotensive, and in pain sufficient opioid dosages to control the pain is good palliative care and not euthanasia (Coyle, 1992).

Clinically significant respiratory depression is always accompanied by other signs of central nervous system (CNS) depression such as sedation and mental clouding and is unusual in the patient receiving chronic opioid therapy unless other contributing factors are present. Pain antagonizes CNS depression, and respiratory effects are unlikely to occur in the presence of severe pain. With repeated administration of an opioid, tolerance develops rapidly to the respiratory depressant effects of the drug (Foley, 1991). Unwarranted fears of respiratory depression should not interfere with appropriate upward titration of opioid drugs to pain relief or the onset of intolerable and unmanageable side effects (Lipman & Gauthier, 1997). Opioid-induced respiratory depression, however, can occur if the patient's pain is abruptly eliminated (e.g., after a neurolytic or neuroablative procedure) and the opioid drug is not reduced. Pain counterbalances the respiratory depressant effects of the opioids. When the pain stimulus is no longer present respiratory depression may occur.

Adjuvant Analgesia

Adjuvant analgesics are those drugs that have a primary indication other than pain but are analgesic in certain pain states (Walsh, 1990). These drugs can be used at any step of the "analgesic ladder." As with the institution of any analgesic regimen, their use is based on a careful assessment of the pain, inferred pain mechanism(s), and analgesic history. Adjuvant drugs in the palliative care setting are typically used to enhance the effects of the opioid drugs, or to allow for dose reduction because of adverse opioid side-effects (Portenoy, 1998). In the palliative care setting, it is useful to classify the adjuvant analgesics into three broad groups: multipurpose adjuvant analgesics, adjuvant analgesics used primarily for neuropathic pain, and adjuvant analgesics used for bone pain. Table 11.14 provides a guide to the commonly used adjuvant drugs. As a general principle, low initial doses with dose titration until symptom relief is achieved is suggested.

Multipurpose Adjuvant Analgesics Used in Palliative Care

Corticosteroids. Corticosteroids are used to treat various types of neuropathic pain resulting from tumor infiltrating or compressing neural structures such as nerve, plexus, root, or spinal cord. Corticosteroids can be extremely useful in the acute management of a pain crisis when neural structures or bone are involved. Dexamethasone (16–24 mg/day), in combination with an opioid, may be used to treat bone pain, neuropathic pain, back pain associated with cord compression, headaches associated with brain tumors, and pain associated with liver capsule distension. Pain relief is assumed to be associated with anti-inflammatory and antiedema effects (Portenoy, 1998). Adverse effects of corticosteroids include hyperglycemia, gastric irritation, dysphoria, delirium, and myopathy. Lower dose corticosteroids (2 to 4 mg dexamethasone) can improve mood and appetite. These drugs should not be used concurrently with a NSAID and their use should be combined with gastroprotective therapy.

Neuroleptics. Few neuroleptics are analgesic. Phenothiazides have not been found to relieve pain or potentiate opioid analgesia (American Pain Society, 1999).

TABLE 11.14 Commonly Used Adjuvant Analgesics

(*Please refer to the PDR for current information as dosing recommendations change. This Table is to be used as a guide only and not to replace a more comprehensive review.)

Class	Indication	Preferred drugs	Dosing schedule	Starting dose (mg/Day)	Usual daily dose (mg/Day)	Comment
Antidepressants	Continuous neuropathic pain	Amitriptyline	q hs	10–25	50–150	If side-effects too great with amitriptyline, try desipramine, or nortriptyline, or paroxetine.
		Imipramine				
		Desipramine				
		Nortriptyline				
		Paroxetine		20	20–60	
Anticonvulsants	Neuropathic pain	Gabapentin	q 8 h	300	2,700	Generally considered first line drug for neuropathic pain.
		Phenytoin	q hs	300	300	
		Valproate	q 8 h	500	750–2,250	
		Clonzepam	q 12 h	0.5	0.5–3	
		Carbamazepine	q 6–8 h	200	600–1,600	
		Topiramate	q 12 h	25	100–400	
		Lamotrigine	q 12 h	25–50	200–400	

(continued)

TABLE 11.14 *(continued)*

Class	Indication	Preferred drugs	Dosing schedule	Starting dose (mg/Day)	Usual daily dose (mg/Day)	Comment
Oral local anesthetics	Neuropathic pain	Mexiletine	q 8 h	300	450–900	May be safer than tocamide and should be tried first.
Alpha-2 adrenergic agonists		Tocainide	q 8 h	600	1,200–1,800	
		Clonidine	q 12 h	.1–.2	.2–.6	
NMDA receptor antagonists		Tizanidine	q 12 h	2–4	4–40	
		dextromethorphan		2–40	up to 1 gm	
		ketamine				Consult with anesthesia colleagues.
		amantadine				
Corticosteroids	Pain from infiltration of neural structures; bone pain; pain in patients with far advanced disease.	Dexamethasone	q 6–8 h	Variable	Variable	Higher doses in cord compression.
Neuroleptics	Pain complicated by delirium or nausea.	Haloperidol	q 6–12 h	0.5–10		
Miscellaneous	For neuropathic pain and muscle spasticity pain.	Lioresal	TID	5–10	120	

TABLE 11.14 (*continued*)

Class	Indication	Preferred drugs	Dosing schedule	Starting dose (mg/Day)	Usual daily dose (mg/Day)	Comment
Antihistamines	Pain complicated by anxiety or nausea.	Hydroxyzine	q 6–8 h	75	200	Hydroxyzine analgesic in controlled trials of high parenteral doses. No evidence of analgesia from oral doses.
Analeptics	To reduce opioid-induced sedation.	methyphenidate	1–2 × day	5	10–40	Higher doses sometimes needed. Last dose before 3 pm.
		dextroamphetamine	1–2 × day	5	10–40	
Bisphosphonates	Bone pain	Pamidronate	60 mg IV every other week	—	—	Inhibit osteoclast activity. Need to monitor blood calcium and phosphate, magnesium, and potassium.

(*continued*)

TABLE 11.14 (*continued*)

Class	Indication	Preferred drugs	Dosing schedule	Starting dose (mg/Day)	Usual daily dose (mg/Day)	Comment
Radiopharmaceuticals	Bone pain	Strontium-89	Single dose			Absorbed at areas of high bone turnover. Marrow toxicity mild.
		Samarium-153				
Miscellaneous	Bone pain	Calcitonin	Daily	25 I.U.	100–200 I.U.	Limited reports of efficacy in bone pain.
	Bowel obstruction	octreotide	100–600 mcg/day s/c bolus or infusion			
		Scopolamine	1.5 mg patch Q 3 days			
		Glycopyrrolate	0.1 mg q 4–6 h prn			

*Table based on clinical experience of the authors and a variety of published sources.
Q = every hour; h = hour.

Adapted from Coyle, N., Cherny, N. I., & Portenoy, R. K. (1995). Pharmacologic management of cancer pain. In D. B. McGuire, C. H. Yarbro, & B. R. Ferrell (Eds.), *Cancer pain management* (2nd ed., pp 118–119). ©1995 Jones & Bartlett Publishers, Boston.

Antihistamines. The antihistamine hydroxycine has analgesic, antiemetic, and mild sedative activity as well as antihistamine effect when given parenterally (Beaver & Feise, 1976; Hupert, Yacoub, & Turgeon, 1980). It is not clear, however, that oral administration has analgesic effects and clinical experience does not support the use of this drug as an adjuvant for cancer pain. Hydroxicine may be helpful to some patients at the end of life who have anxiety, nausea, and or itch associated with their pain (Coyle & Portenoy, 1995).

Benzodiazepines. The use of benzodiazepines as adjuvant analgesics is limited because of their sedative effects compounding that of the opioids. Understanding the etiology and inferred mechanism of pain is therefore important when deciding whether or not to add a benzodiazepine to the patient's analgesic regimen. Clonazepam is sometimes used in an attempt to relieve lancinating neuropathic pain, and diazepam to relieve muscle spasm associated with acute pain (American Pain Society, 1999).

Adjuvant Analgesics Used Primarily for Neuropathic Pain

Antidepressant Drugs. Antidepressant drugs are nonspecific analgesics that are used predominantly for the continuous dysesthesias component of neuropathic pain in the cancer population (Hewitt & Portenoy, 1998; Portenoy, 1991). Analgesia associated with the antidepressants is thought to result from enhancement of neurotransmitter activity in endogenous pain-modulating pathways (Basbaum & Fields, 1984; Besson & Chaouch, 1987). Analgesia can occur in the absence of mood change, and the effective analgesic dose in the palliative care population is usually much lower than that required to treat depression (Max, 1987; Max, Lynch, Muir, Shoaf, & Smoller, 1992; Watson, Evans, & Reed, 1982). Some tricyclic antidepressants have also been shown to increase plasma concentrations of morphine in cancer patients. Common dose-related side effects include sedation, orthostatic hypotension, constipation, dry mouth, and dizziness. Tricyclic antidepressants are relatively contraindicated in patients with coronary disease in whom they can worsen ventricular arrthymias (Portenoy, 1998). In that situation the risk/benefit ratio for the patient needs to be carefully weighed. A tricyclic with less cardiotoxicity potential such as desipramine should be considered. Amitriptyline has the best documented analgesic effect, but is less well-tolerated in many end-of-life patients because of the anticholinergic effects (e.g., dry mouth, urinary retention, constipation, and delirium) (American Pain Society, 1999). Other tricyclic antidepressants have less potent anticholinergic effects and therefore may be better tolerated in palliative care patients (e.g., nortriptyline or desipramine). Desipramine and nortriptyline can produce insomnia and should therefore be administered during the day (American Pain Society, 1999). The starting dose of a tricyclic antidepressant should be low (refer to Table 11.14), with the dose increase every few days. The usual effective dosing range is 50 to 150 mg of amitriptyline, imipramine, doxepin, or desipramine daily. Analgesia is usually achieved in about a week after achieving a therapeutic dosing level (Coyle & Portenoy, 1995). Because of the sedative effects of amitriptyline, most patients prefer to be treated with a single nighttime dose.

Anticonvulsant Drugs.   Anticonvulsant drugs are used to control the sharp, shooting, stabbing quality of neuropathic pain (Swerdlow, 1984). Carbamazepine, phenytoin, valproate, and gabapentin have all been used in the management of neuropathic pain. Their side-effect profile needs to be carefully factored into the benefit of their use. Gabapentin, a newer anticonvulsant, has been found to be useful in the management of both the dysesthetic and electric shock-like components of neuropathic pain (Portenoy, 1998; Rosenberg, Harrell, Ristic, Werner, & deRosayro, 1997; Rowbotham, Harden, Stacey, Berstein, & Magnus-Miller, 1998) and has a more favorable side-effect profile than other anticonvulsants (Goa & Sorkin, 1993). The mechanism of the analgesia produced by anticonvulsant drugs is not clear but most of these drugs reduce neuronal hyperactivity and suppress paraxysmal discharge (Weinberger, Nicklas, & Berl, 1976).

GABAb Agonists.   Baclofen, an agonist at the GABBAb receptor, is primarily used for spasticity but is potentially analgesic for lancinating or paroxysmal pains associated with neural injury of any kind (Fromm, Terrence, & Chattha, 1984; Portenoy, 1998). Baclofen may interfere with mechanisms involved in neuropathic pain (Portenoy, 1998). The starting dose is 5 mg two to three times per day, and the dose can be titrated upwards to a range of 30 to 90 mg per day (Portneoy, 1998). The side-effect profile includes dizziness, somnolence, and gastrointestinal distress. Slow upward dose titration is suggested in the palliative care setting. Abrupt discontinuation following prolonged use can result in a withdrawal syndrome including delirium and seizures (Kofler & Leiss, 1992). Doses should therefore always be tapered before discontinuation.

Alpha-2 Adrenergic Antagonists.   Clonidine is the most commonly used alpha-2 adrenergic antagonist for neuropathic pain refractory to opioids and other adjuvants. Systemic administration of clonidine via the oral or transdermal route or via intraspinal infusions have been used (Eisenach et al., 1995; Portenoy, 1998). Interactions with alpha-2 receptors in the spinal cord or brainstem activate endogenous systems that reduce nociceptive input in the central nervous system thought to be involved in the processing of noxious stimuli (Kayser, Desmeules, & Guilland, 1995).

Local Anesthetics. Local anesthetics are generally considered second line drugs in the management of neuropathic pain, and are considered for use in patients who have failed to respond to the tricyclic antidepressants, anticonvulsants, and baclofen (Coyle & Portenoy, 1995). A brief intravenous infusion of lidocaine or procaine has been used to relieve severe neuropathic pain that has not responded promptly to an opioid and requires immediate relief (Portenoy, 1998). Long-term use of subcutaneous lidocaine has been reported for the relief of refractory neuropathic pain (Brose & Cousins, 1991). Oral local anesthetics used in neuropathic pain include tocainide, mexilitine, and flecainide (Portenoy, 1998). The analgesic effects of local anesthetics is thought to derive from suppression of aberrant electrical activity or hypersensitivity in neural structures involved in the pathogenesis of neuropathic pain (Portenoy, 1998).

Local anesthetics produce dose-dependent adverse effects that involve the central nervous system and cardiovascular system including dizziness, tremor, unsteadiness, parasthesias, nausea, bradycardia, and other arrythmias (Portenoy, 1998). Their use should be avoided in patients with a history of cardiac arrythmias or cardiac insufficiency. Mexilitine is the only commonly used oral local anesthetic in the United States. As with the other adjuvant drugs used in palliative care, low initial doses with gradual titration upwards to reach a balance between favorable effect and adverse side effects is suggested. Mexilitine dosing should start at 150 mg once or twice a day, gradually titrated up to a maximum dose of 300 mg three times a day (Portenoy, 1998). Lidocaine infusions in the medically frail typically start at 2 to 5 mg/kg infused over 20 to 30 minutes (Portenoy, 1998). Anesthesia members of the pain and palliative care team are usually involved in decisions surrounding the use of a lidocaine infusion.

Topical Analgesics. Topical analgesics have a useful place in end-of-life care where patients are typically vulnerable to the side effects of systemically administered drugs. Topical analgesics such as local anesthetic preparations, capsaicin, formulations containing NSAIDs (Rowbotham, 1994) and prostaglandin E1 ointment (Mashimo, Tomi, Pak, Demizu, & Yyoshiya, 1991) have all been used for continuous neuropathic pain with a predominantly peripheral mechanism.

Topical local anesthetics, for example, the eutectic mixture of local anesthetics (EMLA) cream, when applied locally, produce a dense cutaneous local anesthesia that can be very soothing to patients with post herpetic neuralgia (Stow, Glynn, & Minor, 1989). To create a dense sensory loss, EMLA cream needs to be applied thickly and covered with an occlusive dressing such as saran wrap. Clinical experience has demonstrated that some patients gain benefit from using a thin application of EMLA cream without an occlusive dressing. The EMLA cream is usually applied three to four times a day for periods of 20 days, followed by a rest period of 5 days to ensure continued benefit. Topical lidocaine in the form of a 5% lidocaine gel can also be effective in patients with post herpetic neuralgia (Rowbotham, Davies, & Fields, 1995). The risk of toxicity from systemic absorption of a topical local anesthetic appears small (Rowbotham et al., 1995; Stow et al., 1989).

Topical capsaicin may be useful to control the constant, burning, local, dysethetic pain of post herpetic neuralgia, for some patients (Watson, Evans, & Watt, 1988). An unpleasant burning sensation, however, may follow topical application, making its use intolerable for some patients. This burning sensation may lessen or disappear after days or weeks of continued use. Capsaicin is thought to lessen pain by reducing the concentration of small peptides (including substance P) in primary afferent neurons, which activate nociceptive systems in the dorsal horn of the spinal cord (Dubner, 1991).

N-Methyl-D-Aspartate (NMDA) Receptor Antagonists. Neuropathic pain includes a large number of diverse pain syndromes, some of which are thought to be mediated by so-called NMDA receptors in the spinal cord. N-Methyl-D-Aspartate receptors bind excitatory amino acids, such as glutamate, and it is likely that processes that involve the excitation of these receptors lead to neurophysiologic changes that ultimately result in pain and allodynia. (Touch that is not normally experienced as painful is experienced as being extremely painful.) The NMDA receptors are also postulated to be involved in the phenomenon of opioid tolerance (Portenoy, 1998). Drugs that block the NMDA receptor such as dextromethorphan and ketamine, have been shown to reduce some types of neuropathic pain and are now in clinical use (Backonja, Arndt, Gombar, Check, & Zimmerman, 1994; Eide, Jorum, Stubhang, Bremners, & Breiril, 1994; Persson, Alexsson, Hallin, & Gustafsson, 1995; Stannard & Porter, 1993).

A trial of ketamine in the medically frail patient at the end of life is justified in the setting of refractory neuropathic pain. Ketamine can, however, produce psychomometic effects (delirium, nightmares, hallucinations, and dysphoria). Assessment for these symptoms prior to initiating the infusion and on an ongoing basis is necessary. As with an infusion of local anesthetics, anesthesia members of the pain and palliative care team are usually involved in decisions surrounding a ketamine infusion in palliative care. A ketamine trial can be initiated at low doses of 0.1 to 0.15 mg/kg for a brief infusion or 0.1 to 0.15 mg/kg/hr for a continuous infusion (Portenoy, 1998).

Adjuvant Analgesics for Bone Pain

Bone pain can be an extremely troublesome problem for cancer patients at the end of life. As previously described, NSAIDs can be helpful in combination with the opioid drugs (Steps 2 and 3 of the analgesic ladder). Parenteral NSAIDs as well as corticosteroids can produce dramatic relief in difficult cases as previously reviewed, for example, the patient with bone pain who presents in a pain crisis. A concentrated course of radiation should also be considered for patients with focal bone pain.

The *radiopharmaceutical Medastrom* is an analog of calcium and is taken up by the skeleton into active sites of bone metastasis (Porter et al., 1993). Medastrom has been found to reduce disease progression in some patients, decrease new sites of pain, and decrease systemic analgesic use (Porter, EcEwan, & Powe, 1993; Robinson, Preston, & Spicer, 1992). Because of the lag response time following treatment of from two to three weeks, this approach is not appropriate for patients who are very close to death.

Biphosphonate pamidronate disodium inhibits osteoclastic bone resorption and has been shown to reduce pain and skeletal complications such as pathological fractures in patients with breast cancer (Hortobagyi, Theriault, & Porter, 1996) and multiple myeloma (Berenson, Lichtenstein, & Porter, 1996).

Calcitonin is also an inhibitor of osteoclast-induced bone resorption and should be considered for patients with refractory bone pain (Blomquist, Elomaa, & Porkka, 1988; Hindley, Hill, Letland, & Wiles, 1982).

SECTION 2: NONDRUG INTERVENTIONS

In addition to the pharmacologic approach to pain management at the end of life, there are other approaches that may be useful. These nondrug or nonpharmacologic interventions or techniques can complement the treatment of the underlying pain etiology and the mainstay pharmacologic approach to pain management. Nondrug interventions cover a broad spectrum of approaches. These types of interventions can modify the pain experience and give individuals an increased sense of control, decrease anxiety, improve mood, and improve sleep.

Some of the nondrug approaches that will be discussed, such as nerve blocks, are considered mainstream, traditional western medicine. Other nonconventional therapies, fall under the heading of "complementary" or "alternative." Complementary therapies are used in addition to conventional therapies. Alternative therapies are used in place of traditional ones. The term "integrative" is being used more and more to represent the integration of standard, traditional therapies with the nonconventional therapies (Decker, 2000). The nondrug interventions that will be discussed here, either traditional or complementary, are best considered as a part of the overall pain management plan.

As with pain control in general, there are a variety of factors that promote and inhibit the use of nondrug techniques. On their own, patients often initiate nondrug interventions such as application of heat or use of vibration. The different methods chosen by patients are often based on previous use of a particular intervention or on home remedies and may or may not be an optimal method to relieve a particular type of pain. Although the inclusion of pharmacologic interventions are usually a well-thought-out part of the plan, the use of nondrug interventions is often not. There may be little input from an individual's doctor or nurse in initiating an intervention (Rhiner, Ferrell, Ferrell, & Grant, 1993).

Patients using nondrug methods may report reduced distress, a sense of control, improved mood, or more bearable pain (Layman-Goldstein & Altilio, 1993). Some patients strongly believe that nondrug interventions should be used instead of analgesics or to increase the time between doses of analgesics. For most patients, however, the maximum benefit from nondrug interventions is obtained when they are used in addition to analgesics (Layman-Goldstein & Altilio, 1993).

Compared to the extensive studies that support the use of pharmacologic techniques, there is not strong scientific evidence supporting the use of many of these techniques (McCaffery & Pasero, 1999). In 1999, the Center of Complementary and Alternative Medicine was established under the auspices of the National Institutes of Health to establish an information clearinghouse and to establish data for evaluating the clinical usefulness of various nontraditional interventions (Decker, 2000). It is hoped that as more money and energy goes into the rigorous evaluation of integrative techniques, it will be easier to appropriately add these interventions into an individual's plan of care. Yet, despite the current situation, patients express benefit from these methods and there are reasons to pursue their use (Jacox et al., 1994; McCaffery & Pasero, 1999; Rhiner, Ferrell, Ferrrell, & Grant, 1993; Spross & Wolff Burke, 1995).

The five main categories of nondrug approaches to pain management are: 1) psychological interventions; 2) physiatric interventions; 3) neurostimulatory interventions; 4) invasive interventions; and 5) integrative interventions. In the following discussion, various techniques will be placed in the context of these catagories. However, as so aptly pointed out by McCaffery and Passero (1999) and Fernandez (1986), there is no common taxonomy and no uniformly accepted classification system for nonpharmacologic interventions. Often, an intervention may fall into more than one category or subcategory.

When reviewing the nondrug techniques, it useful to consider whether a specific intervention will need high or low levels of patient and caregiver involvement, and whether it is noninvasive or invasive. Some of the interventions, such as acupuncture, are invasive and should only be done by skilled practitioners. Because of this and other factors, it may or may not be possible to facilitate use of some of the nondrug techniques in individuals with advanced disease. The Clinical Practice Guidelines for the Management of Cancer Pain Panel Consensus stated that "with rare exceptions, noninvasive approaches should precede invasive palliative approaches" (Jacox, Carr, Payne, et al., 1994, p. 89).

PSYCHOLOGICAL INTERVENTIONS

A palliative care patient needs a biopsychosocial approach to pain management, one that includes the body, mind, and emotions. Incorporation of these elements into a patient's plan of care can lead to more effective pain management. Psychological interventions can help to do this. These interventions can primarily be classified as psychoeducational, cognitive, behavioral, or psychotherapeutic. They can include such things as patient and family education, distraction, self statements, relaxation techniques, guided imagery and hypnosis, patient pain diaries, and Cognitive-Behavioral Therapy (CBT). Three recent studies supported the use of these approaches, sometimes called cognitive-behavioral techniques, in chronic pain patients (Johansson, Dahl, Jannert, Melin, & Andersson, 1998; McCarberg, & Wolf, 1999). The Clinical Practice Guidelines for the Management of Cancer Pain Panel encouraged the use of psychosocial interventions for pain management early in the course of disease, as part of a multimodal approach (Jacox, Carr, Payne, et al., 1994). The nurse, caring for an individual at the end of his or her life, may find that this person is well versed in using specific psychological approaches and is open to using these techniques to aid in coping with pain and other symptoms. On the other hand, the person that the nurse may be caring for may be too weak, debilitated, and cognitively impaired to be taught or even use a previously taught simple relaxation technique. Assessment is key to developing a realistic plan. The intervention must match the specific problem with an appreciation for the patient's abilities and motivations.

Psychoeducational

Patient and Family Education regarding pain management is an intervention that can increase an individual's sense of control. Ideally, at the end of life, patients, their families, and their caregivers will be well informed about pain management. However, the nurse working with these individuals will often find that this is not the case, especially in individuals who initially present with advanced disease. Whatever the circumstances, it is necessary to maintain ongoing assessment and reinforcement of educational information as the clinical situation and patient's needs change. Lack of knowledge regarding pain management is a well-established barrier to good pain control (McCaffery, 1999).

Knowledge regarding pain management should include: pain and its etiology, the principles and methods of pain management, types of analgesics, potential side effects of analgesics and their management, equipment/devices used to deliver analgesics, the concepts of physical dependence, tolerance, and psychological dependence (often thought of as addiction), nonpharmacologic interventions, and expected participation in pain management (Adelhardt et al., 1995). Knowledge of these concepts will enable an individual and their family to be an active, informed participant in the plan of care. (This necessary information was previously reviewed in Section I). Through education, a patient and family may be able to reframe beliefs concerning the inevitability of pain, addiction, and other cognitive errors (Spross & Wolff Burke, 1995). Knowledge deficits related to pain management encompass all dimensions of learning: cognitive, psychomotor, and affective. It is especially important to allay fears and concerns about opioid use, specifically addiction, tolerance, and physical dependence (refer to Section I for a review of these concepts). Individuals who need equipment to relieve their pain will need special opportunities for their families and themselves to practice with that equipment management (Adelhardt et al., 1995).

There are several well-developed references that elaborate on teaching pain management information to patients, families, and caregivers which can be useful to nurses (Ferrell, Grant, Chan, Ahn & Ferrell, 1995; Grant & Rivera, 1995; McCaffery & Pasero, 1999). Readers are encouraged to review these references for more detailed information. Regardless of the setting, principles of patient/family education are to be adhered to. An evaluation of all learners prior to any educational efforts will help to determine priorities and focus efforts. It is best to wait until pain is adequately controlled before giving patients and their families too much information. Teaching sessions may need to be brief with the most important information presented first and continually repeated. A wide variety of written, audio, and CD learning tools on pain management are available to reinforce information. All educational efforts are to be documented. This will improve continuity of care and provide a mechanism for identifying continuing education needs (Grant & Rivera, 1995).

In the palliative care setting, the inclusion of family, supportive friends, and caregivers is essential in pain management. They also have important educational needs and their role in supporting a successful pain management plan cannot be underestimated. Pain has a significant physical and psychological impact on family members caring for a loved one in pain. A study by Ferrell, Grant, Chan, Ahn, and Ferrell (1995) showed that a structured pain education program improved quality of life outcomes for both elderly patients and their family caregivers.

Ideal outcomes of a successful pain management educational intervention will include the patient, family, or caregivers being able to: notify the MD, NP, PA, or RN of any new or unrelieved pain, change in pain location, quality, or intensity and of any side effects experienced; identify the cause of pain; state the rationale of the prescribed analgesic regimen; identify the medications, doses, route, frequency, and potential side effects of an analgesic regimen; if indicated, use equipment related to pain management properly (such as PCA pump); comply with the analgesic regimen, use nonpharmacologic methods appropriately; and express understanding of the differences between tolerance, physical dependence, and psychological dependence (often thought of as addiction).

Cognitive

Distraction is an intervention that focuses on the cognitive component of the pain experience, and is sometimes referred to as cognitive refocusing or attention diversion. According to McCaffery and Pasero (1999), an individual directs his or her attention and concentration to pleasant or nonthreatening stimuli other than the pain. It is thought that because a person has a limited capacity for processing information, the individual who focuses on something other than the pain has less attention that could be given to the pain. This distraction can be passive or active (Fernandez, 1986). Passive distraction can include such things as listening to music, watching a ball game, or movie. Tapes of things humorous to an individual should be considered. Rhiner et al. (1993) promote the use by patients of a library of various musical and humorous choices when utilizing distraction as a nondrug treatment. Active distraction can include such things as mental problem solving, singing, playing an instrument, or playing a video game. Often, for distraction to be effective, its focus must be of interest to the individual. The distraction strategy for a particular individual will depend upon the individual's ability to concentrate and his or her energy level. At the end of life, one's energy level is not predictable. For example, an individual could start out listening to recorded music but decide to make it a more active diversion by tapping out the rhythm and singing along.

McCaffery and Pasero (1999) review in-depth ways to effectively assist patients in using distraction. They suggest that effective distraction strategies should stimulate the four major sensory modalities of sound, sight, touch, and movement. A distraction strategy that is capable of providing a change in stimuli when pain changes is more likely to be an effective one.

The use of distraction for short periods of time for such things as painful procedures is well established. Its use is thought to increase self-control and pain tolerance, and decrease pain intensity (Jacox, Carr, Payne, et al., 1994; McCaffery & Pasero, 1999; Rhiner, Ferrell, Ferrrell, & Grant, 1993; Spross & Wolff, 1995). It has been associated with positive mood and changes and decreases in pain intensity (McCaffery & Pasero, 1999). The use of distraction for chronic pain is more controversial. McCaffery and Pasero (1999), in their review of the literature found that after using distraction, patients with chronic pain may experience more intense pain. It is uncertain as to why this occurs. It may be that distraction prevents the individual from recognizing that certain activities are causing more pain. Following the use of distraction, an individual may be fatigued, irritable, and more aware of the pain. Also, without education, family and caregivers may feel that the individual utilizing distraction does not have the pain or the degree of pain that he or she says. This can lead to a variety of negative situations including a reluctance to administer analgesics.

Self statements can be helpful in getting one through a painful experience. The use of self-statements is based on Bandura's theory of self-efficacy. This theory focuses on a person's beliefs regarding his or her ability to perform behaviors that will produce certain outcomes. It is hypothesized that a person's expectation of self-efficacy will determine "whether a person will initiate coping behavior, the amount of effort a person will put into it, and how long the person will persist in the face of obstacles" (Dunajcik, 1999, p. 501). Application of this theory involves teaching the patient methods that he or she can use to lessen the severity of pain or improve his or her ability to cope with the pain. Practicing and reinforcement of these methods is important to insure. A health care professional works with a patient to "coach" him or her in the use of self statements.

All people carry on internal dialogues that both manifest and influence their belief systems. By becoming aware of the ongoing self-statements, one can gain insight into perceptions and appraisals. Once an appraisal is accessed, a determination is made concerning the helpfulness of the belief system. Clinicians can help patients to use cognitive coping statements to enhance adaptations and to counteract the maladaptive thought processes (Loscalzo, personal communication, February 10, 2000).

Self-statements are devised to assist the patient to get through a painful situation (Fernandez, 1986). Self-statements are usually of two types. The first is a coping self-statement. This type of statement emphasizes the ability of an individual to get through a painful episode. For example, at the start of a pain flare, instead of focusing on their fear of the pain, a person is taught to say to himself or herself , "I've had this kind of pain before, I can keep it under control. I will do this and this . . . " Another version of this technique is reframing or cognitive reappraisal. To use this, individuals are taught to be alert to negative thoughts they might be having and to replace them with more positive thoughts and images. Use of reframing can increase a person's sense of control. For example, instead of thinking "I've had this kind of pain before and it was awful," an individual could say to him or herself, "I've had this kind of pain before and it has gone away" (Jacox, Carr, Payne, et al., 1994, p. 82).

Reinterpretive statements, another kind of self statement that are utilized less often, are an attempt to modify the unpleasant aspects of the pain experience. Denial or rationalization self-statements regarding the pain are used to help one cope with the experience of pain (Fernandez, 1986). For example, someone with a hot, burning pain might say to themselves, "the heat from my pain feels quite nice." These types of statements are harder to use effectively at the end of life but may be useful to patients who are at earlier points in the disease trajectory. In no way does this mean that the pain would be untreated.

Relaxation Techniques utilize techniques designed to produce a "state of relative freedom from both anxiety and skeletal muscle tension" (McCaffery & Pasero, 1999, p. 400). It is considered an adjunct to pain treatment. It is helpful for people whose pain experience causes them to feel out of control, those who will be experiencing procedures or activities that may be stressful or uncomfortable, and those who have successfully used relaxation techniques in the past, including meditation, yoga, and Lamaze. Through the use of relaxation techniques, a person can be taught behaviors to counteract the physical, emotional, and behavioral changes produced by stressors and to maximize control and cope with stressful situations. The goal is to relax one's physical body and quiet one's mind. This technique gives the patient a tool to use independently or with others (Layman-Goldstein & Altilio, 1993).

There are a few relative contraindications to the use of relaxation techniques. These include individuals with a history of psychosis, individuals experiencing respiratory compromise, and individuals who are experiencing a pain emergency. Only experts, who are very experienced and well-trained in the use of these techniques, should work with individuals with respiratory compromise. The unavailability of these experts or the presence of contraindicated conditions may be a barrier to the use of relaxation techniques at the end of life for some patients. During a pain crisis, relaxation will not be effective and the patient will associate the technique with severe pain instead of the desired outcome, pain relief. It is important not to set up a situation where the patient makes the paired association of severe pain and relaxation techniques. To optimize the patient's learning and effective use of this technique, it is better to wait until the pain is under better control. If you are able to stay with a patient during a pain crisis, you could consider having the patient breathe with you (Layman-Goldstein & Altilio, 1993). Also of concern, is the use of relaxation techniques in individuals with bradycardia or heart block because of the physiologic effects of relaxation. These effects can include decreased pulse, blood pressure, respiratory rate, O_2 consumption, CO_2 production, and basal metabolism (Spross & Wolff Burke, 1995). These effects may interact synergistically to cause adverse physiologic effects. Spross and Wolff Burke (1995) suggest that in the acute-care setting clinicians do a pre- and post-relaxation exercise check on pulse and blood pressure when assisting patients with relaxation techniques.

Rhiner et al. (1993) point out that individuals who have never incorporated relaxation into their lives may have difficulty incorporating it at a time when they are experiencing more stress. In fact, some may find it counter-therapeutic. It is most important to match the intervention to whom the patient is and his or her needs.

The National Institutes of Health (NIH) Technology Panel, which evaluated the effects of relaxation on pain and sleep, divides the relaxation techniques into brief and deep methods. In general, the brief methods take less time to acquire or practice. Very often brief methods are abbreviated forms of a corresponding deep method. The brief methods include deep breathing, focused breathing, paced respiration, and self control. Deep methods include such techniques as Progressive Muscle Relaxation (PMR), autogenic training , and meditation. To use autogenic training, one is taught to imagine a peaceful environment and focus on a "heaviness in the limbs, warmth in the limbs, cardiac regulation, centering on breathing, warmth in the upper abdomen, and coolness in the forehead" (NIH Technology Assessment Panel on Integration of Behavioral and Relaxation Approaches Into the Treatment of Chronic Pain and Insomnia, 1996, p. 314). The use of PMR involves the tensing and then relaxing in sequence of each of the 15 major muscle groups.

As a health professional, it is helpful to practice relaxation techniques on oneself before attempting to assist patients in their use. It is useful to have beginning practitioners practice with each other to gain experience and to provide each other with feedback. In learning the technique, one may consider taping oneself. An exercise that a beginning practitioner can use with patients teaches focused beathing and can be taped so that the patient can use it whenever he or she wants (Layman-Goldstein & Altilio,

1993). Also, in this way, the patient and their family may be conditioned to associate the clinician's voice with support, comfort, and emotional connection in future interactions (Loscalzo, 1996). The reader is referred to several references that teach in detail the use of relaxation techniques (Benson, 1975; Copley Cobb, 1984; Loscalzo, 1996; Mast, Meyers, & Urbnanski, 1987a, 1987b, 1987c; McCaffery & Pasero, 1999).

It is important to set the right tone before instructing individuals in relaxation techniques. Ideally, the environment should be as quiet and as calm as possible. This is often challenging, if not impossible in hospital environments. How one enters the room, what one says, and how one communicates one's sense of competence is important. One may be able to influence a patient's sense of control and ability to cope. It is important when working with patient's families to calm them, increase their confidence, and engage them as collaborators.

Most relaxation techniques necessitate active patient involvement. However, McCaffery and Pasero (1999) describe specific techniques that utilize the patient as a passive recipient. These include superficial massage for relaxation, listening to music pleasing to the patient, and animal companion visits. These later techniques may be effective when individuals are fatigued or are lacking the mental or physical ability to actively participate in relaxation techniques.

Guided Imagery and Hypnosis are related cognitive techniques used to manage pain. Spross and Wolff Burke (1995) define imagery as "a mental process that draws on any or all of the senses to create mental representations of reality in order to achieve a specific goal such as reducing pain" (p. 172). Fanning (1988) thinks of imagery as either process or end-result imagery in which one imagines the act of doing something (process) or achieving a desired end result. A state of positive expectancy regarding a problem is created by the belief that a successful solution exists, the confidence that the needed resources are available, and that the use of imagery will promote healing. Imagery can also be classified as incompatible or transformative (Fernandez, 1986). These categories can be further divided. Incompatible imagery can be incompatible emotive imagery (imagery that evokes emotions such as anger, humor, or self-assertion, which are incompatible with pain) or incompatible sensory imagery (images of "pure" sensations that have no obligatory link to particular emotions, i.e., imagining a cold winter day while experiencing a "hot, burning" pain). Transformative imagery, which is designed to alter specific features of the pain experience, can be classified as either contextual transformative or stimulus transformative.

Imagery can be helpful to patients in a variety of situations to cope with disease and gain control of their lives (Stephens, 1993). The most familiar use is to enhance treatment effects. Patients can also use imagery to distract themselves from the present, cope with limitations (such as immobility), and anticipate the future. The later three are perhaps the most useful for patients with pain who can use imagery to regain control of negative thoughts (Spross & Wolff Burk, 1995). Stephens (1993) views imagery as influencing such potential outcomes as improving problem solving and role relations, increasing sense of control, and reducing anxiety. This, in turn, can influence things such as immune response, motor functioning, pain reduction, and wound healing. Work by Moran (1989) demonstrated that other-guided imagery is more effective than self guided imagery in reducing chronic low back pain .

Although imagery can be a very useful technique, it may not be helpful for all individuals. Individuals who are not candidates for imagery include those with a history of mental illness such as psychosis or those with dementia or delirium (a common problem at the end of life). Unstructured, free-flowing imagery can bring to the surface "intense, latent feelings and unconscious conflicts" (Stephens, 1993, p. 240). It is imperative to monitor an individual for distress, restlessness, or agitation during the use of imagery. Individuals need to be taught that they are in complete control of the situation at all times. If, for any reason, the imagery is unpleasant or distressing, they can simply open their eyes to stop the situation (Stephens, 1993).

A debriefing after the use of imagery can be helpful to identify what did or did not work and to determine how to proceed. Those who have positive experiences may wish to modify the original script to make it more effective. Some will want the therapist to create an audiotape for future use (Spross & Wolff Burke, 1995). Some clients who experience distress may be open to exploring the source of their feelings, some may not.

It is thought that the techniques of relaxation, imagery, and hypnosis do not differ empirically. For this reason, Syrjala, Donaldson, Davis, Kippes, and Carr (1995) relabeled hypnosis as "relaxation and imagery" in order to facilitate patient acceptance of their study entitled "Relaxation and imagery and cognitive-behavioral training reduce pain during cancer treatment: A controlled clinical trial." In this study, it was found that "relaxation and imagery," or hypnosis, reduced cancer treatment-related pain.

Hypnosis has been defined as "a state of heightened awareness and focused concentration that can be used to manipulate the perception of pain" (Jacox, Carr, Payne, et al., 1994, p. 186). It was found by the Management of Cancer Pain Guideline Panel to have the highest strength and consistency of evidence supporting its use. Historically, hypnosis is well-established in the treatment of pain. It both induces deep relaxation and redirects the patient's attention away from his or her pain (Cleeland, 1987). Healthy, intact, individuals vary in their ability to utilize hypnosis. Debilitated individuals, at the end of life may have less than their usual ability to utilize hypnosis, making it suitable for even fewer. Hypnosis should only be done by specially trained professionals and will not be reviewed here in greater depth. It is important that both entry into practice and advanced practice students are aware of the value of hypnosis and consider making a referral to a trained professional if hypnosis is something that a patient wishes to explore.

Behavioral

A *Pain Diary* is a tool that is especially useful for the ambulatory population of patients. Clinicians can review this diary with patients over the phone, at home or on clinic visits. Its use facilitates pain assessment, evaluation of pain management interventions, and need for further education (Grant & Rivera, 1995). It can be as simple or as sophisticated as the patient using it. The amount of information included often is a reflection of the patient's energy level. Essential information includes date and time of events, medication, dose of medication, and pain intensity before and after interventions. It is helpful if patients include their activities, periods of rest and sleep, pain quality, mood, and other symptoms, but, this is up to the individual patient. Some prefer to use preprinted forms provided by pharmaceutical companies or other sources, while others prefer to use their computer or a simple spiral notebook. A pain diary can give a patient a sense of control and puts words to feelings that they can share with the family and others.

Patients with advanced disease may at some point be unable to maintain a pain diary. Often their caregivers can be encouraged to record some of the basic information. Use of a pain diary can help patients or family members identify pain management barriers and successes. Use of this tool can assist some in gaining a sense of control in an overwhelming situation (Grant & Rivera, 1995). Successful use of this tool requires patient/family education and reinforcement of its use.

Psychotherapeutic

Cognitive-Behavior Therapy (CBT) was originally developed by psychologists to treat anxiety, stress, and depression using some of the psychoeducational, cognitive, and behavioral techniques previously described. Cognitive Behavioral Therapy has been used to treat individuals in a variety of situations with the goal of therapy based upon the situation. For the individual with cancer-related pain, the goal of CBT is to enhance the sense of self-efficacy or personal control (Fishman & Loscalzo, 1987). The experience of total pain (see Figure 11.3) can add to an individual's sense of fear, anger, anxiety, hopelessness, and helplessness. Fishman writes of the experience of self disintegration faced by individuals with advanced disease who are often dealing with the frustration of personal and interpersonal needs and aspirations while dealing with multiple symptoms and aggressive cancer treatments (Fishman, 1992). Cognitive and behavioral interventions, such as distraction, relaxation, or use of pain diaries, used as part of the multimodal approach to pain management and described previously in this chapter, are incorporated into CBT. Cognitive and behavioral interventions, "which focus on the interactions of thoughts, feelings, and behaviors of the patient and family," can be taught to patients and families to add to their repertoire of coping skills (Loscalzo, 1996, p. 143). Ideally, this occurs early in the treatment phase of an illness. As disease progresses, an individual may experience cognitive impairment from a variety of causes. It is not possible to employ psychological approaches in an individual who is cognitively impaired. It may be necessary to focus more on the family and caregivers as the disease progresses. In this situation, the goal would still be to maximize their coping skills and increase their sense of control.

Cognitive Behavioral Therapy, a pragmatic psychological approach, and its techniques can be taught to interested clinicians who do not have specialized training in psychology or psychopathology. Nurses and social workers often obtain training in the use of some of these techniques. Fishman and Loscalzo (1987), in an article aimed at the non-mental health clinician, review the principles and application of CBT. Realistically, the beginning staff nurse may be able to learn and apply the specific techniques of relaxation and distraction. More training would be needed for the use of CBT and the techniques of guided imagery and hypnosis, and structured support. Often the nurses who have expertise in using these techniques are advanced practice nurses, especially psychiatric clinical nurse specialists. The practice setting dictates what is possible. A busy, noisy inpatient unit may limit use of some techniques. Often the knowledge that a patient may benefit from CBT and a timely referral to a skilled practitioner is what is most achievable.

The use of CBT works best in a series of structured sessions that are flexible and modifiable, according to the developing needs of the individual. Fishman and Loscalzo (1987) suggest that there be clear and explicit goals for both the series of sessions and for each individual session. These goals are to be developed collaboratively by therapist and patient. They will jointly look at the range of problems present and prioritize them. This list will be reviewed on a regular basis and reprioritized as personal, social, and medical changes develop. Based on this list, appropriate interventions to address these problems will be determined. The purpose of the interventions is to resolve specifically defined current problems, not long-term personality and social relations disturbances. Also, the interventions are to be made in a standard and systematic manner. The use of this flexible, adaptive collaboration is designed to enhance the patient's sense of self-control and sense of coherent purpose (Fishman & Loscalzo, 1987). Certain individuals and their families are more receptive to CBT than to traditional psychological approaches, which they may view as too intrusive (Loscalzo, 1996). Cognitive Behavioral Therapy, a psychotherapeutic approach, provides a structure, which some clinicians find useful, in which to collaborate with patients and their families to apply the nondrug psychological interventions to a pain management plan.

PHYSIATRIC INTERVENTIONS

Physiatric interventions are another kind of nondrug intervention that can be helpful in the pain management plan. The fact that pain is disabling is well established. Palliation and rehabilitation are not incompatible (Cheville, 1999). No matter what the goals of care, the input from a physical rehabilitation expert may be useful to help the individual achieve his or her fullest physical, psychological, social, vocational, avocational, and educational potential (Dietz, 1982). The rehabilitation expert looks at an individual with cancer-related disability from four rehabilitation perspectives: 1) preventive (to minimize the effects of predictive disabilities); 2) adaptive (to assist the individual to adapt to definite changes); 3) maintenance (maintaining the individual at the current level of functioning); and 4) terminal rehabilitation (keeping the individual functioning and involved in the environment). By keeping these four categories in mind, it is easier to set realistic, achievable goals for the individual with pain.

Positioning and Movement

A debilitated individual with pain may find him- or herself in static positions for extraordinary lengths of time. This in itself can exacerbate existing pain or produce new pain, including pressure sores and painful joint conditions. Healthy individuals are unconsciously and continuously initiating pain-relieving movements. A nurse can assist patients and their caregivers to promote positions or postures that maintain or facilitate normal physiologic function of the musculoskeletal system. When properly done, positioning places minimal stress on the joint capsule, tendons, and muscle structure (Spross & Wolff Burke, 1995).

Loose-packed positions, those that place the least amount of stress on a joint, are best. Elbow flexion of 45 degrees, hip flexion of 30 degrees, and hip abduction of 20 degrees are some examples of loose-packed positions.

Anatomically correct positions can be maintained for brief periods of time. Use of rolled towels, small pillows, or foam cut into various shapes can be helpful in maintaining positions (Spross & Wolff Burke, 1995).

Patients who experience pain with movement may need to be premedicated prior to positioning. Care must be taken with patients who have bony disease and a high risk of pathologic fractures. An individual's pain or anxiety should not be increased with positioning. Although repositioning can be a helpful intervention to decrease pain, as death nears, it may be appropriate to do it less often if the patient experiences significant discomfort from this activity.

For the palliative care patient who is not so close to death, range of motion (ROM), either active (AROM) or active assisted (AAROM) or passive (PROM) can promote comfort and maintain or restore the integrity of muscles, ligaments, joints, bones, and nerves used in movement. This, in turn, will hopefully prevent the development of additional complications. An individual who lacks the energy for AROM may attempt AAROM or PROM (for the neurologically impaired or unconscious patient). McCaffery and Wolff (1992) have written a useful review of the use of cutaneous modalities, positioning, and movement to facilitate pain relief in the hospice population.

Supportive Orthotic Devices

In attempting to decrease pain and increase functioning, it may be helpful to consult with a physical therapist or rehabilitation medicine physician to evaluate the possible use of a supportive orthotic device such as a splint, sling, brace, or corset. Their use can immobilize or provide support to painful tissues and maximize the use of weakened tissues to promote functioning. Appropriate use of such a device may decrease incident or mechanical type pain for certain patients (Dunajcik, 1999; Tunkel & Lachmann, 1998). Also, for patients with bone metastasis, use of certain devices may immobilize areas of potential fractures to prevent this painful complication (Jacox et al., 1994).

Assistive Devices

Canes, walkers and wheelchairs when appropriately used can promote mobility, decrease pain, and prevent injury (Tunkel & Lachmann, 1998). Consulting with a rehabilitative specialist to obtain the correct assistive device for an individual patient and teaching the patient and his or her caregivers the proper use of such devices can be invaluable. Often, an evaluation of the home situation will be necessary to recommend the most appropriate device to maximize an individual's rehabilitation efforts.

Other Modalities

The application of heat, cold, vibrations, and massage, also fall under the heading of physiatric methods. Some would argue that these techniques are neurostimulatory because of their activation of the large diameter nerve fibers. The gate control theory proposed that activation of the large diameter fibers inhibited the smaller "pain" fibers and closed the gate to the transmission of stimuli by smaller nerve fibers. As more information about the underlying mechanisms of pain has become known, this theory has gradually been replaced. However, the actual mechanisms that affect pain relief from cutaneous stimulation are unclear. Frequently these techniques are referred to as cutaneous stimulation. Most of the cutaneous interventions are thought to counteract the effects of decreased oxygen and accumulated metabolites associated with musculoskeletal pain and to promote superficial increases in circulation (Spross & Wolff Burke, 1995). These methods are thought to possibly reduce pain, inflammation, and/or muscle spasm. They are noninvasive, relatively low cost, easy to use, and can often be done by the patients themselves or by their caregivers (Jacox et al., 1994). To provide pain relief, these modalities can be applied directly over the site of pain, proximally to the site of pain, distally to the site of pain, or contralaterally to the site of pain (McCaffery & Pasero, 1999).

The use of superficial heating or cooling can cause a decrease in sensitivity to pain. There is a lack of well-controlled studies concerning the use of heat and cold. Most of the information discussed is based on clinical experiences presented in the literature. Despite the lack of firm evidence, the Management of Cancer Pain Guideline Panel (Jacox et al., 1994) recommends the offering of cutaneous stimulation techniques, such as applications of superficial heat and cold, to alleviate pain. Patients with aching muscles, muscle spasm, joint stiffness, low back pain, or itching may benefit from the use of superficial heating or cooling. Their use seems to be most effective for well-localized pain (McCaffery & Passero, 1999). It is important to consider patient safety and comfort when using these interventions. This method should not be used with patients who have bleeding disorders, or pains such as causalgia (which are characterized by a hypersensitivity to touch), or in areas with recent injury, broken skin, open wounds, or skin where a patient is receiving radiation therapy (Jacox et al., 1994; McCaffery & Passero, 1999; Spross & Wolff Burke, 1995). Sites proximal, distal, or contralateral should be considered if the area of pain is contraindicated. Cold should not be used if an individual has a history of peripheral vascular disease (such as Raynaud's disease), connective tissue disease, or reports an "allergy" to cold. Often, those who report an allergy to cold may experience an asthma attack upon exposure to cold air (Bailey, 1999). Heat should not be used with topical menthol products because of the potential for tissue damage (Jacox et al., 1994; McCaffery & Pasero, 1999; Spross & Wolff Burke, 1995).

Most hospitalized individuals will need an order or institutional protocol before initiation of superficial heating or cooling. There are several convenient ways of utilizing these modalities for palliative patients. For example, cold application can be safely done using gel packs kept in the refrigerator, homemade cold packs (sealed plastic bags filled with 1/3 alcohol and 2/3 water placed in freezer), or one pound bags of frozen peas or corn (which has been gently hit to separate contents). Heat can be administered by heating pad, hot packs, immersion in water, or retention of body heat with plastic wraps. Care must be taken with both modalities to protect the skin with at least a layer of terry cloth towel or pillowcase. Moisture increases the intensity of the heat or cold. Patients are to be discouraged from lying on heat sources. The skin must be inspected at regular intervals for irritation, swelling, blistering, excessive redness that does not subside between treatments or bleeding. Some patients develop a "hunting reaction," in which after application of cold, the skin alternatively blanches and turns red. If this occurs, the use of cold should be immediately discontinued. Extreme vigilance is necessary for patients with impaired or decreased sensation, cognitive impairment, or who are unconscious and may be considered a relative contraindication. Treatment should be discontinued if the patient asks or if pain or any form of skin irritation occurs (Jacox et al., 1994; McCaffery & Pasero, 1999; Spross & Wolf Burke, 1995).

Research is lacking concerning the frequency and duration of such treatments. McCaffery and Pasero (1999) suggest a trial and error approach that is individualized to the patient. They suggest that a minimal effective duration for application of hot or cold is 5 to 10 minutes with the usual duration being 20 to 30 minutes. The decision to use heat or cold will depend upon the patient situation. When compared to heat, cold often relieves more pain, and relieves it faster. Often pain relief from cold will last longer. Cold can either relieve or exacerbate joint stiffness. Evaluation of each situation is necessary. It may be useful to alternate between heat and cold. The duration of application may be as short as five to ten seconds or three minutes of heat to one minute of cold for a period of twenty to thirty minutes (Spross & Wolff Burke, 1995; McCaffery & Passero, 1999).

Individuals will often need education on the use of superficial heat and cold as a pain-relieving measure. Educational information that is useful in teaching patients and their family members, and caregivers about the use of superficial heat and cold for pain relief can be found in several sources (McCaffery & Pasero, 1999; Rhiner et al., 1993).

Methods of applying deep heat, diathermy, microwave diathermy, and ultra sound, although helpful for some painful situations will not be discussed in detail. It is thought that they, even more than superficial heat, increase blood flow and metabolic rate. Methods, which deliver deep heat, must be used with caution in patients with active cancer and are not to be used over areas of active tumor (Jacox et al., 1994; Tunkel & Lachmann, 1998). Also, methods which deliver deep heat may be fairly challenging to use with palliative care patients who have advanced disease. Consultation with a physiatrist would be necessary when considering the use of deep heat.

Massage, another form of cutaneous stimulation, uses touch in the various forms of pressure, friction, and vibration to the soft tissues to reduce pain, promote relaxation, and communicate care and concern, especially in patients who have a communication impairment or language barrier. In a nondrug intervention program for pain relief, 63% of cancer patients selected massage/vibration as a nondrug intervention for pain relief (Rhiner et al., 1993). It is thought to decrease pain by increasing superficial circulation and, in some situations, by relaxing muscles. Studies that utilized massage in ill populations showed that brief massages are tolerated and safe (Bauer & Dracup, 1987; Meek, 1993; Tyler, Winslow, Clark, & White, 1990). A meta-analysis of the effects of backrub effleurage suggests that patient comfort and relaxation is enhanced by a simple three-minute backrub. Also, positive changes were demonstrated on heart rate, blood pressure, and respiratory rate. Some variables, such as gender, length of massage, and environmental conditions seem to play a role in effectiveness (Labyak & Metzger, 1997).

Massage is contraindicated over sites of tissue damage (such as open wounds or tissue undergoing irradiation), in patients with bleeding disorders, thrombophlebitis, patients uncomfortable with touch, or those who might misinterpret touch as sexual (although this might be acceptable if the massager was a spouse or close partner). When considering massage, it is important for the nurse to consider the patient's comfort with touch, previous experiences with massage, and preferred techniques (Spross & Wolff Burke, 1995). Massage to the site of pain may or may not serve to decrease pain at that site. Palliative care patients may not be up to an extensive massage, but may find massage of limited sites beneficial and not require much effort on their part. For example, the neck, back, or shoulders may be sufficient to promote comfort. Some may find this to be too strenuous. For these, the nurse could consider massage to the hands or feet. Massage movements can include rhythmic stroking, kneading or circular, distal-to-proximal movements. Effleurage, using slow, smooth, long strokes, is usually done to promote relaxation. The patient should be involved in choosing the sites and massage movements that provide the most comfort along with how long the massage should last. It may be helpful to try different types of strokes with varying degrees of pressure in an effort to find what is most effective for an individual (Jacox et al., 1994; Labyak & Metzger, 1997; McCaffery & Pasero, 1999; Spross & Wolff Burke, 1995). The patient may be sitting in a chair, or lying on their side or prone on a bed or table. It is helpful to determine with the individual if, during the massage, the room will be quiet, if music will be played, or if conversation will take place (McCaffery & Wolff, 1992).

During the actual massage, ideally both the nurse and patient will be as relaxed as possible. The patient should be in a position that is supported and easy to maintain for the duration of the massage. The massager should be in a position that utilizes good body mechanics. Patient comfort and modesty are to be maintained with sheets, blankets, or towels. The use of a warmed, alcohol-free lotion will decrease friction. One hand should be on the patient at all times until the massage is over. For example, the right hand could begin its stroke as the left hand is completing its stroke. Removing both hands can communicate to the patient that the massage is over. Patients may fall asleep during massage (McCaffery & Pasero, 1999; McCaffery & Wolff, 1992). Feedback from the patient, if possible, is useful for future planning. If patients find massage helpful, it should be scheduled on a regular basis. Massage can be quite comforting to dying patients who are often deprived of human touch at the end of life. Family members and caregivers may wish to be instructed or included in this pain-relieving intervention. They should be taught to use the techniques that the patient found to be most helpful (McCaffery & Pasero, 1999). Others, who are overwhelmed, may find this a burden—one more thing for them to do.

Vibration is a form of massage that passes fine tremors either electrically (using a vibrator) or manually (using one's hands) to the skin (Spross & Wolff Burke, 1995). It is thought to increase superficial circulation and stimulate large-diameter fibers (Jacox et al., 1994). It should not be used over sites overlying tumor, where skin has been injured, or areas of thrombophlebitis, with patients who bruise easily, or for migraine headache or headache which is worsened by sound or movement (McCaffery & Passero, 1999). Vibration can be used for itching, muscle spasm, neuropathic pain, phantom pain, and tension headache. It can be used as a substitute for TENS (McCaffery & Pasero, 1999; McCaffery & Wolff, 1992; Spross & Wolff Burke, 1995). By varying the pressure of vibration, one gets different effects. When applied with light pressure, its results are similar to massage. Moderate pressure vibration may act to relieve pain by causing numbness, paresthesias, and/or anesthesia to the stimulated area (McCaffery & Pasero, 1999).

Electric vibrators can be either hand held or stationary. Some are battery powered and some are plugged into an electrical outlet. Many have at least two frequencies, high (100 to 200 Hz) and low (10 to 50 Hz); some have a heat delivery option. Although the high setting is often the more effective frequency, it is advised to initially try the low frequency. Some patients, depending upon the site of pain, are able to administer the vibrator themselves. Use of the vibrator, like other cutaneous stimulation interventions, is often a trial and error situation with the site and duration of treatment up to the patient (McCaffery & Pasero, 1999; Spross & Wolff Burke, 1995). One study looked at the duration of poststimulatory pain relief resulting from brief (1 to 15 minutes) treatments and longer (30 minutes). The relief from the brief intervention was brief while the longer treatment resulted in prolonged relief (Lundeberg, Nordeman, & Ottoson, 1983). In most institutional settings, use of a vibrator will require an order from the health care provider (McCaffery & Pasero, 1999).

NEUROSTIMULATORY INTERVENTIONS

Transcutaneous electrical nerve stimulation, (or TENS) has been defined as "a method of producing electroanalgesia through electrodes applied to the body" (Jacox et al., 1994, p. 188). The TENS system, is a small battery-operated device that is attached by cables to electrodes taped to the skin overlying a nerve. Initiation requires an order from the health care provider. Patients with musculoskeletal, arthrogenic, or neurogenic pain may benefit from use of TENS. It should not be used with patients who are unable to communicate its effects. It is contraindicated in individuals with demand-type pacemakers. Those who have a history of epilepsy, transient ischemia attacks, strokes, epilepsy, or myocardial disease should not have the TENS electrodes placed on the head, neck, or chest. Also, the electrodes should not be placed over the site of tumors, near the carotid sinus, or directly on the eye. It should be started by a health care professional who is trained in its use and who will be able to take the time to instruct the patient in its use. Patients should be informed that it may take various adjustments to the TENS settings, electrode placements, and duration of treatment to find the most effective settings. Their feedback is essential in this process. A body chart can be used to easily document these trials (Spross & Wolff Burke, 1995). Thompson and Filshie (1998) describe the use of TENS in detail.

Acupuncture, a treatment from Traditional Chinese Medicine (TCM), has been shown to effectively treat pain, depression, nausea, and other health problems (Clark, 1999; NIH Consensus Conference, 1998). In this holistic, energy-based approach, thin needles, usually stainless steel, are placed in precise anatomical points (365 specific locations) to balance energy movement along the body's 12 meridians (Decker, 2000). Acupressure is the application of finger pressure to the acupuncture points. Moxibustion is the stimulation of an acupuncture point by heat. This is done by burning a special compressed combustible substance near the acupuncture point. Other variations in acupuncture stimulation of sites include the use of electrical stimulators or lasers. The NIH Consensus Development Panel on Acupuncture (1998) found that the incidence of adverse effects from acupuncture is substantially lower than for many standard medical procedures or medications used for the same conditions.

In Traditional Chinese Medicine (TCM), it is thought that good health depends upon the balance of energy in the body. Energy, termed chi or qi is thought to be constantly circulating in the body. Acupuncture acts to promote circulation of chi. Presently, western medicine classifies acupuncture and acupressure, as neurostimulatory techniques. However, adherents of TCM would probably disagree with this simplistic classification and feel more comfortable thinking of it as a complementary or alternative approach. Acupuncture is based on a holistic, energy focused approach to individuals, not a disease-oriented, diagnostic treatment approach. The fact that acupuncture causes a multitude of biological responses has been clearly demonstrated. Much work is currently underway to better understand the anatomy and physiology of the acupuncture points (NIH Consensus Conference, 1998). Melzack found that 70% of trigger points correspond to acupuncture sites (Spross & Wolff Burke, 1995). These acupuncture points have been found to be highly innervated. Proposed mechanisms of action for pain relief considered by western medicine includes endorphin release, mediation of pain-producing neurotransmitters, and stress-induced analgesia (Spross & Wolff Burke, 1995).

The NIH Consensus Development Panel on Acupuncture, in their review of the data, stated that at present the "data in support of acupuncture are as strong as those for many accepted Western medical therapies" (1998, p. 1520). At present, there is fairly convincing data showing the effectiveness of acupuncture in postoperative dental pain, and in adult postoperative and chemotherapy nausea and vomiting. Some studies indicate that it may be helpful as an adjunct treatment in painful situations such as headache, menstrual cramps, fibromyalgia, myofascial pain, osteoarthritis, and low back pain. Good controlled studies using acupuncture in palliative care patients are lacking. In this population, it may be both difficult and controversial to implement an acupuncture study comparing acupuncture to placebo or sham under controlled conditions, utilizing standardized outcomes. Ideally, as more research is done and acupuncture is further incorporated into the mainstream health care system, more informed decisions regarding the appropriateness of acupuncture for patients in varying situations will be made (NIH Consensus Panel, 1998). As health care professionals, it is important to guide patients from a perspective of evidence, not marketing.

More and more patients are seeking acupuncture treatments. It is gaining more practitioners with western medicine backgrounds and more general support from western practitioners. Some nurses, along with others, are going through extensive training to become licensed practitioners of acupuncture. Issues of training, licensure, and accreditation are in the process of being clarified. In the United States, educational standards have been developed for the training of physician and nonphysician practitioners. An agency recognized by the U.S. Department of Education has accredited many of the acupuncture educational programs. Physician acupuncturists can sit for a nationally recognized exam. Nonphysician acupuncturists can sit for an entry-level competency exam that is offered by a national credentialing agency. Unfortunately, there is much variation from state to state. This includes differences in the requirements to obtain licensure and in the titles conferred. This variation leads to confusion and to less confidence in the qualifications of acupuncture practitioners. It is important that nurses be aware of the requirements and titles conferred in the states in which they practice, so as to guide patients who desire a TCM evaluation for acupuncture to the most qualified, safe practitioners (NIH Consensus Panel, 1998).

A more detailed discussion of acupressure and acupuncture is beyond the scope of this text. Nurse educators desiring to include more information of these techniques in the nursing curriculum are encouraged to seek out licensed practitioners of acupuncture for collaboration. Some schools of nursing have faculty who are also licensed acupuncturists. At this time, most insurance policies do not cover acupuncture or other integrative approaches and most patients and families have to pay out of pocket for these interventions.

INVASIVE INTERVENTIONS

Invasive interventions can be considered for a small percentage of palliative patients whose pain cannot be adequately controlled by pharmacologic means. This population includes individuals whose pain is localized to one or two areas and is expected to persist, and who cannot achieve an acceptable balance between analgesia and intolerable, dose-limiting side effects from these analgesics.

In evaluating patients for invasive approaches, it is important to clarify that all feasible primary therapies that are likely to improve patient outcomes have been initiated, that the opioid dose has been titrated up to the maximal tolerated dose, that side effects have been treated with appropriate medication therapy or through opioid rotation, that appropriate adjuvant analgesics have been considered or tried, and that the appropriate routes of drug administration have been instituted. Other patient-related factors to assess include: presence of active infection, coagulopathy, or use of anticoagulant drugs, coexisting medical conditions that increase risks (Cherney, Arbit, & Jain, 1996), and that the potential rapidity of tumor growth in areas unaffected by the neurodestructive intervention (Schroeder, 1986). Also to be considered is "the likelihood and duration of analgesic benefit, the immediate and long-term risks, the likely duration of survival, the availability of local expertise, and the anticipated length of hospitalization" (Cherney, Arbit, & Jain, 1996, p. 128).

Neurodestructive procedures should be considered irreversible with potentially irreversible side effects (Schroeder, 1986). A dying, bed-bound patient may be willing to accept the possible disabilities of motor weakness, loss of bowel or bladder functions, or loss of position sense as a reasonable "price" to pay for adequate pain relief. However, many are not as hope for life, especially a "normal" one, frequently continues in those who are dying. An ambulatory patient is rarely receptive to the possibilities of these side effects (Swarm & Cousins, 1998). In considering the appropriateness of an intervention Arbit and Bilsky (1998) like to categorize patients as individuals with terminal disease who have a life expectancy of weeks to months and those who potentially have a longevity of months to years. The later group is then evaluated to be either highly functional or functionally impaired.

Neural Blockade, an anesthetic intervention for either temporary or permanent effect is commonly called a nerve block. A local anesthetic (usually lidocaine or bupivacaine) is injected into or around a nerve. Nerve blocks can be considered diagnostic, prognostic, therapeutic, or preemptive/prophylactic. A *diagnostic nerve block* is done to determine the specific pain pathway and to aid in the differential diagnosis. A *prognostic nerve block* is one that is done to predict the efficacy of a permanent ablating procedure. A *therapeutic nerve block* is done to provide temporary pain relief in a pain crisis or to treat painful conditions that respond to these blocks (e.g., a celiac block for the relief of pain due to pancreatic cancer). A *preemptive/ prophylactic nerve block* is done proactively to prevent the development of a chronic pain syndrome. Neurolysis is a permanent procedure that interferes with the transmission of a painful stimulus by injection of a chemical substance such as alcohol or phenol to destroy or ablate the nerve (Saberski, 1998). A successful prognostic nerve block may not always mean a successful neurolysis. This may be due to such things as analgesic and sedating premedications, placebo response, spread of local anaesthetic to adjacent neural structures, or systemic absorption of local anaesthetics. Also, patients near the end of their lives may be unwilling or unable to undergo two blocking procedures, the prognostic followed by the neurolysis. In this situation, the anesthesiologist may decide on a neurolytic procedure without a preceding prognostic block (Swarm & Cousins, 1998). Contraindications to an individual undergoing a nerve block includes: infection, coagulopathies, ineffective prognostic block, inadequate patient/family preparation, patient refusal, inability to understand and sign informed consent, and inability to cooperate during the procedure.

General types of neural blockade are peripheral blocks (including brachial plexus, and cranial, intercostal, and sacral nerves), neuroaxial blocks (including epidural and intrathecal), and sympathetic nerve blocks (including celiac plexus block and superior hypogastric block) (Swarm & Cousins, 1998). Specific nerve blocks are identified by the anatomical location where they are performed. Depending upon the location of the block, some of the risks or complications include fatigue, oversedation (if analgesics are not decreased in relation to decreased pain), sensory loss, motor weakness, altered bowel and bladder function, altered sexual function, intravascular injection, hematoma, and new pain. If sufficient denervation occurs from a somatic block, for example, a deafferentation pain will result. It is estimated that 14 to 30% of individuals undergoing peripheral neurolytic blockade may develop neuropathic pain as a result (Swarm & Cousins, 1998). Side effects from nerve blocks can include Horner's syndrome (characterized by constricted pupil, ptosis, "and decreased sweating resulting from interruption of the sympathetic pathways to the eye" [Goldberg, 1983, p. 86]), numbness, weakness, increased warmth, diarrhea, and lowered blood pressure. These effects are temporary, if done with a local anesthetic, or long lasting or permanent, if done with alcohol or phenol (as with a neurodestructive block). It is the responsibility of nurses caring for individuals undergoing these procedures to be knowledgeable about the side effects and alert to developing complications. Readers are encouraged to review the work of Cherny, Arbit, and Jain (1996), Saberski (1998), Schroeder (1986), Swarm and Cousins (1998), and Eisenberg, Carr, and Chalmer (1995) for more detailed information on neural blockade.

Cordotomy is a neuroablative, neurosurgical procedure that involves making a lesion in the anterior spinothalamic tract, contralaterally to the pain site, either percutaneously or with an open surgical approach to destroy the function of a portion of the particular spinothalamic tract which innervates the site of pain. The spinothalamic tract is important in several ways. Pain and temperature for the contralateral side of the body is mediated through the anterior spinothalamic tract. The area for superficial pain is found in the superficial area of this tract and the area for deep visceral pain and temperature is found in the deeper area (Arbit & Bilsky, 1998). Deliberate damage to the spinothalamic tract, through a neuroablative procedure will affect the dermatomal area innervated by the selected level. Preservation of proprioception and power is often possible with cordotomy, but the level of analgesia may tend to decrease over time (Cherney, Arbit, & Jain, 1996).

Cordatomy is most successful in patients with unilateral pain below C5 (Arbit & Bilsky, 1998; Saberski, 1998). Cordotomy is indicated in pain that is unresponsive to other therapy in patients with a life expectancy of less than one year (Saberski, 1998; Sanders & Zuurmond, 1995). Because of a variety of factors, including progressive disease, it is difficult to ascertain its actual success rate. It is thought that in skilled hands, complete pain relief immediately after cordotomy is as high as 60 to 80% (Saberski, 1998). As time progresses, pain relief drops possibly due to progression of disease and the resulting development of new pain. Saberski (1998) and Sanders and Zuurmond (1995) discuss the possibility of developing a delayed post-cordotomy dysesthesia, "a condition in which a disagreeable sensation is produced by ordinary stimuli" following a lesion in a peripheral or central pathway (Stedman, p. 531, 1995). Arbit and Bilsky (1998) estimate that this occurs sometimes over a year after the procedure in 1% of patients. For this reason, it is advised to avoid this procedure in individuals with an extended life expectancy (Arbit & Bilsky, 1998).

Sometimes the relief of one pain by cordotomy, unmasks a mirror pain in the ipsilateral side. Prior to the procedure, the patient may not be aware of this pain because of the overwhelming contralateral pain. Sometimes, the nociceptive components of a pain may be successfully relieved but not the neuropathic components (Arbit & Bilsky, 1998). A study by Sanders and Zuurmond (1995) demonstrated the effectiveness and safety of percutaneous cervical cordotomy in terminally ill cancer patients. Complications following cordotomy can include dysfunction of autonomic respiration, sleep apnea, Horner's syndrome, arterial hypotension, hemiparesis (usually transient), and bladder dysfunction (Arbit & Bilsky, 1998). The function of the ipsilateral diaphragm can be impaired by cordotomy (Saberski, 1998). Patients with pulmonary disease on the contralateral side of the cordotomy are at risk for respiratory decompensation. It is recommended that patients undergo preoperative pulmonary function tests to help identify individuals at increased risk. Bilateral cordotomy is associated with a higher risk of sleep apnea ("Ondine's curse"), respiratory compromise, and arterial orthostatic hypotension. These conditions may or may not be transient and self-limiting. Their presence is thought to be a major contributing factor to mortality following bilateral procedures. Because of this, the presence of a low ejection fraction or significant preexisting heart disease contraindicates the use of the bilateral procedure (Arbit & Bilsky, 1998). The unilateral percutaneous cordotomy is the preferred procedure. When bilateral lesions are necessary, the open approach may be indicated (Saberski, 1998). As a safety measure, Arbit and Bilsky (1998) suggest waiting at least one week between cordotomies to assess for the development of respiratory compromise from unilateral lesions. Sometimes open cordotomy is done if the percutaneous procedure is not available, or if a patient is unable to lie supine for a percutaneous procedure (Saberski, 1998). An individual's ability to tolerate the actual procedure plays a role in what is done. Often patients with advanced disease may be unable to tolerate multiple sessions to alleviate pain. Ideally, the neurosurgeon can make the most of a single opportunity to relieve the pain (Arbit & Bilsky, 1998).

INTEGRATIVE INTERVENTIONS

Music has been shown to be an effective intervention for pain control through a variety of physiologic and psychologic effects. Affective, cognitive, and sensory processes can be engaged, activated, and altered by music. This is done by processes such as use of prior skills, relaxation, distraction, alteration of mood, and improved sense of control. Physical effects include: increasing or decreasing pulse and blood pressure (Magill-Levreault, 1993). Music therapy, as defined by Spross and Wolff Burk (1995), is "the scientific and systematic use of music to effect beneficial changes in physiologic and psychologic processes that influence experiences of pain and illness" (p. 175).

In using music with an individual, one needs to evaluate the patient's medical situation, general mood state, coping abilities, degree of isolation, and prior musical experiences, in addition to the total pain experience. People are often music listeners, music eventers, or music performers. By understanding someone's prior musical experiences and integrating it into music therapy, the intervention will provide opportunities to regain a sense of identity and sense of control. As with distraction, the use of music can be either a passive or an active experience. The level of involvement often will be related to the energy status of the individual (Magill-Levreault, 1993).

Music listeners can use audiotapes to promote distraction, relaxation, and alter mood disturbances such as anxiety, depression, fear, anger, and sadness (Magill-Levreault, 1993). Music eventers are those who may view music as a backdrop to significant life events. Especially for these individuals, the use of familiar songs can assist in reminiscing, life review, and opening communication between patients and others. Music performers, depending upon their state, can participate in music by tapping out rhythms with their fingers, conducting, or actually performing (Magill-Levreault, 1993).

Music therapists are especially effective in this type of work, facilitating personal growth and enhanced self-expression. Often, they are able to select and perform songs that initially matches the mood and needs of a patient and then use the music as a catalyst to mobilize feelings and open communication (Magill-Levreaul, 1993). Involvement of significant others is encouraged, if the patient desires. In the clinical situation, one should be aware of a patient's personal music preference. Not all types of music are considered universally pleasant (McCaffery & Pasero, 1999; Spross & Wolff Burke, 1995; Magill-Levreault, 1993). A patient's needs may change daily. Because of this, the music selection is best done with the individual on a day-to-day basis. "The aim is always to promote comfort, healing, and a decreased sense of pain. Working in collaboration with other pain modification approaches, music therapy can help soothe pain as well as heal the suffering" (Magill-Levreault, 1993, p. 45). Schroeder-Sheker (1994) explores the use of music in the actively dying.

Therapeutic Touch (TT) is a complementary technique based on systems theory of the multidimensional nature of the individual and the homeostatic concepts of balance and wholeness, which work with energy fields in promoting relaxation states, reducing pain, and promoting healing. It was developed by Dolores Krieger, a nurse physiologist, in conjunction with Dora Kunz, a healer (Owens & Ehrenreich, 1991a). Therapeutic Touch is based on the following four premises: 1) a human being is an open energy system, 2) there is bilateral symmetry in a human being, 3) illness is an imbalance in one's energy field, and 4) a human being has the natural capacity to transform and transcend his or her condition of living (Spross &Wolff Burke, 1995).

Despite its name, TT does not involve physical touching. It involves a conscious intention on the part of the healer to help the client (Spross & Wolff Burke, 1995). The practitioner of TT first centers him or herself in the here and now. Then the practitioner does an assessment of the client's energy field for symmetry by placing his or her hands four to six inches from the body starting at the head and moving towards the feet. The energy field is then "unruffled" by the practitioner performing sweeping motions of the hands to smooth out the energy field. During the next phase, the treatment phase, the practitioner channels energy to areas of the field that the practitioner senses are imbalanced or void. Finally, in the last phase, reassessment, the energy field is reevaluated for repatterning of energy flow (Owens & Ehrenreich, 1991b).

Use of this technique for palliative patients who are interested, may be useful because it involves no effort or expenditure of any energy on the part of the patient. Debilitated patients do not have to learn new skills at a time when they may be unable to do so. Also, there do not seem to be any adverse effects. Anecdotal evidence suggests that TT can be a beneficial adjunct to traditional therapies (Kotora, 1997). A study that looked at the desire for "serenity" by persons nearing death and nursing interventions to facilitate this state found that pain control, TT, and assisting clients to build trust were the three highest ranked interventions both in the frequency of use and in effectiveness (Messenger & Roberts, 1994).

The research base to support the use of TT in clinical practice is not solid. A recent metaanalysis of TT research found that there are many approaches to TT and that the TT practices vary from study to study. These factors may lead to less convincing conclusions when evaluating the effectiveness of TT as a modality. Although a number of studies had mixed or negative results, most studies supported the hypotheses regarding the efficacy of TT (Winstead-Fry & Kijek, 1999). A recent study looked at the effect of TT on the well being of individuals with terminal cancer. The results showed a positive increase in the sensations of well-being following three TT treatments. Well being was measured using the Well-Being Scale, a visual analogue scale that measures pain, nausea, depression, anxiety, shortness of breath, activity, appetite, relaxation, and inner peace (Giasson & Bouchard, 1998). Some of the proponents of TT feel that even if it is determined that TT is basically taking advantage of a placebo effect, from a holistic nursing point of view this is still a beneficial adjuvant nursing intervention. Meehan (1998) expresses the thought that "the potential of TT to enhance the placebo phenomenon requires further exploration but should not be discounted in seeking to relieve discomfort and distress and facilitate healing" (p. 117).

Therapeutic Touch has been taught and researched since the 1970s. However, in recent years, its use has become more controversial. Some feel that TT should be treated as a religious practice. This would require new approaches to the practice and teaching of TT in nursing (Bullough & Bullough, 1998). Mainstream American medicine is unconvinced as to the value of TT. In 1998, a study published in the very major mainstream *Journal of the American Medical Association* concluded that because 21 experienced practitioners of TT were unable to detect the investigator's "energy field" at a rate greater than chance, there was unrefuted evidence that the "claims of TT were groundless and that further professional use is unjustified" (Rosa, Rosa, Sarner, & Barrett, 1998, p. 1005). Some question the validity of this study and the biases inherent in the peer reviewers. However, because this was published in a leading peer-reviewed medical journal, many in mainstream western medicine are unsupportive of the use of TT. Eskinazi and Muesam (1999) point out that conventional journals may have difficulty evaluating integrative techniques fairly due to the fact that some of the concepts implicit in these techniques are outside of the current biomedical framework. Often information and opinions presented by mainstream medicine may be misinformed or based on a misunderstanding of an area of alternative medicine. It is important to explore knowledge outside the existing dogmas to promote real progress (Eskinazi & Muesam, 1999).

How to Integrate Nondrug Interventions into a Comprehensive Pain Management Plan

A successful pain management plan is based on a comprehensive pain assessment and incorporates the components of treating underlying disease, pharmacologic interventions, psychological intervention, physiatric interventions, neurostimulatory interventions, invasive interventions, and integrative interventions. At the end of life, it may or may not be appropriate or feasible to treat underlying disease. Certainly, the patient with advanced disease may not be able to tolerate a surgery to remove a pain-producing tumor. Yet, some interventions aimed at treating underlying disease may be useful. For example, palliative radiation to areas of bony disease may be well tolerated and decrease bone pain (Jacox et al., 1994). Pain caused by infection, such as pelvic abscess or occult infections from ulcerating tumors, may be relieved by treatment with appropriate antibiotics (Cherny & Portenoy, 1994). The importance of pharmacologic interventions, the mainstay of pain relief at the end of life, and how to integrate these interventions into the pain management plan has been well described in the first section of this chapter.

As part of the interdisciplinary team caring for a patient at the end of life, it is important for the nurse to understand how the nondrug interventions (psychological, physiatric, neurostimulatory, invasive, and integrative) are incorporated into the pain management plan. The availability of experienced consultants to perform certain interventions also plays a role. If no one is available to perform a specific intervention, it cannot be offered as an option in the pain management plan for that individual at that point in time. A Palliative Care team may need to work on system issues to improve access to specialists that may be helpful to their patients. The use of any intervention is based upon the assessment of the patient. It is important to carefully evaluate the individual and apply what is appropriate for that individual in a particular situation. After the initiation of systemic analgesic therapy and treatment of underlying disease (if appropriate), the next step would be to consider the addition of psychological, physiatric, neurostimulatory, or integrative techniques to improve control and possibly improve the balance between analgesia and side effects (Cherny & Portenoy, 1994; Rhiner et al., 1993). If these measures prove to be suboptimal, the consideration of the use of invasive techniques is appropriate (Cherny & Portenoy, 1994). Finally, if it is impossible to find the balance between pain relief and side effects, then, sedation at the end of life (as described in the first section of this chapter) must be considered. Figure 11.6 shows the flow of this process.

THE ROLE OF THE NURSE IN IMPLEMENTING NONDRUG INTERVENTIONS

The nurse caring for patients at the end of life has both collaborative and independent functions in implementing nondrug interventions. First, the nurse must be aware of which interventions, he or she is able to perform. Factors to consider when making this determination include education in the use of particular techniques, comfort in teaching or implementing a particular technique, patient/family educational materials available, availability/affordability of specific necessary devices/materials, and time available to an individual nurse to initiate a particular intervention. Psychological interventions that an individual nurse must be comfortable initiating include patient/family education, and ideally cognitive interventions such as distraction, self-statements, and brief method relaxation techniques, and behavioral interventions such as a pain diary. Physiatric interventions that an individual nurse might initiate for an end-of-life patient's pain control could include postioning and movement, use of superficial heat or cooling, massage, or vibration. The use of music, an integrative technique, may also be initiated by an individual nurse. If the nurse has had additional training, he or she may consider the use of Therapeutic Touch, deep relaxation methods, or Cognitive Behavioral Therapy. In addition, the nurse needs to know which members of the immediate primary team can perform nondrug interventions that may be useful as part of a comprehensive pain management plan. Also to be determined, is the availability of special consultants, such as neurosurgeons, anesthesiologists, hypnotherapists, or acupuncturists, for consultation and intervention as necessary. The nurse may need to assist in making appropriate referrals to these consultants. Finally, as part of the team, it may be necessary to educate other team members as to the efficacy of nondrug methods so that these techniques can be more efficiently integrated into the pain management plan (Rhiner et al., 1993).

Only after it is determined who is capable and available to teach or perform a particular nondrug interventions, can the nurse and his or her team realistically consider its use for an individual patient based upon the pain assessment. As with the pharmacological interventions, the nondrug interventions need to be directed at etiologic factors. For example, vibration, a physiatric modality, when applied with moderate pressure, can help to relieve pain by decreasing sensation to a painful area and may act to decrease tension in muscles (Rhiner, Ferrel, Ferrel, & Grant, 1993). This would make

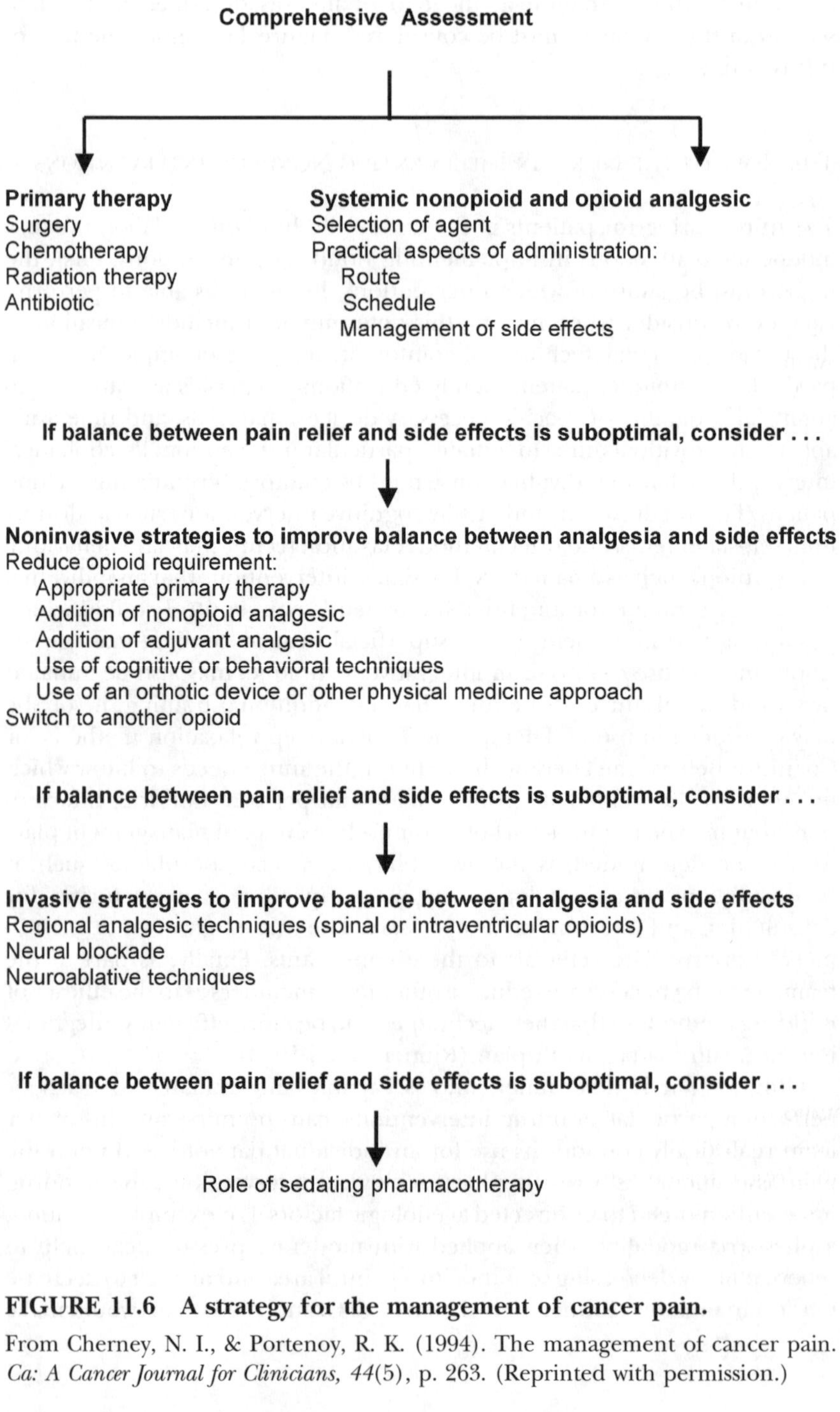

Comprehensive Assessment

Primary therapy
Surgery
Chemotherapy
Radiation therapy
Antibiotic

Systemic nonopioid and opioid analgesic
Selection of agent
Practical aspects of administration:
    Route
    Schedule
    Management of side effects

If balance between pain relief and side effects is suboptimal, consider . . .

Noninvasive strategies to improve balance between analgesia and side effects
Reduce opioid requirement:
    Appropriate primary therapy
    Addition of nonopioid analgesic
    Addition of adjuvant analgesic
    Use of cognitive or behavioral techniques
    Use of an orthotic device or other physical medicine approach
Switch to another opioid

If balance between pain relief and side effects is suboptimal, consider . . .

Invasive strategies to improve balance between analgesia and side effects
Regional analgesic techniques (spinal or intraventricular opioids)
Neural blockade
Neuroablative techniques

If balance between pain relief and side effects is suboptimal, consider . . .

Role of sedating pharmacotherapy

FIGURE 11.6   A strategy for the management of cancer pain.

From Cherney, N. I., & Portenoy, R. K. (1994). The management of cancer pain. *Ca: A Cancer Journal for Clinicians, 44*(5), p. 263. (Reprinted with permission.)

this approach a useful addition to the pharmacologic regimen already in place for an individual found to have pain from muscle spasm.

It is also important to consider whether a patient or their family has the physical, mental, or emotional energy necessary to participate in a particular intervention. Nondrug interventions that need a high level of patient involvement may not be possible when an individual is debilitated. Assessment needs to include a patient's ability to concentrate and follow directions, level of fatigue, and cognitive status (McCaffery & Passero, 1999). In the assessment, also include an individual's previous experience and attitude towards nondrug interventions (Rhiner et al., 1993; McCaffery & Pasero, 1999). Determine which methods may be not useful due to religious or cultural issues or concerns or because they counter an individual's usual coping style (McCaffery & Pasero, 1999).

The next step is active collaboration by the nurse with the patient to choose a nondrug intervention that may be useful (Spross & Wolff Burke, 1995). As with CBT, it is useful to review with the patient the pain-related problems present, assign priorities to the problems, focus on the priority problems, set goals and implement an intervention designed to address the priority problem (Fishman & Loscalzo, 1987). As part of this process, the nurse needs to be aware of what is realistically possible with the individual patient at that moment in time, given his or her medical condition (Loscalzo, 1996). Spross and Wolff Burke (1995) recommend focusing on only one or two nondrug interventions at a time. At this point, the patient's family, friends and caregivers need to be asked if they wish to be involved in the nondrug intervention (McCaffery & Pasero, 1999; Spross & Wolff Burke, 1995). Some will want to be actively involved. Others will feel too overburdened (McCaffery & Pasero, 1999). Obstacles to the use of the selected nondrug intervention will need to be anticipated along with the development of strategies to overcome these obstacles (Spross & Wolff Burke, 1995).

Patient/family/caregiver education follows. Even if the patient's family, friends, or caregivers are not actively involved, they will need information as to the role of the nondrug intervention in the pain management plan (Spross & Wolff Burke, 1995). This helps to elicit their cooperation and promote successful use of the intervention (Rhiner et al., 1993). Written and audio materials that reinforce verbal information are useful (McCaffery & Pasero, 1999; Spross & Wolff Burke, 1995). It is important to emphasize that nondrug interventions are not a replacement for analgesics (McCaffery & Pasero, 1999). The patient and their family will need opportunities to develop skills using the nondrug intervention (Spross & Wolff Burke, 1995). Ideally, they will be able to actually use the intervention with the nurse present before utilizing it independently.

It is useful to debrief a patient and their caregiver following the use of a nondrug intervention. In this debriefing, the effect on pain and other outcomes, and the need for more assistance needs to be assessed (Spross & Wolff Burke, 1995). If a nondrug intervention is assessed to be ineffective, then it should be modified or replaced (Spross & Wolff Burke, 1995).

SECTION 3: SPECIAL POPULATION CONCERNS AT THE END OF LIFE

The principles discussed in Sections 1 and 2 of this chapter, concerning the assessment of the patient in pain, and the use of pharmacologic and nonpharmacologic interventions in the comprehensive pain management plan can be applied to all patients. However, there are issues specific to special populations that play a role in their pain assessment and pain management plan at end of life. The Management of Cancer Pain Panel advocates for clinicians to give special attention to the assessment and treatment of pain in special populations (Jacox et al., 1994). The purpose of this section is to briefly highlight end-of-life pain-related issues in four populations as an example of some of the concerns in special populations and is not intended as a comprehensive approach. The following section will look at issues specific to the following four groups; 1) those with a history of substance abuse, 2) those with impaired communication, 3) older adults, and 4) pediatrics. These four groups were chosen because they are frequently encountered. Cultural factors and religious factors play a role in the pain management of certain groups. Sometimes there is a mismatch between the normative values of the patient and the health care provider. It is the practice setting that frequently determines which populations a nurse cares for. It is the responsibility of the nurse to know the needs and special concerns of the populations that he or she cares for most often.

SPECIAL CONSIDERATIONS IN THOSE WITH A HISTORY OF SUBSTANCE ABUSE

The prevalence of substance abuse in the United States and the association between drug abuse and life-threatening diseases such as AIDS, Hepatitis C, and some types of cancer make it likely that nurses caring for patients at the end of life will work with some individuals who have a history of substance abuse (Passik & Portenoy, 1998). As a group, it is very heterogeneous with very diverse clinical problems (Passik, Portenoy, & Ricketts, 1998a). It will include individuals who are living drug-free lives, those in methadone maintenance programs, and those who are currently abusing drugs (Fultz & Sonay, 1975). It is not uncommon to find individuals with addictive disease who also have a concurrent psychiatric illness such as anxiety, depression, bipolar disorder, or schizophrenia (Compton, 1999). Changes in comorbid physical and psychosocial factors, which drugs an individual has abused, and with what frequency, can further complicate issues that clinicians face (Passik, Portenoy, & Ricketts, 1998a).

The challenge is to provide humane, high quality care to people at the end of life who have a history of drug abuse in a society context that often views addiction from a moral or criminal perspective (Compton, 1999). The field of addiction medicine is a newly developing science that is based upon recent neuroscience advances that include identification of the brain mechanisms involved with addiction vulnerability and nociception (Portenoy et al., 1997). Despite this developing scientific understanding of the disease of addiction, individuals with a substance addiction are rarely cared for in an approach that draws upon this knowledge and their pain is frequently undertreated (Compton, 1999). This is true even in the area of palliative care. Recent formal involvements by experts from the fields of pain management and chemical dependency are working to remedy this problem (Portenoy et al., 1997).

The following points are helpful to keep in mind when working with dying persons who have a history of substance abuse:

- In order to maintain an objective, nonjudgmental approach, be aware of one's own reaction when asked to administer an opioid to a patient with a history of substance abuse.
- Individuals with a history of substance abuse, past or present, will be tolerant to opioids and will require higher doses of opioid to effectively treat pain than those with no history of drug abuse (Passik & Portenoy, 1998).
- Staff may be reluctant to administer opioids in adequate amounts to relieve pain because of concerns of worsening or "readdicting" an addiction disorder contribute to the problem of undermedication (Gonzales & Coyle, 1992).
- Identify whether the individual has a far distant history of drug abuse, is in a methadone maintenance program (MMP), or is actively abusing substances (Jacox et al., 1994).
- Patients who have a far distant history of drug abuse or who are in MMP may be reluctant to take opioids because of fear of readdiction (Gonzales & Coyle, 1992).
- Patients who are actively abusing substances are the most challenging of the three groups to work with. An interdisciplinary team that emphasizes clear communication is most effective in addressing the multiple

medical, psychosocial, and administrative problems present (Passik & Portenoy, 1998).

- If a patient is currently in a MMP, permission must be obtained to contact the program and coordinate therapy. Some MMP providers wish to remain actively involved at the end of life, others do not (Passik & Portenoy, 1998).
- For MMP patients at the end of life, it may be useful to incorporate the equianalgesic daily methadone dose into their analgesic regimen. Some patients, however, prefer to keep the methadone dose taken for addiction separate from whatever medication is taken to control pain as long as they are able to swallow.
- Methadone may be stigmatized as an analgesic in patients who have a history of substance abuse. Patients and their families and friends may need education as to the effectiveness of methadone as an analgesic.
- Providers need to be aware of the need for more frequent dosing of methadone when given for analgesia, usually at least every six hours (Passik, Portenoy, & Ricketts, 1998b).
- One nurse practitioner or physician should be identified to write all analgesic orders or prescriptions. This needs to be communicated to all caring for the patient.
- Individuals with a history of substance abuse frequently have difficulties handling stress and will need extra support at the end of life. Psychiatric symptoms and comorbidities, such as anxiety, depression, and bipolar disorders are frequently encountered and are to be treated (Passik & Portenoy, 1998).
- Nondrug methods can be employed, as appropriate, in any pain management plan for dying patients, but they should not be used as substitutes for medications to treat pain, depression, anxiety, or other symptoms (Passik & Portenoy, 1998).
- Individuals with a history of substance abuse who want to die at home need a careful assessment of their home environment to ensure adequate pain management and safety at home.

SPECIAL CONSIDERATIONS IN THOSE WITH IMPAIRED COMMUNICATION

Impaired communication can be due to a language barrier where the patient's primary language is not that spoken by the nurse or caregivers. The impaired communication can also be from an organic or functional etiology. This can include sensory impairment, cognitive impairment, aphasia, etc. This impairment may or may not be a result of the life threatening illness the patient is experiencing. Because of the difficulties that these patients have with communication, they may not report their pain in an accurate or timely fashion. This may cause their pain to be undertreated. Other factors that can impede the communication of pain is the religious or cultural background of a patient. Cultural or linguistic differences may impair adequate assessment of pain and also may inhibit the patient's willingness to accept treatment for pain (Adelhardt et al., 1995).

The American Pain Society (1999) recommends that patients who are unable to communicate and who undergo a procedure that would be painful for others are to be treated presumptively for pain. The Acute Pain Management Guidelines Panel (1992) recommends that if pain is suspected, an analgesic trial can be made to diagnose pain as well as treat it. Terminally ill patients with pain who are unable to speak and who are known to have pain are likely to continue to have pain and should have continuing pain treatment (Levy, 1985).

In caring for dying individuals with impaired communication the following is useful:

- Identify the communication deficit that is impeding the patient's ability to report pain and pain relief and to comply with the pain management plan.
- Obtain the appropriate pain assessment tools and place at the patient's bedside.
- If the patient and his or her caretakers do not speak the same language, identify the patient's language and identify available translators. Obtain a pain scale in the patient's language and review it with the patient and translator. It is helpful to write key words or phrases in both the patient's language and the corresponding translations in the caretaker's language (Adelhardt et al., 1995).
- Provide more frequent pain assessments if a patient is unable to ask for pain medication, or does not reliably ask for pain medication.
- If the patient cannot communicate, it is useful to collaborate with the patient's family and caregivers to determine what behavioral activities may indicate pain for this patient (Adelhardt et al., 1995). This may be such things as grimacing, pacing, restlessness, moaning, lying still, or guarding (American Pain Society, 1999).
- Document possible pain behaviors and any tools needed for pain assessment in the patient's record to assist other caregivers in providing continuity of care.
- If the patient is to die at home, issues related to impaired communication need to be addressed in the home setting (Adelhardt et al., 1995). Family members and other caregivers may need extra education and support. In some communities, it may be possible to obtain nurses or

home health aides who speak the patient's language if language barrier is an issue.

Special Considerations for Older Adults

The probability that the elder patient will experience pain at the end of life is high. Pain prevalence increases significantly with age and is due to both malignant and nonmalignant causes (Hewitt & Foley, 1997). Aggressive pain management is as necessary for the elderly as for younger individuals (Jacox et al., 1994). In the elderly, pain is frequently undertreated across all practice settings. The dying elder patient may be cared for at home, in a nursing home, or in a hospital. In any setting, untreated pain can lead to loss of function and psychological complications in this vulnerable population.

Misconceptions regarding pain in the older adult can interfere with good pain management. Ferrell and Ferrell (1995) reported that common misconceptions may include such things as: 1) pain is a normal or expected part of aging; 2) if individuals do not complain of pain, they must not have much pain; and 3) the side effects from opioids make them too dangerous to use with elderly people. Nurses need to reinforce that pain is not an inevitable part of aging. Pain in the elder patient is to be evaluated and treated (Hewitt & Foley, 1997).

In treating pain in the elderly, it is important to be aware of the effects of age on the pharmacokinetic and pharmacodynamic responses to analgesic medications including risk of drug accumulation (Hewitt & Foley, 1997; Jacox et al., 1994). The general rule for using medications with the elder is to "start low and go slow." Miaskowski, in her review of the literature suggests that a starting dose of one-half to one-third the usual adult dose is appropriate (Hill et al., 1999). The reader is referred to several thoughtful detailed texts on this and other information relevant to the care of the elderly patient in pain at the end of life (Ferrell, 1998; Ferrell & Ferrell, 1995; Herr & Mobily, 1991; Hewitt & Foley, 1997; Hofmann, Farnon, Javed, & Posner, 1998; Shimp, 1998). Nurses caring for dying elder patients with pain need to be aware of the following:

- Pain assessment can be disproportionately confounded by cognitive impairment or dysfunction, memory difficulties, depression, and abuse of alcohol (Ferrell, Ferrell, Ahn, & Tran, 1994; Pasero, Reed, & McCaffery, 1999).
- The presence of polypharmacy, multiple diagnosis, and complex symptoms from comorbid conditions may further complicate the pain experience (Ferrell, Ferrell, Ahn, & Tran, 1994).

- The patient's ability to independently self medicate and participate in the pain management plan may be affected by functional factors such as impaired vision, impaired fine motor skills of hands, memory problems, and cognitive impairments.
- Identify the caregiver. (The caregiver may be elderly or the patient may live alone.) Evaluate the ability, availability, and desire of the caregiver and of other family and friends to assist with care, administer pain medications, and participate in the pain management plan (Adelhardt et al., 1995).
- Assess the role of the dying elder patient in their environment. Because of pain or disease, they may no longer be able to function in roles that they had previously performed, such as care of a spouse or family member. The nurse may need to facilitate planning within to redistribute responsibilities.

SPECIAL CONSIDERATIONS IN PEDIATRIC PATIENTS

Until recently, the dying child with pain was not viewed as a significant problem. Children were not considered to feel pain as intensely as adults and were therefore considered not to need aggressive pain management. Fortunately, since the 1970s, the literature on pediatric pain has expanded significantly and pediatric pain is viewed as a specialty in its own right. Nurses have played a significant role in this development (Eland, 1990). The nurse caring for the dying child needs to be well versed in how to manage pain in children using a multidimensional approach with an awareness of issue specific to the pediatric population. More detailed information on assessment and management of pain in children at the end of life can be found in Eland (1990), Finley and McGrath (1998), Frager (1997), Patterson (1992), Roy (1996), Siever (1994), Solomon and Saylor (1995), and the WHO (1998).

The following pointers are helpful in working with the children with pain at the end of life:

- The child and family are the unit of care.
- Parents and caregivers must be incorporated into the pain management plan as part of the therapeutic alliance, which also includes the child and the health care providers (Jacox et al., 1994).
- Address family concerns regarding the risk of addiction in the medically ill child (Walco, Cassidy, & Schechter, 1994).
- A child's self report of pain is considered the most reliable and valid indicator for estimate of pain location and intensity (Jacox et al., 1994).

- It is helpful to initiate discussions about pain and to learn the individual child's word for pain (Adelhart et al., 1995).
- Developmentally appropriate tools exist to evaluate the child in pain. It is important to consider the child's age, cognitive level, verbal capabilities, type of pain and context when selecting a developmentally appropriate measure (Stevens, 1997).
- Behavioral observation is the primary assessment measure for preverbal or nonverbal children. Observed pain behaviors may include vocalizations; facial expressions; body movements; autonomic responses; or changes in daily activities, usual behaviors, appetite, or sleep (Jacox et al., 1994).
- The goal of pain management in children is to prevent as much pain as possible and to treat procedural pain aggressively (WHO, 1998).
- The pharmacologic management principles, by the ladder, by the clock, by the appropriate route, and by the child, are similar to those used with adults with the exception that the starting doses are determined by weight. The child is frequently assessed and doses are titrated to effect (WHO, 1998).
- The oral route is the desired route whenever possible (Jacox et al., 1994).
- Avoid IM injections and utilize the intravenous or subcutaneous route when parenteral administration is necessary (Miser, Moore, Greene, Gracely, & Miser, 1986).

CONCLUSION

Management of pain in the dying underscores the need to integrate assessment and treatment strategies to the needs of the individual patient. The basic principles of assessment and pharmacologic management and use of nondrug interventions must be incorporated into undergraduate nursing education. Nurses are expected to care for the dying from the moment they graduate. The delivery of optimal therapy depends on an understanding of the clinical pharmacology of the analgesic drugs and comprehensive assessment of the pain, the patient's medical condition, psychosocial state, and goals of care. Although the nurse will usually be part of an interdisciplinary team, he or she will often be the one responsible for assessing pain, administering analgesics, monitoring for adequacy of pain relief and presence of side effects, and communicating with other members of the team. Unless knowledgeable in the basic principles of pain assessment and management these responsibilities cannot be met.

ACKNOWLEDGMENTS

We would like to gratefully thank the following individuals for their thoughtful review of various sections of this chapter: Didi Loseth, RN, MS; Susan Derby, RN, MA; Angela Racolin, RN, MA; Karen Holritz, RN, MS; Matthew Loscalzo, LCSW-C; Russel Portenoy, MD; Gilbert Gonzales, MD; and Kathleen Foley, MD.

Education Plan 11.1 Plan for Achieving Competencies: Pain Assessment and Management

Knowledge Needed	Attitude	Skills	Undergraduate Behavioral Outcomes	Graduate Behavioral Outcomes	Teaching/Learning Strategies
The significance of unrelieved pain at the end of life: —Barriers to pain management.	*Acknowledge the fear of patients and families related to unrelieved pain. *Consider students'/nurses' own personal attitudes toward pain management.		*Recognize patient, clinician, and institutional barriers that interfere with adequate pain management. *Educate patients and families regarding the significance of unrelieved pain.	*Educate patients, families, clinicians, and administration regarding the importance of effective pain management to overcome related barriers.	*In the classroom, post-conference, or seminar, ask students/nurses to reflect on a personal experience of pain and its significance to their sense of physical, emotional, social, and spiritual well-being. Compare and contrast responses. *Within the context of a clinical setting, identify patient, clinician/self, and institutional barriers that interfere with adequate pain management.

Education Plan 11.1 *(continued)*

Knowledge Needed	Attitude	Skills	Undergraduate Behavioral Outcomes	Graduate Behavioral Outcomes	Teaching/Learning Strategies
Basic principles of pain assessment at the end of life: —Definition of pain; —Need for a multidimensional and interdisciplinary approach; —Clinical assessment of pain: *Types of pain; *Temporal patterns of pain; *Pain history: • onset • location/site	*Accept the importance of the nurses' role and responsibilities in the interdisciplinary assessment of pain. *Accept that pain is what the patient says it is. *Affirm the importance of pain assessment as a nursing priority. *Consider the multidimensional aspects of pain.	*Obtain a comprehensive pain history to determine the type and temporal pattern of the patient's pain. *Determine the severity of pain using a pain assessment tool. *Conduct a physical examination based on the patient's history and knowledge of the disease process.	*Contribute to the interdisciplinary management of pain through comprehensive history and physical assessment.	*Coordinate the interdisciplinary team efforts related to the comprehensive assessment of pain. *Role model comprehensive assessment skills. *Educate other health professionals regarding the assessment of level of pain and need for pain management prior to their interventions.	*Role play a patient-clinician interaction to obtain a pain history, conduct a physical exam, and utilize a pain assessment instrument. *Analyze a written or videotaped case study to evaluate the comprehensiveness of the pain history and physical examination. *Role play clinician-clinician interaction regarding pain assessment and a need for change in interaction

Education Plan 11.1 *(continued)*

Knowledge Needed	Attitude	Skills	Undergraduate Behavioral Outcomes	Graduate Behavioral Outcomes	Teaching/Learning Strategies
• quality • severity • exacerbating and relieving factors • impact of pain on psychological well-being • history of treatment • responses to previous and current analgesic regimens. —Physical examination —Use of pain assessment tools.					*In the clinical setting, complete a health history and physical examination of a patient and document the findings in the clinical record.

Education Plan 11.1 *(continued)*

Knowledge Needed	Attitude	Skills	Undergraduate Behavioral Outcomes	Graduate Behavioral Outcomes	Teaching/Learning Strategies
Components of Pain Management: • WHO Analgesic Ladder • NSAIDS • Mechanisms of action; • Adverse effects and management; • Drug selection; • Choice of starting dose and titration; • Opioids • Mechanisms of actions; • Principles of opioid administration;	*Affirm the importance of effective pain management. *Emphasize the need to suspend clinician bias related to use of opioids. *Dispel myths related to pharmacological management of pain.	*Demonstrate competence in managing pain using NSAIDS, opioids, and adjuvant therapies. *Set up accurately the equipment needed for parenteral infusions of pharmacologic agents for pain management. *Accurately titrate doses of pharmacological agents to achieve pain relief. *Correctly calculate opioid conversions using equianalgesic dose tables.	*Administer appropriate pharmacological therapies to achieve maximal relief of pain. *Assess for side effects and adverse effects of pharmacological pain therapies. *Administer appropriate therapies to relieve side effects of analgesics. *Educate patients and families regarding the use of opioids and other analgesics as it relates to tolerance, addiction, and physical dependence.	*Determine a comprehensive plan to treat and manage pain and related symptoms. *Coordinate interdisciplinary team efforts to execute comprehensive pain therapies. *Educate other health care providers regarding effective and comprehensive pain management.	In the clinical laboratory, have a faculty demonstration and students'/nurses' return demonstration of the set-up and titration of opioids using a PCA pump, or other infusion equipment.

Education Plan 11.1 *(continued)*

Knowledge Needed	Attitude	Skills	Undergraduate Behavioral Outcomes	Graduate Behavioral Outcomes	Teaching/Learning Strategies

• Choice of a starting dose and dose titration.
• Managing a pain crisis;
• Sedation at the end of life;
• Tolerance, physical dependence, and psychological dependence;
• Opioid side effects and their management;
• Adjuvant analgesia:
  • Corticosteroids
  • Benzodiazepines
  • Antidepressants
		*Effectively manages adverse effects of analgesics.			*Based on case studies, determine the appropriate pharmacological management, using the WHO analgesic ladder, and calculate the titration and conversion of opioids.
					*Based on case studies, evaluate the appropriateness of various pain management plans based on type of illness, etiology of pain, pain history and assessment, patient preference, health status, goals

Education Plan 11.1 *(continued)*

Knowledge Needed	Attitude	Skills	Undergraduate Behavioral Outcomes	Graduate Behavioral Outcomes	Teaching/Learning Strategies
• Anticonvulsants • GABAB Agonists • Alpha 2-Adrenergic antagonists • Local anesthetics • Topical analgesics • NMDA receptor antagonists • Radiopharmaceuticals • Biphosphonates					of care, and mechanism of action, and pharmaco-therapeutic properties of pharmacological agents. *In the clinical setting, implement a plan of care for pain management of a select patient. In postconference, discuss the barriers to effective pain management, the patient's response to pain

Education Plan 11.1 *(continued)*

Knowledge Needed	Attitude	Skills	Undergraduate Behavioral Outcomes	Graduate Behavioral Outcomes	Teaching/Learning Strategies
					management, side effects experienced by the patient due to opioid use, and recommended changes, if needed, in the plan of care. *Have students develop pain management protocol or practice guidelines for a specific patient population. Develop the protocol based on empirical evidence through critiquing related research studies and in collaboration with members of the interdisciplinary team.

Education Plan 11.1 *(continued)*

Knowledge Needed	Attitude	Skills	Undergraduate Behavioral Outcomes	Graduate Behavioral Outcomes	Teaching/Learning Strategies
Nondrug interventions for pain management: —Benefits —Development of scientific evidence regarding efficacy of nonpharmacological agents.	*Verify the use of nonpharmacological interventions as complementary therapies to the pharmacological management of pain. *Support the use of nonpharmacological interventions that have been empirically validated as effective in pain management.		*Critique scientific research to determine the value and appropriate utilization of nonpharmacological interventions in pain management.	*Participate in research studies to determine the efficacy of nonpharmacological interventions in the pain management, particularly related to palliative care.	*Conduct a review of the research literature to analyze the efficacy of various nonpharmacological interventions in pain management. Present the findings in a written paper or class presentation.

Education Plan 11.1 *(continued)*

Knowledge Needed	Attitude	Skills	Undergraduate Behavioral Outcomes	Graduate Behavioral Outcomes	Teaching/Learning Strategies
Nondrug Interventions for Pain Management: • Psychological; • Psychiatric; • Neurostimulatoryinterventions for • Invasive; • Integrative.	*Respect patients' opinions, preferences, and desires/requests regarding nonpharmacological interventions for pain management.	*Demonstrate skill in the administration of select nonpharmacological interventions for pain management.	*Educate patients and families, and other health professionals about nonpharmacological approaches to pain management, including techniques, benefits, and contraindications. *Accurately and appropriately administer basic nonpharmacological interventions for effective pain management, such as education, distraction, self-statements, relaxation techniques, guided imagery, use of a pain	*Accurately and appropriately administer advanced nonpharmacological interventions for effective pain management, such as hypnosis, cognitive behavioral therapy, and accupressure if educationally prepared. *Advocate for the availability of specialists who are prepared to administer selected nonpharmacological interventions for pain management.	*Invite a guest speaker to class to discuss and demonstrate selected nonpharmacological interventions for pain management. *Demonstrate selected nonpharmacological interventions with a return demonstration by students/nurses. Discuss the experience as the provider and recipient of the intervention.

Education Plan 11.1 *(continued)*

Knowledge Needed	Attitude	Skills	Undergraduate Behavioral Outcomes	Graduate Behavioral Outcomes	Teaching/Learning Strategies
			diary, positioning, movement, support-ive and assistive devices, heat and cold, massage, vibration, use of TENS unit, music therapy, and therapeutic touch. *Seek referral to appropriate specialists for nonpharmacological interventions for pain management.	*Develop a comprehensive plan of care that includes the use of pharmacological and nonpharmacological therapies for pain management.	*View the video series available through the Holistic Nurses Association, which discusses and demonstrates various nonpharmacological interventions. *Based on case studies, evaluate the appropriateness of a pain management plan utilizing nonpharmacological interventions based on type of illness, etiology of pain, pain history and assessment, patient preference, health status, and goals of care.

Education Plan 11.1 *(continued)*

Knowledge Needed	Attitude	Skills	Undergraduate Behavioral Outcomes	Graduate Behavioral Outcomes	Teaching/Learning Strategies
					*In the clinical setting, implement a plan of care for pain management of a select patient utilizing nonpharmacological interventions. In postconference, discuss the barriers to the use of nonpharmacological interventions, the patient's response to the intervention, side effects experienced by the patient, and recommended changes, if needed, in the plan of care.

Education Plan 11.1 *(continued)*

Knowledge Needed	Attitude	Skills	Undergraduate Behavioral Outcomes	Graduate Behavioral Outcomes	Teaching/Learning Strategies
Special Populations Concerns at the End of Life: —Patients with a history of substance abuse; —Patients with impaired communication; —Elder patients; —Pediatric patients.	*Consider the special needs of patients who have a history of substance abuse, have impaired communication, are older adults, or children. *Acknowledge personal attitudes and misconceptions toward patients with a history of substance abuse or the older adult and how those attitudes may affect compassionate and effective care, including the relief of pain.	*Demonstrate accurate pain assessment skills for patients from special populations.	*Provide effective pain management for those frequently undertreated for pain, specifically individuals with a history of substance abuse, those with impaired communication, the older adult, and children. *Seek referral from consultants when necessary for appropriate pain management in special populations.	*Educate patients, family, and health professionals regarding the pain assessment and management for individuals of special populations. *Establish protocols and clinical practice guidelines to insure compassionate and effective pain management of special patient populations.	*Explore with students/nurses their assumptions regarding patients with a history of substance abuse, those with impaired communication, older adults, and children. *Have each student/nurse analyze a past clinical experience in which they cared for a patient in a special population described above with regard to the adequacy of pain assessment and management. Discuss the barriers and facilitators to effective pain management in the case.

473

Education Plan 11.1 (*continued*)

Knowledge Needed	Attitude	Skills	Undergraduate Behavioral Outcomes	Graduate Behavioral Outcomes	Teaching/Learning Strategies
					*Select a particular patient scenario with regard to medical diagnosis, discuss how the assessment and treatment would differ if the patient had a history of substance use, had impaired communication, was an elder or a child. *Assign students to care for a patient within the special populations described, and develop a plan of care for effective pain management. Evaluate the plan of care in class or post-conference.

REFERENCES

Acute Pain Management Guidelines Panel (1992). *Acute pain management: operative or medical procedures and trauma. Clinical practice guideline.* AHCPR Pub. No. 92-0032. Rockville, MD: Agency for Health Care Policy and Research, Public Health Services, U.S. Department of Health and Human Services.

Adelhardt, J., Byrnes, M., Derby, S., Holritz, K., Layman-Goldstein, M., Racolin, A., & Staniewicz, J. (1995). *Care of the patient in pain: Standard of oncology nursing practice.* New York: Memorial Sloan-Kettering Cancer Center.

Ahles, T. A., Ruckdeschel, J. H., & Blanchard, E. B. (1984). Cancer related pain—11. Assessment with visual analogue scales. *Journal of Psychosomatic Research, 28,* 121–124.

American Cancer Society (1999). *Cancer Facts and Figures—1999.* Atlanta, GA: American Cancer Society, Inc.

American Nurses Association (1990). *Position paper on the promotion of comfort and relief of pain in dying patients.* Washington, DC: American Nurses Association.

American Pain Society (1999). *Principles of analgesic use in the treatment of acute pain and cancer pain* (4th ed.). Glenview, IL: American Pain Society.

American Pain Society (1995). Quality Improvement Guidelines for the treatment of acute pain and cancer pain. *JAMA, 274*(23), 1874–1880.

Arbit, E., & Bilsky, M. H. (1998). Neurosurgical approaches in palliative care. In D. Doyle, G. W. C. Hanks, & N. MacDonald (Eds.), *Oxford textbook of palliative medicine* (2nd ed.) (pp. 414–420). Oxford: Oxford University Press.

Backonja, M., Arndt, G., Gombar, K. A., Check, B., & Zimmerman, M. (1994). Response of chronic neuropathic pain syndromes to ketamine: A preliminary study. *Pain, 56,* 51–57.

Bailey, P. P. (1999). Asthma. In T. M. Buttaro, J. Trybulski, P. P. Baily, & J. Sandberg-Cook (Eds.), *Primary care: A collaborative practice* (pp. 283–308). St. Louis: Mosby.

Basbaum, A. L., & Fields, H. L. (1984). Endogenous pain control systems: Brainstem spinal pathways and endorphin circuitry. *Annals Review Neuroscience, 7,* 309–338.

Bauer, W. C., & Dracup, K. A. (1987). Physiological effects of back massage in patients with acute myocardial infarctions. *Focus Critical Care, 14*(6), 42–46.

Beaver, W. T., & Feise, G. (1976). Comparison of the analgesic effect of morphine, hydroxyzine and their combination in patients with postoperative pain. In J. J. Bonica & D. Albe-Fessard (Eds.), *First International Congress on Pain. Advances on Pain Research and Therapy* (pp. 553–557). New York: Raven Press.

Benson, H. (1975). *The relaxation response.* New York: William Morrow.

Berenson, J. R., Lichtenstein, A., & Porter, L. (1996). Efficacy of pamidronate in reduction of skeletal events in patients with advanced multiple myeloma. *New England Journal of Medicine, 334,* 488–493.

Besson, J. M., & Chaouch, A. (1987). Peripheral and spinal mechanisms of nociception. *Physiology Review, 67,* 167–186.

Billings, J. A., & Block, S. D. (1996). Slow euthanasia. *Journal of Palliative Care, 12,* 21–30.

Blomquist, C., Elomaa, I., & Porkka, L. (1988). Evaluation of salmon calcitonin treatment in bone metastases from breast cancer: A controlled trial. *Bone, 9,* 45–51.

Bookbinder, M., Coyle, N., Kiss, M., Layman-Goldstein, M., Holritz, K., Thaler, H., Gianella, A., Derby, S., Brown, M., Racolin, A., Ho, M. N., & Portenoy, R. K. (1995). Implementing national standards for cancer pain management: Program model and evaluation. *Journal of Pain and Symptom Management, 12,* 334–347.

Breitbart, W., Bruera, E., Chochinov, H., & Lynch, M. (1995). Neuropsychiatric syndromes and psychological symptoms in patients with advanced cancer. *Journal of Pain and Symptom Management, 10,* 131–141.

Brescia, F., Portenoy, R. K., Ryan, M., Drasnoff, L., & Gray, G. (1992). Pain, opioid use and survival in hospitalized patients with advanced cancer. *Journal of Clinical Oncology, 10*, 149–155.

Brose, W. G., & Cousins, M. J. (1991). Subcutaneous lidocaine for treatment of neuropathic cancer pain. *Pain, 45*, 145–148.

Bruera, E., Macmillan, K., & MacDonald, N. (1989). The cognitive effects of the administration of narcotic analgesics in patients with cancer pain. *Pain, 39*, 13–26.

Bruera, E., Miller, L., McCallion, J., Macmillan, K., & Hanson, J. (1992). Cognitive failure in patients with terminal cancer, a prospective study. *Journal of Pain and Symptom Management, 7*, 192–195.

Bruera, E., Suarez-Almozor, M., Velasco, A., Bertolino, M., MacDonald, S. M., & Hanson, J. (1994). The assessment of constipation in terminal cancer patients admitted to a palliative care unit: A retrospective review. *Journal of Pain and Symptom Management, 9*, 515–519.

Bullough, V. L., & Bullough, B. (1998). Should nurses practice therapeutic touch? Should nursing schools teach therapeutic touch? *Journal of Professional Nursing, 14*(4), 254–257.

Burt, R. A. (1997). The Supreme Court speaks: Not assisted-suicide but a constitutional right to palliative care. *New England Journal of Medicine, 337*, 1234–1236.

Byock, I. (1997). *Dying well: The prospect of growth at the end of life.* New York: Riverhead Books.

Carver, A. C., Vickrey, B. G., & Bernat, J. L. (1999). End of life care: A survey of US neurologists' attitudes, behavior and knowledge. *Neurology, 53*(2), 284–293.

Cavanaugh, T. A. (1996). The ethics of death-hastening or death-causing palliative analgesics administered in the terminally ill. *Journal of Pain and Symptom Management, 12*, 248–54.

Cherny, N., & Catane, R. (1995). Professional negligence in the management of cancer pain. *Cancer, 76*, 2181–2184.

Cherny, N., & Coyle, N. (1994). Suffering in the advanced cancer patient: A definition and taxonomy. *Journal of Palliative Care, 10*(2), 57–70.

Cherny, N., & Coyle, N. (1999). Ethical principles in the management of cancer pain. In G. M. Aronoff (Ed.), *Evaluation and treatment of chronic pain* (3rd ed.) (pp. 643–654). Baltimore, MD: Williams & Wilkins.

Cherny, N., & Portenoy, R. K. (1994). Practical issues in the management of cancer pain. In P. D. Wall & R. Melzack (Eds.), *Textbook of pain* (3rd ed.) (pp. 1437–1467). Edinburgh: Churchill Livingstone.

Cherny, N., & Portenoy, R. K. (1994). Sedation in the management of refractory symptoms: Guidelines for evaluation and treatment. *Journal of Palliative Care, 10*, 31–38.

Cherny, N. I., Arbit, E., & Jain, S. (1996). Invasive techniques in the management of cancer pain. *Hematology/Oncology Clinics of North America, 10*(1), 121–137.

Cherny, N. I., & Portenoy, R. K. (1994). The management of cancer pain. *Ca: A Cancer Journal for Clinicians, 44*(5), 262–303.

Cheville, A. L. (1999). Cancer rehabilitation and palliative care. In Conference Course Syllabus Abstract of *Cancer rehabilitation in the new millennium: Opportunities and challenges* (pp. 125–128). R. Payne & A.L. Cheville, course directors. New York: Memorial Sloan-Kettering Cancer Center.

Christie, J. M., Simmonds, M., Patt, R., Coluzzi, P., Busch, M. A., Nordbrock, E., & Portenoy, R. K. (1998). Dose titration: A multicenter study of oral transmucosal fentanyl citrate for the treatment of breakthrough pain in cancer patients using transdermal fentanyl for persistent pain. *Journal of Clinical Oncology, 16*, 3238–3245.

Clark, C. C. (1999). *Encyclopedia of complementary health practice.* New York: Springer Publishing Co.

Cleeland, C. E. (1989). Pain control: Public and physicians' attitudes. In C. S. Hill & W. S. Fields (Eds.), *Drug treatment of cancer pain in a drug-oriented society. Advances in Pain research and Therapy* (Vol. 11, pp. 81–89). New York: Raven Press.

Cleeland, C. S. (1987). Nonpharmacological management of cancer pain. *Journal of Pain and Symptom Management, 2*(2), S23–S28.

Cleeland, C. S., Gonin, R., Hatfield, A. K., Edmonson, J. H., Blum, R. H., Stewart, J. A., & Pandya, K. J. (1994). Pain and its treatment in outpatients with metastatic cancer. *New England Journal of Medicine, 330,* 592–596.

Clissold, S. P. (1986). Aspirin and related derivatives of salicylic acid. *Drugs, Suppl. 4, 32,* 70–77.

Compton, P. (1999). Substance abuse. In M. McCaffery & C. Passero (Eds.), *Pain: Clinical manual* (2nd ed.) (pp. 428–466). St. Louis: Mosby.

Copley Cobb, S. (1984). Teaching relaxation techniques to cancer patients. *Cancer Nursing, 7,* 157–161.

Coyle, N. (1992). The euthanasia and physician-assisted suicide debate: Issues for nursing. *Oncoogy Nursing Forum, 19,* 41–46.

Coyle, N. (1995). Suffering in the first person. In B. R. Ferrell (Ed.), *Suffering.* Boston: Jones and Bartlett.

Coyle, N., Adelhardt, J., Foley, K. M., & Portenoy, R. K. (1990). Character of terminal illness in the advanced cancer patient: Pain and other symptoms in the last four weeks of life. *Journal of Pain and Symptom Management, 5,* 83–93.

Coyle, N., Cherny, N. I., & Portenoy, R. K. (1994). Subcutaneous infusions at home. *Oncology, 8,* 21–32.

Coyle, N., & Portenoy, R. K. (1995). Pharmacologic management of cancer pain. In D. B. McGuire, C. H. Yarbro, & B. R. Ferrell (Eds.), *Cancer pain management* (2nd ed.) (pp. 89–130). Boston: Jones & Bartlett.

Curtis, E. B., Krech, R., & Walsh, T. D. (1991). Common symptoms in patients with advanced cancer. *Journal of Palliative Care, 7,* 25–29.

Daut, R. L., Cleeland, C. S., & Flanery, R. C. (1983). Development of the Wisconsin Brief Pain Questionnaire to assess pain in cancer and other diseases. *Pain, 17,* 197–210.

De Conno, F., Caraceni, A., Gamba, A., Mariani, I., Abbattista, A., Brunelli, C., La Mura, A., & Ventafridda, V. (1994). Pain measurements in cancer patients: A comparison of six methods. *Pain, 57,* 151–166.

De Conno, F., Groff, L., & Brunelli, C. (1996). Clinical experience with oral methadone administration in the treatment of pain in 196 advanced cancer patients. *Journal of Clinical Oncology, 14,* 2836–2842.

De Stoutz, N., Bruera, E., & Suarez-Almazor, M. E. (1995). Opioid rotation for toxicity reduction in terminal cancer patients. *Journal of Pain and Symptom Management, 10,* 378–84.

Decker, G. M. (2000). An overview of complimentary and alternative therapies. *Clinical Journal of Oncology Nursing, 4*(1), 49–52.

Dietz, H. (1982). *Rehabilitation oncology.* New York: John Wiley & Sons.

Dixon, R., Crews, T., Inturrisi, C. E., & Foley, K. M. (1983). Levorphanol: Pharmacokinetics and steady-state plasma concentrations in patients with pain. *Research Communications in Chemistry, Pathology and Pharmacology, 41,* 3–17.

Dubner, R. (1991). Topical capsaicin therapy for neuropathic pain. *Pain, 48,* 383–390.

Dunajcik, L. (1999). Chronic nonmalignant pain. In M. McCaffery & C. Pasero (Eds.), *Pain: Clinical manual* (2nd ed.) (pp. 467–521). St. Louis: Mosby, Inc.

Eide, P. K., Jorum, E., Stubhang, A., Bremners, J., & Breivil, H. (1994). Relief of postherpetic neuralgia with the N-methyl-D-aspartic receptor antagonist ketamine: A double blind, cross-over comparison with morphine and placebo. *Pain, 58,* 347–354.

Eisenach, A. B., Du Penn, S., Dubois, M., Mignel, R., & Allin, D. (1995). Epidural clonidine analgesia for intractable cancer pain. *Pain, 61,* 391–400.

Eisenberg, E., Carr, D. B., & Chalmer, T. C. (1995). Neurolytic celiac plexus block for treatment of cancer pain: A meta-analysis. *Anesthesia and Analgesia, 80,* 290–295.

Eland, J. M. (1990). Pain in children. *Nursing Clinics of North America, 25*(4), 871–84.

Elliot, K., & Foley, K. M. (1988). Neurologic pain syndromes in patients with cancer. *Neurologic Clinics, 7,* 333–360.

Eskinazi, D., & Muehsam, D. (1999). Is the scientific publishing of complimentary and alternative medicine objective? *Journal of Alternative and Complimentary Medicine, 5*(6), 587–594.

Ettinger, Vitale, P. J., & Trump, D. L. (1979). Important clinical pharmacologic considerations in the use of methadone in cancer patients. *Cancer Treatment Reports, 63,* 457–459.

Fainsinger, R., Schoeller, T., & Bruera, E. (1993). Methadone in the management of cancer pain, a review. *Pain, 52,* 137–47.

Fanning, P. (1988). *Visualization for change.* Oakland, CA: New Harbinger Publications.

Fernandez, E. (1986). A classification system of cognitive coping strategies for pain. *Pain, 26,* 141–151.

Ferrell, B. A. (1998). Supportive care in elderly people. In A. Berger, R. K. Portenoy, & D. E. Weissman (Eds.), *Principles and practice of supportive oncology* (pp. 853–859). Philadelphia: Lippincott—Raven Publishers.

Ferrell, B. R., & Ferrell, B. A. (1995). Pain in elderly persons. In D. B. McGuire, C. Henke Yarbro, & B. R. Ferrell (Eds.), *Cancer pain management* (2nd ed.) (pp. 273–287). Boston: Jones and Bartlett Publishers.

Ferrell, B. R., Ferrell, B. A., Ahn, C., & Tran, K. (1994). Pain management for elderly patients with cancer at home. *Cancer (Supplement), 74*(7), 2139–2146.

Ferrell, B. R., Grant, M., Chan, J., Ahn, C., & Ferrell, B. A. (1995). The impact of cancer pain education on family caregivers of elderly patients. *Oncology Nursing Forum, 22*(8), 1211–1218.

Ferrell, B. R., Rhiner, M., Cohen, M. Z., & Grant, M. (1991). Pain as a metaphor for illness. Part 1: Impact of pain and family caregivers. *Oncology Nursing Forum, 18,* 1303–1309.

Ferrell, B. R., Virani, R., & Grant, M. (1999). Analysis of end-of-life content in nursing textbooks. *Oncology Nursing Forum, 26,* 869–876.

Finley, G. A., & McGrath, P. J. (Eds.) (1998). *Measurement of pain in infants and children. Progress in pain research and management* (Vol. 10). Seattle: IASP Press.

Finns, J. J. (1999). Acts of omission and commission in pain management: The ethics of naloxone use. *Journal of Pain and Symptom Management, 17*(2), 120–124.

Fishman, B. (1991). The treatment of suffering in patients with cancer pain: Cognitive behavioral approaches. In K. M. Foley, J. J. Bonica, & V. Ventafridda (Eds.), *Advances in pain research and therapy* (Vol. 16, pp. 301–316). New York: Raven Press.

Fishman, B. (1992). The cognitive behavioral perspective of pain management in terminal illness. *Hospice Journal, 8*(1–2), 73–88.

Fishman, B., & Loscalzo, M. (1987). Cognitive-behavioral interventions in management of cancer pain: Principles and applications. *Medical Clinics of North America, 71*(2), 271–287.

Fishman, B., Pastenak, S., Wallenstein, S., Houde, R., Holland, J. C., & Foley, K. M. (1986). The Memorial Pain Assessment Scale: A valid instrument for the assessment of cancer pain. *Cancer, 60,* 1151–1157.

Foley, K. M. (1989b). The decriminalization of cancer pain. In C. S. Hill & W. S. Fields (Eds.), *Drug treatment of cancer pain in a drug oriented society. Advances in Pain Research and Therapy* (Vol. 11, pp. 5–18). New York: Raven Press.

Foley, K. M. (1991). The relationship of pain and symptom management to patient requests for physician-assisted suicide. *Journal of Pain and Symptom Management, 6,* 289–297.

Foley, K. M. (1993). Changing concepts of tolerance to opioids: What the cancer patient has taught us. In C. R. Chapman & K. M. Foley (Eds.), *Current and emerging issues in cancer pain: Research and practice* (pp. 331–50). New York: Raven Press.

Foley, K. M. (1996). Pain syndromes in patients with cancer. In R. K. Portenoy & R. M. Kanner (Eds.), *Contemporary neurology series: Pain management: Theory and practice* (Vol. 48, p. 215). Philadelphia: F. A. Davis.

Foley, K. M. (1998). Pain assessment and cancer pain syndromes. In D. Doyle, G. W. C. Hanks, & N. MacDonald (Eds.), *Oxford textbook on palliative medicine* (2nd ed.) (pp. 310–331). Oxford: Oxford University Press.

Frager, G. (1997). Palliative care and terminal care of children. *Children and Adolescent Psychiatric Clinics of North America, 6*(4), 889–909.

Fromm, G. H., Terrence, C. F., & Chattha, A. S. (1984). Baclofen in the treatment of trigeminal neuralgia: Double-blind study and long-term follow-up. *Annals of Neurology, 15*, 240–244.

Fultz, J. M., & Sonay, E. C. (1975). Guidelines for the management of hospitalized narcotic addicts. *Annals of Internal Medicine, 82*(6), 815–818.

Galer, B. S., Coyle, N., & Pasternak, G. W. (1992). Individual variability in the response to different opioids: Report of five cases. *Pain, 49*, 87–91.

Giasson, M., & Bouchard, L. (1998). Effect of therapeutic touch on the well-being of persons with terminal cancer. *Journal of Holistic Nursing, 16*(3), 383–398.

Goa, K. I., & Sorkin, E. M. (1993). Gabapentin: A review of its pharmacological properties and clinical potential in epilepsy. *Drugs, 46*, 409–427.

Goldberg, S. (1983). *Clinical neurology made ridiculously simple.* Miami: MedMaster, Inc.

Gonzales, G. R., & Coyle, N. (1992). Treatment of cancer pain in a former opioid abuser: Fears of the patient and staff and their influence on care. *Journal of Pain and Symptom Management, 7*, 246–249.

Goodwin, J. S., & Regan, M. (1982). Cognitive dysfunction associated with naproxen and ibuprofen in the elderly. *Arthritis and Rheumatism, 25*, 1013–1015.

Gourlay, G. K., Plummer, J. L., Cherry, D. A., & Purser, T. (1991). The reproducibility of bioavailability of oral morphine under fed and fasted conditions. *Journal of Pain and Symptom Management, 6*, 431–436.

Grant, M. M., & Rivera, L. M. (1995). Pain education for nurses, patients, and families. In D. B. McGuire, C. Henke Yarbro, & B. R. Ferrell (Eds.), *Cancer pain management* (2nd ed.) (pp. 289–319). Boston: Jones and Bartlett Publishers.

Groenwald, S. L., & Thaney, K. (1987). Rehabilitation. In S. Groenwald (Ed.), *Cancer nursing: Principles and practices* (pp. 740–758). Boston: Jones and Bartlett Publishers.

Grond, S., Zech, D., Diefenbach, C., Radbruch, L., & Lehmann, K. (1996). Assessment of cancer pain: A prospective evaluation of 2266 cancer patients referred to a pain Service. *Pain, 64*, 107–114.

Grossman, S. A., Sheidler, V. R., Swedeen, K., Mucenski, J., & Piantadosi, S. (1991). Correlation of patient and caregiver ratings of cancer pain. *Journal of Pain and Symptom Management, 6*, 53–7.

Hanks, G. W. (1996). Morphine in cancer pain: Modes of administration. *British Medical Journal, 312*, 823–826.

Hanks, G. W., & Cherny, N. (1998). Opioid analgesic therapy. In D. Doyle, G. W. C. Hanks, & N. MacDonald (Eds.), *Oxford textbook of palliative medicine* (2nd ed.) (pp 331–355). Oxford: Oxford University Press.

Hawkey, C. J. (1990). Non-steroidal anti-inflammatory drugs and peptic ulcers. *British Medical Journal, 300*, 278–284.

Hawkey, C. J., & Yeomans, N. D. (1998). Evolving strategies for managing non-steroidal anti-inflammatory drug associated ulcers. *American Journal of Medicine, 104* (suppl. 3A), 1S–96S.

Herr, K. A., & Mobily, P. R. (1991). Pain assessment in the elderly. *Journal of Gerontological Nursing, 17*(4), 12–19.

Hewitt, D. J., & Foley, K. M. (1997). Pain and pain management. In C. K. Cassel, H. J. Cohen, E. B. Larson, D. E. Meier, N. M. Resnick, L. Z. Rubenstein, & L. B. Sorenson (Eds.), *Geriatric medicine* (3rd ed.) (pp. 865–882). New York: Springer-Verlag New York, Inc.

Hewitt, D. J., & Portenoy, R. K. (1998). Adjuvant drugs for neuropathic pain. In R. K. Portenoy & E. Bruera (Eds.), *Topics in palliative care* (Vol. 2, pp. 41–62).

Hill, C. S., Audell, L. G., Kanner, R., Miaskowski, C., Paice, J., & Rogers, A. G. (1999). A roundtable discussion: The management of pain in special populations of cancer patients. *Primary Care & Cancer, 19*(3), 16, 27, 32–34.

Hindley, A. C., Hill, E. B., Letland, M., & Wiles, A. E. (1982). A double-blind controlled trial of salmon calcitonin in pain during malignancy. *Cancer Chemopharmacolgy, 9*(2), 71–74.

Hofmann, M. T., Farnon, C. U., Javed, A., & Posner, J. D. (1998). Pain in the elderly hospice patient. *American Journal of Hospice and Palliative Care, 15*(5), 259–265.

Hortobagyi, G. N., Theriault, R. L., & Porter, L. (1996). Efficacy of pamidronate in reducing skeletal complications in patients with breast cancer and lytic bone metastases. *New England Journal of Medicine, 335,* 1785–1791.

Houde, R. W. (1986). Clinical analgesic studies of hydromorphone. In K. M. Foley & C. E. Inturrisi (Eds.), *Advances in pain research and therapy* (Vol. 8, pp. 129–36).

Hunt, G., & Bruera, E. (1995). Respiratory depression in patients receiving oral methadone for cancer pain. *Journal of Pain and Symptom Management, 10*(5), 401–404.

Hupert, C., Yacoub, M., & Turgeon, L. R. (1980). Effects of hydroxyzine on morphine analgesia for the treatment of postoperative pain. *Anesthesia Analgesia, 59,* 690–696.

Ingham, J., & Coyle, N. (1997). Team work in end-of-life care: A nurse physician perspective in introducing physicians to palliative care concepts. In D. Clark, S. Ahmedzai, & J. Hockley (Eds.), *New themes in palliative care* (pp. 225–274). London: Open University Press.

Inturrisi, C. E., Colburn, W. A., Kaiko, R. F., Houde, R. W., & Foley, K. M. (1987). Pharmakokinetics and pharmacodynamics of methadone in patients with chronic pain. *Clinical Pharmacology and Therapeutics, 41,* 392–401.

Inturrisi, C. E., Portenoy, R. K., Mz, M. B., Colburn, W. A., & Foley, K. M. (1990). Pharmacokinetic-pharmacodynamic (PK-PD) relationships of methadone infusions in patients with cancer pain. *Clinical Pharmacology and Therapeutics, 47,* 565–570.

Jacox, A., Carr, D. B., Payne, R., Berde, C. B., Breithart, W., Cain, I. M., Chapman, C. R., Cleeland, C. S., Ferrell, B. R., & Finley, R. S. (1994). *Management of Cancer Pain. Clinical Practice Guideline No. 9.* AHCPR Publication No. 94-0592. Rockville, MD: Agency for Health Care Policy and Research, U.S. Department of Health and Human Services, Public Health Services.

Jaffe, J. H., & Martin, W. R. (1990). Opioid analgesics and antagonists. In A. G. Gilman, T. W. Rall, A. S. Nies, & P. Taylor (Eds.), *The pharmacological basis of therapeutics* (8th ed.) (pp. 485–521). New York: Permagon Press.

Jenkins, C. A., & Bruera, E. (1999). Nonsteroidal anti-inflammatory drugs as adjuvant analgesics in cancer patients. *Palliative Medicine, 13,* 183–196.

Johansson, C., Dahl, J., Jannert, M., Melin, L., & Anderson, G. (1998). Effects of a cognitive-behavioral pain-management program. *Behavior Research and Therapy, 36*(10), 915–930.

Joranson, D. E., Cleeland, C. S., & Weissman, D. E. (1992). Opioids in chronic pain and non-cancer pain: A survey of state medical board members. *Federal Bulletin: Journal of Medical Licensure and Discipline, 79,* 15–49.

Kaiko, R. F. (1983). Central nervous system excitatory effects of meperidine in cancer patients. *Annals of Neurology, 13,* 180–185.

Kayser, V., Desmeules, J., & Guilland, G. (1995). Systemic clonidine differentially modulates the abnormal reactions to mechanical and thermal stimuli in rats with peripheral mononeuropathy. *Pain, 60,* 275–285.

Kofler, M., & Leis, A. A. (1992). Prolonged seizure activity after baclofen withdrawal. *Neurology, 42,* 697.

Kotora, J. (1997). Therapeutic touch can augment traditional therapies. *Oncology Nursing Forum, 24*(8), 1329–1330.

Latimer, E. J. (1991). Ethical decision-making in the care of the dying and its application to clinical practice. *Journal of Pain and Symptom Management, 6,* 329–336.

Layman-Goldstein, M., & Altilio, T. (1993). *Cancer pain: Cognitive and behavioral approaches to cancer pain management—relaxation training.* New York: Memorial Sloan-Kettering Cancer Center, video script.

Levin, D. N., Cleeland, C. S., & Dar, R. (1985). Public attitudes towards cancer pain. *Cancer, 56,* 2337–2339.

Levy, M. (1985). Pain management in advanced cancer. *Seminars in Oncology, 12,* 384–410.

Levy, M. H. (1989). Integration of pain management into comprehensive cancer care. *Cancer, 63,* 2328–2335.

Lipman, A. G., & Gauthier, M. E. (1997). Pharmacology of opioid drugs. In R. K. Portenoy & E. Bruera (Eds.), *Topics in palliative care* (Vol. 1, chapter 7). New York: Oxford University Press.

Loew, K. P., Smith, M. T., Williams, B., & Cramond, T. (1992). Single-dose and steady—state pharmacokinetics and pharmacodynamics of oxycodone in patients with cancer. *Clinical Pharmacology and Therapeutics, 52,* 487–495.

Loscalzo, M. (1996). Psychological approaches to the management of pain in patients with advanced cancer. *Hematology/Oncology Clinics of North America, 10*(1), 139–155.

Lundeberg, T., Nordeman, R., & Ottoson, D. (1984). Pain alleviation by vibratory stimulation. *Sep, 20*(1), 25–44.

Lynn, J., Teno, J. M., Phillips, R. S., Wu, A. W., Desbiens, N., & Harrold, J. (1997). Perceptions of family members of the dying experience of older and seriously ill patients. *Annals of Internal Medicine, 126,* 97–106.

Magill-Levreault, L. (1993). Music therapy in pain and symptom management. *Journal of Palliative Care,* Winter (4), 42–48.

Managing caner pain in adults (1999) [CD ROM]. New York: Memorial Sloan-Kettering Cancer Center.

Manfredi, P. L., Borsook, D., Chandler, S. W., & Payne, R. (1997). Intravenous methadone for cancer pain unrelieved by morphine and hydromorphone: Clinical observations. *Pain, 70,* 99–101.

Manfredi, P. L., Ribeiro, S. W., & Payne, R. (1996). Inappropriate use of naloxone in cancer patients with pain. *Journal of Pain and Symptom Management, 11,* 131–134.

Mashimo, T., Tomi, K., Pak, M., Demizu, A., & Yyoshiya, I. (1991). Relief of causalgia with prostaglandinE1 ointment. *Anesthesia Analgesia, 72,* 700–701.

Mast, D., Meyers, J., & Urbanski, A. (1987a). Relaxation techniques: A self-learning module for nurses: Unit I. *Cancer Nursing, 10*(3), 141–147.

Mast, D., Meyers, J., & Urbanski, A. (1987b). Relaxation techniques: A self-learning module for nurses: Unit II. *Cancer Nursing, 10*(4), 217–225.

Mast, D., Meyers, J., & Urbanski, A. (1987c). Relaxation techniques: A self-learning module for nurses: Unit III. *Cancer Nursing, 10*(5), 279–285.

Max, M. (1987). Amitriptyline relieves diabetic neuropathy pain in patients with normal or depressed mood. *Neurology, 37,* 589–596.

Max, M., Lynch, S. A., Muir, J., Shoaf, S. E., Smoller, B., & Dubner, R. (1992). Effects of desipramine, amitrityline and fluoxetine on pain in diabetic neuropathy. *New England Journal of Medicine, 326,* 1250–1256.

McCaffery, M. (1999). Pain management: Problems and progress. In M. Caffery & C. Pasero (Eds.), *Pain: Clinical manual* (2nd ed.) (pp. 1–14). St. Louis: Mosby, Inc.

McCaffery, M., & Pasero, C. (1999). Practical nondrug approaches to pain. In M. McCaffery & C. Pasero (Eds.), *Pain: Clinical manual* (2nd ed.) (pp. 399–427). St. Louis: Mosby, Inc.

McCaffery, M., & Wolff, M. (1992). Pain relief using cutaneous modalities, positioning, and movement. *Hospice Journal, 8,* 121–154.

McCarberg, B., & Wolf, J. (1999). Chronic pain management in a health maintenance organization. *Clinical Journal of Pain, 15*(1), 50–57.

McGrath, P. (1990). *Pain in children: Nature, assessment and treatment.* New York: Guildford Press.

McGuire, D. B. (1995). The multiple dimensions of cancer pain: A framework for assessment and management. In D. B. McGuire, C. H. Yarbro, & B. R. Ferrell (Eds.), *Cancer pain management* (2nd ed.) (pp. 1–17). Boston: Jones and Bartlett.

Meehan, T. C. (1998). Therapeutic touch as a nursing intervention. *Journal of Advanced Nursing, 28*(1), 117–225.

Meek, S. S. (1993). Effects of slow stroke back massage on relaxation in hospice clients. *Image: Journal of Nursing Scholarship, 25,* 17–21. Memorial Sloan-Kettering Cancer Center. (1999).

Merskey, H. (1986). Classification of chronic pain: Descriptions of chronic pain syndromes and definition of pain terms. *Pain, Suppl, 3,* S217.

Messenger, T., & Roberts, K. T. (1994). The terminally ill: Serenity nursing interventions for hospice clients. *Journal of Gerontological Nursing, 20*(11), 17–22.

Miser, A. W., Moore, L., Greene, R., Gracely, R. H., & Miser, J. S. (1986). Prospective study of continuous intravenous and subcutaneous morphine infusions for therapy-related pain in children and young adults with cancer. *Clinical Journal of Pain, 2,* 101–106.

Moran, K. J. (1989). The effects of self-guided imagery and other-guided imagery on chronic low back pain. In S. D. Funk, E. M. Tornquist, M. T. Champagne, L. A. Coop, & R. A. Wiese (Eds.), *Key aspects of comfort: Management of pain, nausea, and fatigue.* New York: Springer.

Morris, J. N., Mor, V., Goldberg, R. J., Sherwood, S., Greer, D. S., & Hiris, J. (1986). The effect of treatment setting and patient characteristics on pain in terminal cancer patients: A report from the National Hospice Study. *Journal of Chronic Disease, 39,* 47–62.

NIH Consensus Conference (1998). Acupuncture. *JAMA, 280*(17), 1518–1524.

NIH Technology Assessment Panel on Intergatration of Behavioral and Relaxation Approaches into the Treatment of Chronic Pain and Insomnia (1996). Integration of behavioral and relaxation approaches into the treatment of chronic pain and insomnia. *JAMA, 276*(4), 313–318.

Owens, M. K., & Ehrenreich, D. (1991a). Literature review of nonphamacologic methods for the treatment of chronic pain. *Holistic Nursing Practice, 6*(1), 24–31.

Owens, M. K., & Ehrenreich, D. (1991b). Application of nonphamacologic methods of managing chronic pain. *Holistic Nursing Practice, 6*(1), 32–40.

Paice, J. A. (1999). Symptom management. In C. Miaskowski & P. Buchsel (Eds.), *Oncology nursing: Assessment and clinical care.* St Louis: Mosby, Inc.

Passik, S. D., & Portenoy, R. K. (1998). Substance abuse issues in palliative care. In A. Berger, R. K. Portenoy, & D. E. Weissman (Eds.), *Principles and practice of supportive oncology* (pp. 513–529). Philadelphia: Lippincott-Raven Publishers.

Passik, S. D., Portenoy, R. K., & Ricketts, P. L. (1998a). Substance abuse issues in cancer patients. Part 1: Prevalence and diagnosis. *Oncology, 12*(4), 517–521, 524.

Passik, S. D., Portenoy, R. K., & Ricketts, P. L. (1998b). Substance abuse issues in cancer patients. Part 2: Evaluation and treatment. *Oncology, 12*(5), 729–734.

Patterson, K. L. (1992). Pain in the pediatric oncology patient. *Journal of Pediatric Oncology Nursing, 9*(3), 119–130.

Payne, R., Chandler, S. W., & Einhaus, E. (1995). Guidelines for the clinical use of transdermal fentanyl. *Anti-cancer Drugs, 6,* 50–53.

Payne, R., & Gonzales, G. R. (1998). Pathophysiology of pain in cancer and other terminal diseases. In D. Doyle, G. W. C. Hanks, & N. MacDonald (Eds.), *Oxford textbook of palliative medicine* (2nd ed.) (pp. 299–310). Oxford University Press.

Pereira, J., Hanson, J., & Bruera, E. (1997). The frequency and clinical course of cognitive impairment in patients with terminal cancer. *Cancer, 79,* 835–842.

Persson, J., Axelsson, G., Hallin, R. G., & Gustafsson, L. L. (1995). Beneficial effects of ketamine in a chronic pain state with allodynia, possibly due to central sensitization. *Pain, 60,* 217–222.

Portenoy, R. K. (1991). Plasma morphine and morphine-6-glucoronide during chronic morphine therapy for cancer pain: plasma profiles, steady state concentrations and consequences of renal failure. *Pain, 47,* 13–19.

Portenoy, R. K. (1992). Cancer pain: Pathophysiology and syndromes. *Lancet, 339,* 1026–1031.

Portenoy, R. K. (1994). The management of common side effects during long-term therapy of cancer pain. *Annals of Academy of Medicine Singapore, 23,* 160–170.

Portenoy, R. K. (1998). Adjuvant analgesics in pain management. In D. Doyle, G. W. C. Hanks, & N. MacDonald (Eds.), *Oxford textbook of palliative medicine* (2nd ed.) (pp. 361–390). Oxford: Oxford University Press.

Portenoy, R. K., Dole, V., Joseph, H., Lowinson, J., Rice, C., Segal, S., & Richman, B. L. (1997). Pain management and chemical dependency: Evolving perspectives. *JAMA, 278*(7), 592–593.

Portenoy, R. K., & Hagen, N. A. (1990). Breakthrough pain: Definition, prevalence and characteristics. *Pain, 41,* 273.

Portenoy, R. K., Thaler, H. T., Inturrisi, C. E., Friedlander-Klar, H., & Foley, K. M. (1992). The metabolite morphine-6-glucoronide, contributes to the analgesia produced by morphine infusion in pain patients with normal renal function. *Clinical Pharmacology and Therapeutics, 51,* 422–431.

Portenoy, R. K., Thaler, H. T., Kornblith, A. B., Lepore, J. M., Friedlander, K. H., & Coyle, N. (1994). Symptom prevalence, characteristics and distress in a cancer population. *Quality of Life Research, 3,* 183–189.

Porter, A. T., EcEwan, A. J., & Powe, J. E. (1993). Results of a randomized phase-111 trial to evaluate the efficacy of strontium-89 adjuvant to local field external beam irradiation in the management of endocrine resistant metastatic prostate cancer. *International Journal of Radiation Oncology and Biologic Physics, 25,* 805–813.

Porter, J., & Jick, H. (1980). Addiction rare in patients treated with narcotics. *New England Journal of Medicine, 302,* 123 (letter).

Posner, J. (1995). *Neurological complications of cancer.* Philadelphia: F. A. Davis Company.

Rawlins, M. D. (1998). Non-opioid analgesics. In D. Doyle, G. W. G. Hanks, & N. MacDonald (Eds.), *Oxford textbook of palliative medicine* (2nd ed.) (pp. 355–361). Oxford: Oxford University Press.

Rhiner, M., Ferrell, B. R., Ferrell, B. A., & Grant, M. M. (1993). A structured nondrug intervention program for cancer pain. *Cancer Practice, 1*(2), 137–143.

Ripamonti, C., Groff, L., Brunelli, C., Polastri, D., Stravrakis, A., & DeConno, F. (1998). Switching from oral morphine to oral methadone in treating cancer pain: What is the equianalgesic dose ratio? *Journal of Clinical Onoclogy, 16,* 3216–3221.

Robinson, R. G., Preston, D. F., & Spicer, J. A. (1992). Radionuclide therapy of intractable bone pain: Emphasis on strontium-89. *Seminars Nuclear Medicine, 22,* 28–32.

Rosa, L., Rosa, E., Sarner, L., & Barrett, S. (1998). A close look at therapeutic touch. *JAMA, 279*(13), 1005–1010.

Rosenberg, J. M., Harrell, C., Ristic, H., Werner, R. A., & de Rosayro, A. M. (1997). The effect of gabapentin on neuropathic pain. *Clinical Journal Pain, 13,* 251–255.

Roth, S. A. (1988). Non-steroidal anti-inflammatory drugs: Gastropathy, deaths and medical practice. *Annals of Internal Medicine, 109,* 353–354.

Rowbotham, M. C. (1994). Topical analgesic agents. In H. Field & J. C. Liebeskind (Eds.), *Pharmacological approaches to the treatment of chronic pain: New concepts and critical issues* (pp. 211–299). Seattle: IASP Press.

Rowbotham, M. C., Davies, P. S., & Fields, H. L. (1995). Topical lidocaine gel relieves postherpetic neuralgia. *Annals of Neurology, 37,* 246–253.

Rowbotham, M. C., Harden, N., Stacey, B., Berstein, P., & Magnus-Miller, L. (1998). Gabapentin for the treatment of postherpetic neuralgia. A randomized controlled trial. *Journal of the American Medical Association, 280,* 1837–1842.

Roy, D. (1996). When children have to die . . . pediatric palliative care. A special thematic issue. *Journal of Palliative Care, 12*(3), 3–59.

Saberski, L. R. (1998). Interventional approaches in oncologic pain management. In A. Berger, R. K. Portenoy, & D. E. Weissman (Eds.), *Principles and practice of supportive oncology* (pp. 93–107). Philadelphia: Lippincott-Raven Publishers.

Sanders, M., & Zuurmond, W. (1995). Safety of unilateral and bilateral percutaneous cervical cordotomy in 80 terminally ill cancer patients. *Journal of Clinical Oncology, 13*(6), 1509–1512.

Schroeder, M. E. (1986). Neurolytic nerve block for cancer pain. *Journal of Pain and Symptom Management, 1*(2), 91–94.

Schroeder-Sheker, T. (1994). Music for the dying: A personal account of the new field of music thanatology history, theories, and clinical narratives. *Journal of Holistic Nursing, 12*(1), 83–99.

Shimp, L. A. (1998). Safety issues in the pharmacologic management of chronic pain in the elderly. *Pharmacotherapy, 18*(6), 1313–1322.

Sibinga, N. E. S., & Goldstein, A. (1988). Opioid peptides and opioid receptors in cells of the immune system. *Annals Rev Immunology*, 219–249.

Siever, B. A. (1994). Pain management and potentially life-shortening analgesia in the terminally ill child: The ethical implications for pediatric nurses. *Journal of Pediatric Nursing, 9*(5), 307–312.

Solomon, M., O'Donnell, L., Jennings, B., Guilfoy, V., Wolf, S. M., Nolan, K., Jackson, R., Koch-Weser, D., & Donnelley, S. (1993). Decisions near the end-of-life: Professionals views of life-sustaining treatments. *American Journal of Public Health, 83*(1), 14–23.

Solomon, R., & Saylor, C. D. (1995). *National Cancer Institute's pediatric pain management: A professional course.* East Lansing, MI: Michigan State University.

Spross, J. A., & Wolff Burke, M. (1995). Nonpharmacological management of cancer pain. In D. B. McGuire, C. Henke Yarbro, & B. R. Ferrell (Eds.), *Cancer pain management* (2nd ed.) (pp. 159–205). Boston: Jones and Bartlett Publishers.

Stannard, C. F., & Porter, G. E. (1993). Ketamine hydrochloride in the treatment of phantom limb pain. *Pain, 54*, 227–230.

Stedman, T. L. (1995). *Stedman's medical dictionary* (26th ed.). Baltimore: Williams & Wilkins.

Stein, C. (1995). The control of pain in peripheral tissues by opioids. *New England Journal of Medicine, 332*, 1685–1690.

Stephens, R. L. (1993). Imagery: A strategic intervention to empower clients part II—a practical guide. *Clinical Nurse Specialist, 7*(5), 235–240.

Stevens, B. (1997). Pain assessment in children—birth through adolescence. *Children and Adolescent Psychiatric Clinics of North America, 6*(4), 725–744.

Stow, P. J., Glynn, C. J., & Minor, B. (1989). EMLA cream in the treatment of postherpetic neuralgia: Efficacy and pharmacokinetic profile. *Pain, 39*, 301–305.

Streisand, J., Busch, M. A., Egan, T. D., Gaylord Smith, B., Gay, M., & Pace, N. L. (1998). Dose proportionality and pharmakokinetics of oral transmucosal fentanyl citrate. *Anesthesiology, 88*, 305–309.

Sunshine, A., & Olson, N. Z. (1993). In P. D. Wall & R. Melzack (Eds.), *Textbook on pain* (3rd ed.) (p. 927). New York: Churchill, Livingston.

SUPPORT (1995). A controlled trial to improve care for seriously ill hospitalized patients. *JAMA, 274*, 1591–1598.

Swarm, R. A., & Cousins, M. J. (1998). Anaesthetic techniques for pain control. In D. Doyle, G. W. C. Hanks, & N. MacDonald (Eds.), *Oxford textbook of palliative medicine* (2nd ed.) (pp. 390–414). Oxford: Oxford University Press.

Swerdlow, M. (1984). Anticonvulsant drugs and chronic pain. *Clinical Neuropharmacology, 7*, 51–82.

Sykes, N. P. (1998). Constipation and diarrhea. In D. Doyle, G. W. C. Hanks, & N. MacDonald (Eds.), *Oxford textbook on palliative medicine* (2nd ed.) (pp. 513–526). Oxford: Oxford University Press.

Syrjala, K. L., Donaldson, G. W., Davis, M. W., Kippes, M. E., & Carr, J. E. (1995). Relaxation and imagery and cognitive-behavioral training reduce pain during cancer treatment: A controlled clinical trial. *Pain, 63,* 189–198.

Szczeklik, A. (1986). Analgesics, allergy and asthma: Non-narcotic analgesics today, benefits and risks. *Drugs, Suppl 4, 32,* 148–163.

Szeto, H. H., Inturrisi, C. E., Houde, R., Saal, R., Cheigh, J., & Reidenberg, M. M. (1977). Accumulation of normeperidine an active metabolite of meperidine, in patients with renal failure or cancer. *Annals of Internal Medicine, 86,* 738–741.

Thompson, J. W., & Filshie, J. (1998). Transcutaneous electrical nerve stimulation (TENS) and acupuncture. In D. Doyle, G. W. C. Hanks, & N. MacDonald (Eds.), *Oxford textbook of palliative medicine* (2nd ed.) (pp. 421–437). Oxford: Oxford University Press.

Tiseo, P. J., Thaler, H. T., Lapin, J., Inturrisi, C. E., Portenoy, R., & Foley, K. M. (1995). Morphine-6-Glucoronide concentrations and opioid related side effects: A survey of cancer patients. *Pain, 61,* 47–54.

Tunkel, R. S., & Lachmann, E. A. (1998). Rehabilitative medicine. In A. Berger, R. K. Portenoy, & D. E. Weissman (Eds.), *Principles and practice of supportive oncology* (pp. 681–690). Philadelphia: Lippincott-Raven Publishers.

Twycross, R., & Lack, S. A. (1983). *Symptom control in the far advanced cancer patient.* London: Pitman Books.

Twycross, R., & Lichter, I. (1998). The terminal phase. In D. Doyle, G. W. C. Hanks, & N. MacDonald (Eds.), *Oxford textbook on palliative medicine* (2nd ed., pp. 984–992). Oxford: Oxford University Press.

Tyler, D. O., Winslow, E. H., Clark, A. P., & White, K. M. (1990). Effects of a 1 minute back rub on mixed venous oxygen saturation and heart rate in critically ill patients. *Heart Lung, 19*(5, pt 2), 562–565.

Umans, J. G., & Inturrisi, C. E. (1982). Antinociceptive activity and toxicity of meperidine and normeperidine in mice. *Journal of Pharmacology and Experimental Therapeutics, 223,* 203–206.

Ventafridda, V., Ripamonti, C., DeConno, F., Tamburini, M., & Cassileth, B. R. (1990). Symptom prevalence and control during cancer patients' last days of life. *Journal of Palliative Care, 6,* 7–11.

Von Roenn, J. H., Cleeland, C. S., Gonin, R., Hatfield, A. K., & Pandya, K. J. (1993). Physician attitude and practice in cancer pain management. A survey from the Eastern Cooperative Oncology Group. *Annals of Internal Medicine, 119,* 121–126.

Walco, G. A., Cassidy, R. C., & Schechter, N. L. (1994). Sounding board: pain, hurt, and harm. The ethics of pain control in infants and children. *The New England Journal of Medicine, 331*(8), 541–544.

Wallace, K., Reade, B., Pasero, C., & Olsson, G. (1995). Staff nurses' perception of barriers to effective pain management. *Journal of Pain and symptom Management, 10,* 204–213.

Wallenstein, S. L., Rogers, A. G., Kaiko, R. F., & Houde, R. W. (1986). Clinical analgesic studies of levorphanol in acute and chronic pain. In K. M. Foley & C. E. Inturrisi (Eds.), *Advances in pain research and therapy* (Vol. 8, pp. 211–215). New York: Raven Press.

Walsh, T. D. (1990). Prevention of opioid side effects. *Journal of Pain and Symptom Management, 5,* 363–367.

Ward, S. E., Goldberg, N., Miller-McCauley, V., Mueller, C., Nolan, A., & Pawlik-Plank, D. (1993). Patient related barriers to management of cancer pain. *Pain, 52,* 319–324.

Watson, C. P. N., Evans, R. J., & Reed, K. (1982). Amitriptyline versus placebo in postherpetic neuralgia. *Neurology, 32,* 671–673.

Watson, C. P. N., Evans, R. J., & Watt, V. R. (1988). Postherpetic neuralgia and topical capsaicin. *Pain, 33*, 333–340.

Weinberger, J., Nicklas, W. J., & Berl, S. (1976). Mechansim and action of anticonvulsants. *Neurology, 26*(2), 162–166.

Weissman, D. E., Burchman, S. L., Dinndorf, P., & Dahl, J. L. (1990). *Handbook of cancer pain management* (2nd ed.). Milwaukee: Wisconsin Cancer Pain Initiative.

Whitcomb, D. C., & Block, G. D. (1994). Association of acetaminophen toxicity with fasting and ethanol use. *Journal of the Medical Association, 272*, 1845–1850.

Wilkie, D. J. (1995). Neural mechanisms of pain: A foundation for cancer pain assessment and management. In D. B. McGuire, C. Henke Yarbro, & B. Rolling Ferrell (Eds.), *Cancer pain management* (2nd ed., pp. 61–87). Boston: Jones and Bartlett Publishers.

Winstead-Fry, P., & Kijek, J. (1999). An integrative review and meta-analysis of therapeutic touch research. *Alternative Therapies in Health Medicine, 5*(6), 58–67.

World Health Organization (WHO) (1986, 1990, 1996). Cancer pain relief and palliative care. Report of a WHO Expert Committee (WHO Technical Support Series, No. 804). Geneva: World Health Organization.

World Health Organization (1998). *Cancer pain relief and palliative care in children.* Geneva: World Health Organization.

Yaksh, T. L., Dirig, D. M., & Malmberg, A. B. (1998). Mechanism of action of non-steroidal anti-inflammatory drugs. *Cancer Investigation, 16*, 509–527.

12

Peri-Death Nursing Care

Marianne LaPorte Matzo

AACN Competencies

#7: Use scientifically based standardized tools to assess symptoms (e.g., dyspnea, constipation, anxiety, fatigue, nausea/vomiting, and altered cognition) experienced by patients at the end of life.

#8: Use data from symptom assessment to plan and intervene in symptom management using state-of-the-art and traditional approaches.

#9: Evaluate the impact of traditional, complementary, and technological therapies on patient-centered outcomes.

#10: Assess and treat multiple dimensions, including physical, psychological, social, and spiritual needs, to improve quality of care at the end of life.

> It is death that endows life with deepest, most profound meaning.
> —Bruno Bettelheim

As an experiential process, dying and death for the individual, their family, and the health care provider can be one of the most profound and significant events experienced. The last hours of life, specifically the symptoms and experiences right before the death occurs, the actual death, and the care of the body after death can be conceptualized as the peri-death period requiring intensive holistic nursing care.

The purpose of this chapter is to relate the role of the nurse during this phase of life and convey the core knowledge necessary so that the nurse can help facilitate a "good" death. The information in this chapter should be considered a requirement for nurses educated at a basic level. The role of the advanced practice nurse regarding peri-death nursing includes mentoring and modeling appropriate behaviors for the novice nurse. Additionally the role includes supporting the novice nurse through the dying experience, and, support of the family during the decision-making process regarding autopsy and funeral arrangements.

SYMPTOM ASSESSMENT AND MANAGEMENT IN THE LAST HOURS OF LIFE

Any, all, or none of the following symptoms may occur during the final stages of the dying process. In-depth nursing interventions for the person with advanced disease can be found in the previous chapters of this book. The focus here is on the physiological changes that occur as death is imminent and the nursing interventions that are appropriate at this time.

PAIN

As the body begins to shut down and dies the need for pain medication may change or decrease. Drugs most often used to manage pain at the end of life are MS Contin, Morphine Sulfate Instant Release (MSIR), Oxycontin, and Oxycodone (IOM, 1997). The liver conjugates these drugs and active metabolites remain in the body exerting a pharmacological effect until they are cleared by the kidneys. As the body is dying, renal and hepatic function is compromised and the drugs are cleared from the system very slowly. This results in an increase in serum opioid concentrations, which results in increased drowsiness or mild confusion. A nursing priority should be to keep the patient pain free and comfortable but with the understanding that the dosage to accomplish this may be considerably less than what had been previously needed for effective pain management.

Patients, health care providers, and family need an understanding of the importance and value of pain management during the dying process. The patient may seek pain relief or may view pain as a way to atone for sins and refuse to be medicated. Health care professionals may worry that using too high a dose of morphine will result in hastening or causing the death of the patient. Like the nurse, the family may fear being the person to give the "last dose" of morphine before the patient dies. Not adequately medicating for pain, though, can interfere with the memories that the family will carry with them for the rest of their lives. They will remember the death of their loved one as a time of agony and pain rather than a time that could have been used for more meaningful conversations and memories.

The role of the nurse in pain management is to assess the level of pain the patient is having, the patient and family's attitudes toward pain, and assure patients and families that comfort and alleviation of pain is a priority. Encouraging patients to report their pain before it becomes intense will prevent unbearable suffering. Determining the adequacy of the pain control and its duration are important assessment data so those dosages can be appropriately adjusted. Given that pain medications frequently cause constipation, nurses must be vigilant in assessing for constipation. Caregivers should be encouraged to continue prophylaxis bowel regimens to prevent or alleviate its associated discomfort.

Other non-pharmacological interventions that alleviate pain are a calm environment, soothing music, and aromatherapy. Simple human touch or therapeutically intended touch, such as Reike or therapeutic touch, can relieve stress, be a source of comfort or support, and overcome fear of abandonment.

ANOREXIA/DEHYDRATION

As patients approach the end of life, they may say that they are "not hungry" which is a normal pre-death finding. Decreased eating results in a metabolic imbalance where the energy a patient takes in does not cover the energy that they expend and results in a state of dehydration. Although healthy people experiencing dehydration will report pain, abdominal cramps, nausea, vomiting, and dry mouth, patients who are terminally ill do not report such symptoms. At the end of life, patients typically only complain of having a dry mouth which is often unrelated to hydration status and most often is the result of medication side effects, increased respiration, or mouth breathing.

In many cases, artificial hydration and nutrition provide an opportunity to "do something" at a time when the mistaken perception is that there is little else the nurse can do for them. Intravenous fluids given to a person who is actively dying increases urinary output, which may result in the necessity for a Foley catheter. It may increase respiratory secretions that may require suctioning and increase cough as well as increasing gastrointestinal fluids leading to abdominal distension and nausea/vomiting. Increasing the intra-vascular volume in the presence of decreasing renal function can further result in peripheral edema and increase the incidence of decubitus ulcers. Pain can result from the IV site and restraints may become necessary to prevent the patient from removing the tubing. The presence of the IV may act as a physical barrier to the family and may be a cause of anxiety to them. In essence, artificial nutrition and hydration at this stage may lead to symptoms of congestive heart failure, increased tracheal and bronchial secretions, nausea and vomiting, painful edema, and diarrhea (Gates & Fink, 1997), rather than improving symptoms or prolonging life.

In contrast, there are many benefits to the patient in withholding food and fluids as death nears. With calorie deprivation comes an increased production of ketones, which results in an elevation of naturally occurring opioid peptides or endorphins which provide analgesia. An electrolyte imbalance, if present, will also result in increased analgesia. Decreased fluid intake will result in fewer pulmonary fluids, which eases respiration, lessens coughing, and reduces drowning sensations. If a tumor is present dehydration may make it smaller in size by reducing the edematous layer around the tumor resulting in less pressure and pain.

Nursing interventions focus on meticulous mouth care to alleviate mouth dryness and prevent sores, dental problems, and infections. Scrupulous cleaning and moistening of the mouth can be one of the most important interventions to prevent suffering in a patient nearing death (Fields & Cassell, 1997). The mouth and teeth can be cleaned with a soft-bristled toothbrush or sponge-covered oral swabs. To maintain moisture in mucosal membranes the mouth should be rinsed frequently with water. A spray bottle can be used to mist the mouth often; a room humidifier is also very helpful. Commercial salivary substitutes or supplements such as Salivart, Oral Balance, Salagen, and MoiStir can also help keep the patient comfortable. Chamomile tea is also very soothing and can be used to clean the mouth or offered to the patient to sip on. Generously applying lip lubricant can prevent dry, chapped lips and alleviate associated discomfort.

If the patient is experiencing oral pain, morphine or morphine elixir can be used if the pain is severe or during mouth care and meals. Topical agents for mouth pain include Viscous Xylocaine 2% solution, 5–15 ml, swish and spit every 2 to 4 hours as needed. KBX solution (Kaopectate, Benadryl, Xylocaine viscous in equal parts), 5–15 ml, swish for 1 minute, then spit or swallow every 2 to 4 hours as needed may also be ordered. The Xylocaine provides topical anesthesia; the Benadryl is a short-acting anesthetic; and the Kaopectate (Mylanta may be substituted) serves as an alkalizing agent (Gates & Fink, 1997).

If the patient is still sipping fluids, encourage those fluids that contain salt to help prevent electrolyte imbalance. Fluids such as bullion soup, tomato juice, or sport drinks like Gatorade may be well-tolerated. Avoid citrus juices or foods that may irritate the mouth, as well as temperature extremes of foods. It is important not to force food or fluids at this point and to support the family who may have a difficult time accepting the patient's refusal to eat or drink. Families can be reminded that even in the case of acute illness, such as the flu, food and fluids can create additional distress.

As death approaches patients often lose their ability to swallow due to weakness or a decrease in neurological function. The gag reflex may diminish and secretions will tend to accumulate in the tracheo-bronchial tree. Positioning is important to prevent the accumulation of secretions in the back of the throat and upper airways (Ferrell, Virani, & Grant, 1999). Scopolamine transdermal patches can be used to decrease secretion production and decrease the occurrence of the "death rattle," which although does not distress the patient, can be very upsetting to the family.

WEAKNESS AND FATIGUE

Fatigue is a primary complaint of patients in the last 4 weeks of life (Gorman, 1998). The tiredness may be a result of both the disease and the treatment for the disease, as well as malnutrition and disrupted sleep patterns. Fatigue may interfere with a person's ability to move, bathe, or toilet (Fields & Cassell, 1997).

The nurse should be aware that while the patient is at high risk for a pressure ulcer, turning and positioning should be done as frequently as possible but only as often as comfort permits. Bony prominences should be padded and supported if this is comfortable for the patient. If any of these interventions result in increased pain or suffering, they should not be implemented. Initially, this may be difficult for the novice nurse to support, as it is contrary to the basic nursing skills that they have been taught. When a patient is actively dying, intervention goals should focus on comfort; any intervention that compromises this goal should be discontinued.

DYSPNEA

Dyspnea is a common symptom experienced at the end of life and results from the lung's inability to function in proportion to the metabolic demands of the body (Fields & Cassell, 1997). When a person experiences difficulty in breathing, there must either be an increase in ventilation or a decrease in activity. Changes in respiration are normal prior to death. The breathing pattern can become irregular and include shallow breathing altered with apnea lasting 5 to 60 seconds (Cheyne-Stokes breathing). Fluids can accumulate in the back of the throat resulting in what is known as a "death rattle" (Ferrell et al., 1999).

Nursing interventions include positioning the patient with the head of the bed raised and/or turning the person on one side. For opioid naive patients, low dose opiates, such as Morphine 5mg PO every 4 hours, can alleviate the sensation of breathlessness. If Morphine is already being used for pain, an increase of 2.5 mg times their regular dose is generally effective. Oxygen is typically only effective if the dyspnea is secondary to hypoxia (e.g., COPD, pulmonary fibrosis) although it may provide a placebo effect (Horn, 1992). A fan blowing a gentle breeze toward the patient's face can also be very effective. Suctioning is usually not recommended as it may incidentally increase secretion production. Emotion focused interventions such as relaxation techniques, prayer and meditation, and distraction may alleviate the anxiety often associated with dyspnea (Horn, 1992).

MULTISYSTEM FAILURE

As the body is shutting down, there is a decrease in blood perfusion and a resulting shutdown of the major organs (e.g., renal and hepatic). Decreased cardiac output and intravascular volume result in tachycardia and hypotension. Additionally, the body will conserve blood volume for vital organs, which results in peripheral cooling (as the body conserves heat) and peripheral and central cyanosis. The skin may therefore become mottled and discolored, which is normal before death.

Urine output is greatly diminished and there can be a loss of sphincter control resulting in urinary and/or fecal incontinence. It may be a good idea to insert a urinary catheter to reduce the need for frequent bedding changes and to prevent skin breakdown. The catheter also helps the continent patient conserve energy by removing the need to use a bedpan or urinal.

Neurological dysfunction is a result of multiple, concurrent, and nonreversible organ failure. Consequently the patient may experience reduced cerebral perfusion, hypoxemia, metabolic imbalances, acidosis, accumulation of toxins from renal and hepatic failure, and sepsis (Ferrell et al., 1999). The net effect of these changes may be a decreased level of consciousness or terminal delirium.

TERMINAL DELIRIUM

Terminal delirium can be manifested as confusion, anxiety, agitation, or restlessness. Confusion is a mental state in which a person reacts inappropriately to their environment because they are confounded or disoriented. It may be the side effect of medications or caused by the dying process itself

(Fields & Cassell, 1997). Anxiety is the biological and emotional reaction to stressful situations including the approach of death. The patient may experience dread, danger, or tension with somatic complaints that includes shortness of breath, nausea, or diarrhea (Fields & Cassell, 1997). Moaning and grimacing can accompany agitation and restlessness and may be misinterpreted by the nurse as pain (Ferrell et al., 1999). The patient may be restless and make repetitive motions (e.g., pulling on clothing or the sheets).

Nursing interventions to manage terminal delirium should focus on the treatment of the underlying physical cause if it is practical and possible. Antianxiety agents like benzodiazepines (Lorazepam, Diazepam, Alprazolam) and neuroleptics (Haldol) can help to quiet distressing symptoms. The family is in need of education and support regarding the cause and the irreversible nature of the behavior. Maintenance of a calm environment, spiritual comfort, and emotional support are vital at this time.

The family can be advised to continue to talk to the patient and calm them with their words. Light massage of the arms, back, or forehead can be very soothing. Soft music and low lights can also be effective. It may be suggested that the number of people in the room be decreased if there is a lot of activity. Refraining from asking the patient many questions can diminish agitation.

Eventually the patient's level of consciousness will decrease and they may even become un-arousable. This is a very upsetting time for families because the patient may seem unresponsive and withdrawn, but it is a normal aspect of the dying process. At this time the patient is starting to "let go" in preparation for his/her death and detaching from his/her relationships and physical environment. They may ask to be with only one person toward the end or seem distracted from their family. A dying person may talk about seeing people who have already died or talk about taking a trip with a long deceased relative. They may describe feeling separate from their body. This is a normal experience and is not considered a hallucination.

Even if the patient is unresponsive, encourage family members to talk with them. Assume that the patient hears everything; this is the time for loved ones to say "good-bye," "I'm sorry," "I love you," or "thank you." The patient may have difficulty letting go and the nurse may need to encourage the family to give the patient permission to die. Encourage the family to show affection to the patient, touch them, and let them know that they will be missed.

AFFIRMING LIFE AND MAINTAINING HOPE

Two very important goals of palliative care nursing are to help the patient live until they die and to encourage hope. First, the nurse can help the patient live until they die by encouraging socialization, listening, being honest, and helping them finish any unfinished business. By offering patients choices regarding routines, food, and activities, nurses promote continued independence and the ability to help maintain control over their lives. Of course, the degree of independence depends on their energy level and ability (Birchenall & Streight, 1997). Furthermore, patient's wishes should be respected even if the choices that they are making are inconsistent with the family or health care provider's values.

Secondly, hope is an important component of the emotional stages of dying and death. It has been a factor in helping the patient and family continue through the difficult months and years leading up to the death. Hope is what maintains a person's spirit and helps them to go on; as the person is dying *what* they hope for may change, but it does not go away. There may be hope for a "miracle" where they will be completely cured; it is not acceptable for the nurse to take this hope away or to tell the patient and family to be "realistic." Their hopes may change from that of cure to the hope of a full night's sleep, a visit from an important person, or for less pain. Persons with hope have been found to live longer and have a greater quality of life than those who are hopeless (Birchenall & Streight, 1997). What is important is for the nurse to be present for the patient and family wherever they are in this process and support the feelings that are experienced. The "rights" of the dying can be found in Table 12.1. Listening and caring for their needs are important nursing functions at this time of life.

FAMILY SUPPORT DURING THE LAST HOURS OF LIFE

Supporting the family during the last hours of the patient's life is an important nursing role. When possible, one nurse should be assigned to be with the family through the last phase of life. Enough time with the dying person should be given to the family so that they have the opportunity to resolve any final interpersonal issues. If the death is occurring at home the family should have access to a "Symptom Relief Kit" with detailed, easy to understand instructions for its use (Appendix 1). Depending on cultural and religious considerations the family should be afforded privacy and clergy support. The primary nurse should communicate with the family regarding what they can expect the dying process to be like and how they will know when the person has died.

Many people have not been with someone who is actively dying and do not know what to expect. Even though no two deaths are alike, it helps to give significant others an idea of what the final stage of life may be like and the symptoms that they may see during this period. Table 12.2 (Final stages

TABLE 12.1   The Dying Person's Bill of Rights

- I have the right to be treated as a living human being until I die.
- I have the right to maintain a sense of hopefulness, however changing its focus may be.
- I have the right to be cared for by those who can maintain a sense of hopefulness, however challenging this might be.
- I have the right to express my feelings and emotions about my approaching death, in my own way.
- I have the right to participate in decisions concerning my care.
- I have the right to expect continuing medical and nursing attention even though "cure" goals must be changed to "comfort" goals.
- I have the right not to die alone.
- I have the right to be free from pain.
- I have the right to have my questions answered honestly.
- I have the right not to be deceived.
- I have the right to have help from and for my family accepting my death.
- I have the right to die in peace and dignity.
- I have the right to retain my individuality and not be judged for my decisions, which may be contrary to the beliefs of others.
- I have the right to discuss and enlarge my religious and/or spiritual experiences, regardless of what they may mean to others.
- I have the right to expect that the sanctity of the human body will be respected after death.
- I have the right to be cared for by caring, sensitive, knowledgeable people who will attempt to understand my needs and will be able to gain some satisfaction in helping me face my death.

Sorrentino, S. A. (1999). *Assisting with Patient Care* (p. 843). Mosby, St. Louis.

of dying) is an information sheet written for the general population regarding the dying process and is a good handout for students.

SIGNS OF DEATH

Signs of death include cessation of a heartbeat and respiration, release of bowel and bladder, eyelids slightly open and not blinking, pupils fixed and dilated, drop in body temperature, as the blood settles body color turns to a waxen pallor, jaw relaxed and slightly open, and no response from the patient. These signs do not occur in order and it may take a few minutes for the body to completely stop (Ferrell et al., 1999). If the death occurs at home the family should be told that it is not an emergency situation but

TABLE 12.2 VNA Hospice Manchester, NH FINAL STAGES—DYING PROCESS

When a person enters the final stage of the dying process, two different dynamics are at work. On the physical plane, the body begins the final process of shutting down, which will end when all the physical systems cease to function. Usually this is an orderly, progressive series of physical changes that are not medical emergencies. These physical changes are the natural way in which the body prepares itself to stop. The most appropriate kinds of responses are comfort-enhancing measures.

The other dynamic of the dying process is emotional and spiritual in nature. The "spirit" of the dying person begins the final process of release from the body, its immediate environment and all attachments. This release also tends to follow its own priorities, which may include the resolution of whatever is *unfinished* of a practical nature and exercising permission from family members to "let go." The most appropriate kinds of responses to the emotional/spiritual changes are those which support and encourage this release and transition.

When a person's body is ready and wanting to stop, but the person is still unresolved or is not reconciled about some important issue or relationship, the person may tend to linger in order to finish whatever needs finishing. On the other hand, when a person is emotionally/spiritually resolved and ready for this release, but his/her body has not completed its final physical process, the person will continue to live until the physical shutdown is completed.

The experience we call "death" occurs when the body and the spirit complete the natural process of shutting down, reconciling and finishing. These processes need to happen in a way appropriate and unique to the values, beliefs and lifestyle of the dying person.

The physical and emotional/spiritual signs and symptoms of impending death which follow are offered to help you understand the natural kinds of things that may happen and how you can respond appropriately. Not all these signs and symptoms will occur with every person, nor will they occur in this particular sequence. Each person is unique and needs your full acceptance, support and comfort.

The following signs and symptoms are indicative of how the body prepares itself for the final stage of life:

Coolness: The person's hands, arms, feet and legs may be increasingly cool. At the same time, the color of the skin may change. The underside of the body may become darker and the skin mottled or discolored. This is a normal indication that the circulation of blood is decreasing to the body's extremities and being reserved for the most vital organs. Keep the person warm with a blanket, nonelectric.

TABLE 12.2 *(continued)*

Sleeping: The person may spend an increasing amount of time sleeping and appear to be uncommunicative or unresponsive, at times difficult to arouse. This normal change is due in part to changes in the metabolism of the body. Sit with your loved one, speak softly and naturally. Plan to spend time when the person seems most alert and awake. Try not to talk as if the person were not there. Speak directly as you normally would, even though there may be no response. Never assume the person cannot hear; hearing is the last of the senses to be lost.

Fluid and Food Decrease: The person may have a decrease in appetite and thirst, wanting little or no food or fluid. The body will naturally begin to conserve energy that would be expended on these tasks. Do not try to force food or drink into the person. To use guilt or manipulation only makes the person more uncomfortable. Small chips of ice, frozen Gatorade or juice may be refreshing in the mouth. If the person is able to swallow, fluids may be given in small amounts by syringe (ask the Hospice nurse for guidance). Glycerin swabs may help keep the mouth and lips moist and comfortable. A cool, most washcloth on the forehead may also increase physical comfort.

Incontinence: Control of urine and/or bowels may be lost as the muscles in that area begin to relax. Discuss with your Hospice nurse what can be done to protect the bed and keep your loved one clean and comfortable. If it would make the person more comfortable, the nurse may suggest a catheter to drain the bladder into a collection bag. The person's normal urine output may decrease and become dark due to the decrease in circulation through the kidneys.

Congestion: The person may have gurgling sounds coming from the chest as though marbles were rolling around inside. These sounds may become very loud. This normal change is due to the decrease of fluid intake and the inability to cough up normal secretions. The sound of the congestion does not indicate the onset of severe or new pain. Suctioning usually increases the secretions. The nurse or home health aide can show you how to keep the mouth clean with "touthettes."

Breathing Pattern Change: The person's regular breathing pattern may change and become irregular, e.g., shallow breaths with periods of no breathing for 5 to 30 seconds and up to a full minute. This is called "Cheyne-Stokes" breathing. The person may also experience periods of rapid shallow panting. Elevating the head and/or turning the person on one side may bring comfort. Use your hands to touch and soothe. Speak gently.

Disorientation: The person may seem to be confused about the time, place, and identity of people, including those close and familiar. This is due in part to metabolism changes. Identify yourself by name before you speak rather than asking the person to guess who you are. Speak softly, clearly, and truthfully when you need to communicate something important, such as, "It's time to take your medication," and explain the reason for the communication, such as, "So you won't begin to hurt." Never use this method to try to manipulate the person to meet your own needs or values. It may be difficult to make this distinction.

(continued)

TABLE 12.2   *(continued)*

Restlessness: The person may make restless and repetitive motions, such as pulling at bed linen or clothing. This often happens and is due to the decrease in oxygen circulation to the brain and to metabolism changes. Do not interfere with or try to restrain such motions. Occasionally the person may twitch or make jerking motions. This may have to do with medication or the disease itself. Sometimes other medication helps decrease this twitching.

To have a calming effect, speak in a quiet, natural way, lightly massage the forehead, back, or arms, read to the person, or play some soothing music. Try to decrease the number of people around the person. Asking a lot of questions may increase the person's agitation.

EMOTIONAL SYMPTOMS AND RESPONSES

Withdrawal: The person may seem unresponsive, withdrawn, or in a comatose-like state. This indicates preparation for release, a detaching from surroundings and relationships and a beginning of "letting go." Since hearing remains almost all the way to the end, now is the time to say whatever you need to say that will help the person "let go." The person may only want to be with a very few or even just one person. This is another sign of preparation for release. If you are not part of this "inner circle" at the end, it does not mean you are not loved or are unimportant. It means you have already fulfilled your tasks, and it is time for you to say, "Good-bye."

Vision-like experiences: The person may speak or claim to have spoken to persons who have already died, or to see places not presently accessible or visible to you. This does not indicate hallucinations or a drug reaction. The person is beginning to detach from this life and is preparing for the transition. Do not contradict, explain, belittle, or argue about what the person claims to have seen or heard. Affirm the experiences. They are normal and natural.

Letting Go: The person may continue to perform repetitive and restless tasks. This may indicate that something is still unresolved or unfinished and preventing the letting go. The Hospice team can assist you in identifying what may be happening and help the person find release from tension or fear. As hard as it might be, you need to give the person permission to let go.

Saying Good-Bye: When the person is ready to die, and you are able to let go, saying "Good-bye" is your final gift of love. It achieves closure and makes the final release possible. It may be helpful to hold or touch and say the things you want to say. It may be as simple (or as complicated) as saying, "I love you." It may include recounting favorite memories, places, and activities you shared. It may include saying "I'm sorry for whatever I've done to cause any tensions or difficulty." You may also want to say "Thank you." Tears are a normal and natural part of saying "Good-bye." You don't need to apologize for them or try to hide them. They are a natural expression of your sadness and loss. It is all right to say, "I will miss you so much."

TABLE 12.2 *(continued)*

How will you know when death has occurred?

Although you may be prepared for the dying process, you may not be prepared for the actual moment. It may be helpful for you and your family to think about and discuss what you would do if you were alone when the death occurs. The death of a Hospice patient is expected and is not an emergency. Nothing must be done immediately. The signs of death include such things as:

- No heartbeat
- Release of bowel and bladder
- No response
- Eyelids slightly open
- Pupils enlarged
- Eyes fixed on a certain spot
- No blinking
- Jaw relaxed and mouth slightly open

You may now notify a Hospice nurse or the On-call nurse as you have been instructed. The nurse will make the pronouncement and notify your physician. The body does not have to be moved until you are ready. The nurse can call the Funeral Home, but you or a member of your family will probably need to speak with the Funeral Director.

Later On

Hospice staff and volunteers continue to be available to support you and your family through the Bereavement Program. We will contact you a week or so after the death has occurred, after all the "busyness" is over and the visitors have gone. If you need or want to communicate with us before then, please do not hesitate to call. Even if you just need a place to go for comfort and support, call or stop in.

We salute you for all you have done during this difficult time. We know it has been an enormous commitment and a true act of love. We feel honored to have shared this experience with you in spite of your pain. You accompanied someone you love as far as you could on life's final journey. We hope you feel good about what you've done. We hope this feeling will sustain you, give you courage, and allow you eventually to go on with your life.

---

given a number to call to inform hospice staff or their physician of the death. The body does not have to be moved immediately so the family should not feel rushed or pressured to act.

Peri-Death Rituals and Customs

Throughout the dying process, and particularly at the very end of life, the nurse must be aware of cultural and religious values, practices, and traditions

of the patient and the family. Customs and rituals have tremendous significance in the healing process following death and the grief response is often
structured by these rituals. The nurse's role is to help the family carry out
the rites and practices that provide solace and support. The nurse should
be open-minded and understanding of the physical and psychosocial and
spiritual needs of the dying patient and his/her family and, offer them
respect and privacy (Purnell & Paulanka, 1998).

Roman Catholic priests will give the "Sacrament of the Anointing of the
Sick" which in the past was called the "Last Rights." The sacrament is for
those who are seriously ill; the family, friends, and priest gather at the
bedside to pray for healing. If it is God's will that the person not recover
from their illness, then the prayer is that God will accompany the dying
person toward the rewards of heaven (Miller, 1993). The nurse can ask the
family if they would like the priest to be called. The priest would hear the
patient's confession of sins, absolve him/her, and offer the Sacrament of
the Sick. The comfort that this ritual can bring to the dying Catholic and
his/her family cannot be underestimated.

Cuban Americans who are dying are usually attended by large groups of
family and friends. Depending on their religious affiliation a Catholic priest,
Protestant minister, rabbi, or *santero* may be called to perform death rites.
For followers of *santero* these rites may include animal sacrifice, ceremonial
displays, and chants (Purnell & Paulanka, 1998). After the death, candles
are lit to light the path of the spirit to the afterlife. Burial is the common
custom although there is no restriction to cremation.

A Hindu who is dying may also request holy rites before death; readings
and hymns from holy books are also comforting. Some may wish to lie on
the floor to symbolize their closeness to the earth. A Hindu priest would
administer the holy rites which may include tying a thread around the wrists
or neck of the dying person, sprinkling blessed water from the Ganges, of
placing a sacred tulsi leaf in their mouth. Some Hindus may wish to return
to India to die, especially to the holy city of Banaras. Many believe that to
die in Banaras insures a rebirth in Heaven or even a release from continued
rebirth. At a minimum, a Hindu will request to die at home because death
in the hospital is very distressing. A Hindu should only touch the dead body;
if it is necessary for a non-Hindus to touch it, disposable gloves should be
worn. Sacred threads, jewelry, and other religious objects should not be
removed. The body should not be washed but only wrapped in a plain sheet.
Washing of the body is a part of the funeral rite and is typically carried out
only by family members; a mixture of milk and yogurt is used to cleanse
the body. In India, a funeral would take place within 24 hours; adult Hindus
are cremated although young children and infants may be buried (Green,
1989a, b, & c).

The dying person of the Muslim faith may wish to lie or sit facing Mecca. If it is possible, the bed should be positioned to accommodate this wish. The Islam believes that the body belongs to God and therefore autopsies are forbidden unless ordered by the Coroner. Likewise, organ donation and cremation are not acceptable. In Iran, a person is immediately placed in a casket if they have died during the day. If they die at night, a copy of the Koran should be placed on their chest and a lighted candle at their head (Iserson, 1994); the body is watched during the night by a person reading the Koran.

Following the death, non-Muslims should wear gloves when touching the body. If there are no family available to carry out post-mortem care, the nurse may carry out the preparation of the body. However, the body is not washed and hair or nails are not cut; wear gloves when administering care and close the eyes. The "normal Muslim procedure is that the body is straightened immediately after death. This is done by flexing the elbows, shoulders, knees and hips first, before straightening them. This is thought to ensure that the body does not stiffen, thus facilitating the washing and shrouding of it. Turn the head towards the right shoulder. This is so the body can be buried with the face towards Mecca" (Green, 1989d, p. 57). The body is then covered with a sheet that cloaks the whole body until a Muslim is available to perform the ritual bath. The body is usually washed three times, first with lotus water, then camphor water, and lastly with plain water (Iserson, 1994). This bathing is done from head to toe and front to back. All body orifices are closed and packed with cotton (to prevent body fluid leakage that is considered unclean). Prayers from the *Qu'ran* are read (especially verses of hope and acceptance) and the body is wrapped in a special cotton shroud. This shroud is made from three pieces of white, unsewn cloth, 9 yards long that are wrapped above, below, and around the mid-section. Muslims are buried in a brick or cement-lined grave with their head facing Mecca. In Iran, the body is buried directly in the earth with the shroud removed from the face and one side of the face turned to be in contact with the earth (Purnell & Paulanka, 1998).

The Jew who is dying may want to hear or recite special prayers, such as the Shema, which confirms one's belief in one God, or psalms, in particular Psalm 23, The Lord is my Shepherd, as well as holding the written prayer in his/her hand (Green, 1989e). A relative remains with the dying person to ensure that the soul does not leave the body when s/he is alone; it is a sign of disrespect to leave the body alone. Even after death, the body is not left alone until the funeral, so that the body is not left defenseless (Purnell & Paulanka, 1998). The eyes should be closed after death, preferably by a child of the deceased; the body should be covered and left untouched (Green, 1989e). Autopsies are not permitted, although organ transplants are. The body should be handled as little as possible by non-Jews and burial should take place within 24 hours. Burial is usually only delayed for the Sabbath. Embalming and cosmetics are not a part of traditional practice. Orthodox Jews are always buried, although more liberal Jews may select cremation. The body is wrapped in a shroud and a prayer shawl. The casket is made of wood, so that the body and the casket decay at the same rate. There is no wake or viewing of the body. At the funeral, the prayer for the dead is said (the *Kaddish*) which praises God and reaffirms faith (Purnell & Paulanka, 1998).

For the Buddhist an important consideration is the state of mind at the time of death; dying thoughts and desires are crucial in determining their next rebirth. A Buddhist monk or minister should be notified at the time of death. The length of time between death and burial can vary between 3 and 7 days depending on the Buddhist tradition. Family members plan the burial; the tradition is to wear white to the funeral.

Native Americans have different traditions in each tribe. There is a belief that the spirit of the deceased remains where the person has died, therefore family may not want the person to die at home. At the same time, it is considered inappropriate for the person to die alone. If the person dies at home, the house must be abandoned or a ceremony is held to cleanse it. Families gather together at the time of death and material possessions are dispersed. When a person dies, a cleansing ceremony is performed or else the spirit of the deceased may try to take over someone's spirit. Those who work with the dead must also have a ceremonial cleansing to protect themselves from the dead person's spirit. No embalming is used; the deceased are buried in sacred ground with their shoes on the wrong feet, rings on their index fingers, and with many gifts surrounding them, or the body is cremated (Purnell & Paulanka, 1998).

Church members of the same gender who have permission to be admitted into the temple dress deceased members of the Church of Jesus Christ of the Latter-Day Saints (Mormons). The body is dressed in white undergarments that are covered by a robe, cap, and apron. Prior to burial white caps are placed on the men and women's faces are veiled (Iserson, 1994).

For Appalachians, a death is an important event, even for extended family. The funeral is a significant social occasion and family and friends will come from long distances to be in attendance. The body is displayed for long periods of time so all that wish to see the body, can. The deceased is buried in his/her best clothes and some people have custom-made clothes for burial (Purnell & Paulanka, 1998). At the funeral home, personal possessions are displayed and it is common to bury these items with the person. Gravesites are typically on hillsides because of the fear that they will be flooded out in low-lying areas (Purnell & Paulanka, 1998).

Subgroups from China, Vietnam, Laos, Thailand, and Burma together are called the Hmong. The Hmong believe that proper burial and worship of the dead and other ancestors directly affects the safety, health, and prosperity of the family. The belief is that the spiritual world coexists with the physical world and that the spirits are able to influence human life. The preference is to die at home because they believe that their soul will wander for all of eternity without a resting place if they were to die elsewhere. There are some groups who believe that death should take place in the hospital so as not to bring bad luck into the home. Autopsy and cremation are acceptable practices to some families. For these groups, burial occurs in the afternoon.

The Chinese will place a coin in the deceased's mouth so that they have money to pay anyone who interferes in their journey. In northern China the body is placed in burial clothes and an unpadded quilt is used as a shroud. The face is covered with cloth or paper and the feet are tied with colored string. The wife or oldest son wipes the corpse's eyes with cotton floss before the coffin is closed. Instead of being buried immediately after the funeral the body may be stored so that a husband and wife can be buried together (Iserson, 1994).

The Japanese bathe their dead, shave some of the hair, and dress the person in white. The corpse wears a ceremonial hat or triangular piece of white paper tied to the forehead. Koreans use perfume to wash the body and dress the body in silk or hemp clothes tied in seven places that correlate with the seven stars in the Ursa Major constellation (Iserson, 1994).

Mexican Americans may take turns sitting vigil over the dying person; dying in a hospital is not desirable because the spirit may become "lost." Spiritual amulets, rosary beads, or other religious artifacts are kept near the patient. Typically, organ donation or autopsy is not allowed. When death occurs, family and friends will often come from long distances for the funeral. A *velorio* is a festive watch of the deceased body before burial. Traditional families my exhibit hyperkinetic shaking and seizure-like activity called *ataque de nervios* which is a way to release emotions related to grieving. Family may erect altars in their homes in honor of the anniversary of their relative's death and may include candles, decorations, and having the deceased's favorite meal at a grave-side picnic (Purnell & Paulanka, 1998).

African Americans generally prefer to have people with terminal illness cared for in the home, but prefer death to occur in the hospital for fear of bad luck being brought to the home. Grief is expressed openly and publicly. Autopsy is acceptable, although organ donation is not.

WHEN DEATH HAS OCCURRED

Post-death nursing care involves preparing the body for the morgue or funeral home and helping the family through decisions regarding autopsy and burial. When death has occurred, the blood will begin to pool in the areas of the body closest to the ground; if the corpse were supine this would be the back and buttocks. A purple-red discoloration of the skin is evident and results from the blood accumulating in the dependent vessels; this is called *livor mortis*. The body begins to cool and this fall in body temperature after death is called *algor mortis* (Kastenbaum & Kastenbaum, 1989). Initially, at the time of death, the muscles in the body relax but within 2 to 6 hours *rigor mortis* begins. Rigor mortis is the stiffening of all muscle groups beginning with the eyelids, neck, and jaw. During the next 4 to 6 hours, it will spread to the other muscles including the internal organs. Rigor mortis will usually last between 24 and 48 hours depending on the temperature where the body is; after this time the muscles relax and secondary flaccidity develops (Iserson, 1994).

Care of the body by the nurse should include closing the eyes, inserting dentures and closing the mouth, and elevating the head of the bed so that the blood does not drain into the face and discolor it. If there is an IV or a catheter, they can be removed at this time, and the physical environment should be straightened. Removal of tubes and equipment is dependent on institutional protocol. Follow the agency protocol regarding jewelry; if there is a wedding ring secure it on the finger with tape. The body should be bathed in plain water and dried, a bed protector should be placed under the body. If there are dressings on wounds they should be replaced with clean ones. The hair should be combed and the extremities straightened and the right great toe tied with an identification tag (Sorrentino, 1999).

If the family wants to participate in the preparation of the deceased for the funeral home, they should be encouraged to do so. The family should also be offered the opportunity to bathe and dress the body if they wish. Some people find comfort in giving the last bath and it helps them to believe that no one else will touch the body in this way again.

When the body and the room have been prepared, family and those close to the patient can be encouraged to say a final good-bye. Within the confines of cultural, personal, and religious practices, the family can be invited to touch or hold the person's body and to take the time that they need. This time spent with the deceased can help to promote the transition from acute grief to a new stage of the grieving process (Ferrell et al., 1999). The body should not be transported to the morgue or mortuary until the family is prepared and they have given their permission. The family's wishes should be respected regarding their presence during the removal of the body.

When the family has given permission for the body to be moved the nurse should follow the institutional protocol regarding shrouding the body. If a person has died at home and it is an expected death, the undertaker is called and they remove the body as it is. In a hospital or nursing home setting, the body is wrapped in a shroud or body bag. The shroud should be secured with safety pins or ties and a second identification tag is attached to the shroud or body bag. The body is then taken to the morgue (Sorrentino, 1999).

The nurse can offer help with making personal phone calls to give the family time to become accustomed to the immediate loss. The physician should be notified of the death and the nurse should be certain to follow agency protocol regarding the removal of medications and equipment. If the family wishes support from their clergy or bereavement professionals can be offered.

In many states, the nurse can sign the death certificate if the death occurs in the hospital or nursing home, or at the family home if hospice is involved. Once the death certificate is signed, the family can contact the mortuary and the body can be transported to the funeral home/crematorium. If the nurse or physician is unwilling to sign the death certificate because of a suspicious nature of the death, the medical examiner is called and they assume responsibility for the body (Iserson, 1994). If the death is sudden and unexpected or if it occurs at home the medical examiner must be notified and they will decide if an autopsy is required. The family has no authority to stop an officially mandated autopsy (Lynn & Harrold, 1999).

The next of kin may request an autopsy even if the medical examiner declines to do one. The nurse should be available to educate the family about the autopsy and assist them in their decision-making process. An autopsy will help determine the cause of death but the family may be charged a fee for this service (the cost may be as much as $2,000). Autopsies also serve other purposes (Table 12.3).

The word autopsy comes from the Greek *autopsia* which means seeing with one's own eyes. Pathologists, who are physicians that have specialized in human anatomy, perform them. Organs are removed and inspected, and body fluids are analyzed. There are three degrees of autopsy: complete, limited, and selective. A complete autopsy exposes all body cavities (including the head) for examination; limited autopsy usually excludes the head; and selective autopsy involves examination of only one or more organs specific to the nature of the illness (Iserson, 1994).

If the deceased has requested that their organs be donated, the nurse is often the person responsible for notifying the proper agencies for organ and tissue harvesting. Organ donation is the practice of giving a part of the deceased body for transplantation into another person. A person designates their wish to donate their organs by signing the back of their driver's license indicating their preferences, specifying organ donation in an advance directive, or by filling out an organ donor card (1-800-24-DONOR). Even

TABLE 12.3   The Uses of Autopsies

Explain unknown or unanticipated medical complications
Assist development/quality assurance of new technology, procedures, drugs, and therapy
Education
Provide information about the nature of disease
Classify and explain sudden, unexpected, and/or unnatural deaths
Understand what damages organs
Identify infectious and contagious diseases
Identify and monitor occupational and environmental health hazards
Quality control in medicine
Provide a source of organs and tissues for medical and scientific purposes
Provide materials and hypotheses for research
Improve accuracy, and therefore usefulness, of vital statistics
Advance clinical knowledge
Assist grief process
Discover genetic diseases within family
Assist in genetic counseling and identification of family health risks
Provide information for insurance/death benefits

Adapted from Iserson. K. V. (1994). *Death to dust* (p. 119). Tucson, AZ: Galen Press, Ltd. and the Massachusetts Medical Society (1996–1998).

with the proper documentation, the family may refuse to allow a relative's organs to be donated. In the United States, at least 5,000 human organs are buried because relatives refuse donation. Persons less than 18 years of age must have the consent of their parents or guardians to sign an organ donor card. Unless the deceased has specified that they do not want their organs donated, the senior next-of-kin may donate all or part of a relative's body (Iserson, 1994).

Depending on what organ is being donated the time for organ removal is variable. Eyes must be removed within 4 hours of the death but once they are in a preservative they can wait 10 to 14 days to be transplanted. Tissue (e.g., bone, skin, and tendons) can wait 12 to 24 hours to be removed from the deceased and can be preserved (depending on the method of preservation) for 3 to 5 years. If the body has been refrigerated within 4 hours of the death, saphenous veins can be harvested in the following 10 hours and heart valves within 24 hours (Iserson, 1994). Approximate cold ischemic times (allowable time from procurement to transplant) are found in Table 12.4.

Once the organs are removed from the body, it is ready for embalming or cremation. Embalming is the process by which the corpse is preserved and

TABLE 12.4 Time between Recovery of Organs and Tissues to Transportation

Tissue Specific:

- Heart Valves: 10 years

- Saphenous Vein: 10 years

- Bone: 5 years or more

- Corneas: 5–7 days

- Bone Marrow: up to 3 years

Organ Specific:

- Kidney: 48–72 hours

- Heart: 4–6 hours

- Liver: Up to 24 hours

- Lung: 4–6 hours

- Pancreas: 12–24 hours

Gift of Life Trust Fund 1998

prepared for viewing. "Basically, the embalmer is a creator of illusions—of pleasant illusions which banish the traces of suffering and death and present the deceased in an attitude of normal, restful sleep. In the practice of embalming this illusion is called a "memory picture" (Strub & Frederick, 1967, p. 133). There is no legal requirement that the body be embalmed, even if it is going to be viewed. The average cost for embalming is about $350 (Iserson, 1994).

There are four embalming methods that all involve the injection of chemicals to preserve the body. Arterial embalming injects the chemicals into the blood vessels; cavity embalming injects the chest and abdomen; hypodermic embalming injects under the skin; and surface embalming is the application of chemicals in gel or liquid form onto the body surface (Iserson, 1994). The size of the body, age, water content, temperature, decomposition, condition of the body's blood vessels, and pre-mortem medication regime (e.g., gentamycin inactivates embalming fluid) will dictate the types, solution strengths, and injection rates of the embalming chemicals. Primarily formaldehyde and methyl alcohol are used as preservative chemicals because they change the cell proteins to prevent putrefaction. Embalmers inject these chemicals into the body using a centrifugal pump that pushes the fluids into the body with 5–10 psi of pressure. At the same time blood and fluid are drained from the body by gravity or electrical aspirators. The embalmer will look for evidence that the chemicals have reached the hands and face and facilitate this process by massaging and repositioning the corpse. When the embalming fluid reaches the hands they are placed in their final position over the chest or abdomen and the fingers are held together by using cyanoacrylate (e.g., SuperGlue). The muscles will gradually harden over the 8- to 12-hour period following the embalming; once they are set, the body's position will not be able to be moved.

If there is going to be a viewing at the funeral home the body is prepared for this with the use of cosmetics. The hair is styled and the corpse is dressed. The body is then "casketed" in the coffin; typically the right shoulder is lower than the left so the body does not look like it is flat on its back.

An increasingly popular alternative to embalming and burial is cremation. Cremation is a process to reduce the "corpse and its container to ashes and small bone fragments" (Iserson, 1994, p. 236). Intensive heat is used to burn the body which evaporates water (70%–80% of non-bone tissue), burns soft tissue, and reduces the average-sized adult to 4 to 8 pounds of ash (cremains). It takes about an hour and a half to cremate a body and what is left are grey ash and bone fragments (cremains). The cremains are then processed through an electric grinder to pulverize the bone fragments into an even consistency. The costs for this service ranges between $500 and $1000.

Prosthetic devices do not burn (e.g., dental gold, metal plates, and screws) and are removed with a magnet from the ashes. Pacemakers with lithium batteries will explode when burned and are removed before cremation. The body does not have to be embalmed before cremation nor does the family need to purchase a coffin. The only requirement is that the body is burned in a combustible container (e.g., cardboard or particleboard). Typically there is a 24- to 48-hour waiting period after the death before cremation can legally take place.

Crematories are the facilities that contain the oven or retorts where the cremation will take place. It is becoming increasingly common for funeral homes to build crematories on the site and to offer a wide range of disposal options. Some cemeteries will have a columbarium for the internment of the urn containing the cremains. Memorial Gardens are also available for the ashes to be scattered or buried and gives visitors a place to visit or place a marker. Some people will divide the cremains to bury, scatter, keep in an urn, share among family members, or even wear in specially designed jewelry.

Burning the corpse as a way to dispose of the dead dates back to prehistoric times. Our primitive ancestors who believed that they could return to their corpse and harm the living feared the dead; destroying the corpse removed that danger. Ancient civilizations believed that cremation would provide the dead with heat and warmth in the next world and protected the body from mutilation by animals or other humans. Native Americans believe that souls are conveyed to paradise by means of fire.

FUNERALS AS A CEREMONY OF DEATH

Across cultures, people accept a responsibility to care for, respect, and honor their dead. For most ethnic groups and religious groups, the process of physically preparing the body for the funeral and burial are handled by persons outside of the family. The undertaker, a person who "undertook" the responsibility to keep the body safe and make the funeral arrangements, has been a part of society since ancient times. The general public interchangeably refers to the person who prepares the body for burial and conducts all aspects of the funeral service as the undertaker, mortician, embalmer, or funeral director (Iserson, 1994).

The funeral director in modern society coordinates all of the details of the funeral for the family. They supervise preparation of the body for viewing or burial, oversee embalming procedures if embalming is desired, coordinate cremation planning, instruct and support the pallbearers, arrange the transportation of the family and the deceased to the cemetery, place death notices in the newspaper, and otherwise facilitate the family's burial decisions. Most funeral directors in the United States have at least a bachelor's degree and about 85% of all funeral homes are family operated (Iserson, 1994). Employed by funeral homes are embalmers, cosmetologists, hairdressers, and hearse and limousine drivers.

The funeral director therefore orchestrates all aspects of the funeral. Those who work in the funeral industry know that the funeral must be perfectly organized and executed because they will not get a second chance to make things right. It was originally believed that the funeral merely held theological value, but for many people the funeral is one of the first steps of successful grieving. The funeral is "*of* the person who has died. . . . It is *for* those who survive" (Raether, 1993, p. 211).

For families that have a wake, this is the first component of post-death ritual. It may be one of the few times that the entire family will reassemble for an event. It is a time for family and friends to view the dead body and to pay their final respects. Seeing the dead body emphasizes the fact that the person is dead, declining to see the body may delay grieving. "I was recently again reminded of how valuable and legitimate a funeral service can be. I accompanied a friend to the funeral of his mother. She had died of a chronic and wasting illness and I had been present at her deathbed.

My friend experienced a deep and profound consolation seeing his mother with the lines of suffering erased from her face and lying at peace" (Raether, 1993, p. 211).

The second component of post-death rituals is the funeral. It is a ceremonial service typically consisting of music, prayers, poetry, eulogies, and it may be part of a funeral mass where communion is celebrated. Some people will plan their funeral before they die which can be comforting to both the dying person and their family (Raether, 1993).

Last is the committal service, the concluding funeral rite. It is the final act of caring for the deceased and is celebrated at the grave, tomb, or crematorium. This service is a "symbolic demonstration that the kind of relationship which has existed between the mourner and the deceased is now at an end" (Raether, 1993, p. 212).

Eight specific therapeutic values have been assigned to the funeral process as delineated by Raether (1993, p. 209). First, the "therapy of direct expression" denotes that the funeral furnishes the setting and opportunity for the bereaved to physically express their grief. Funerals offer "therapy of language" by providing the bereaved an opportunity to talk about what has happened, voice their feelings, and begin to feel relief in the telling.

The "therapy of sharing" is the coming together of the family and significant others to provide emotional and physical support to each other. Time spent with the bereaved is an important aspect of burying the dead. Immersion in the many aspects of the funeral process also encompasses the "therapy of activity." The routine of greeting mourners at the funeral home or interacting with those who offer their sympathy prevents the bereaved from withdrawing and focuses their energy in the immediate post-death period. The funeral also provides the "therapy of ceremony" that is both glorifying and ennobling. The liturgical aspect of the funeral ceremony encompasses the views of the meaning of life and the nature of life hereafter. Given that accepting the reality of the death is difficult for many people, the "therapy of viewing" establishes a final and amended view of the deceased. This revised image replaces those composed during the illness or at the time of death and may bring comfort to the mourner. Lastly, the "therapy of suffering" addresses the guilt that mourners may be experiencing and provides the occasion to verbalize what had been previously left unsaid.

Another important aspect of the post-death experience for the bereaved is the formation of a new identity within their community. The role of widow, no longer having a child, or losing a parent brings with it a change in how the bereaved interact and corresponds to society at large. Social groups may shrink, volunteer opportunities may be lost, and favorite activities may be forfeited due to the loss of the deceased. Nurses need to be aware of the difficulties inherent in these role shifts and offer alternatives and community support referrals during this transitional stage.

When the nurse is providing end-of-life care, the unit of care is the dying person and their family. When the death occurs, the family is still in need of nursing care and interventions. The goal of post-death nursing care is to promote optimal adjustment and to help the family and significant others with the tasks of bereavement. Bereavement is an important developmental stage; the nurse should provide interventions that offer the opportunity for healing and growth, a redefinition of self, and opportunities to make new plans. Follow-up is important during the bereavement period as well as encouraging memorial rituals commemorating the deceased's life and death. Unique opportunities exist in peri-death nursing to support the dying patient and their family in making what is a painful and difficult process also one that is priceless.

Education Plan 12.1 Plan for Achieving Competencies: Peri-Death Nursing Care

Knowledge	Attitude	Skills	Undergraduate Behavioral Outcome	Graduate Behavioral Outcomes	Teaching/Learning Strategies
In the last hours of life: —Symptom assessment and management; —Spiritual goals; —Family support; —Signs of death.	*Value patient and family comfort as a priority. *Appreciate the importance of presence during the active phase of dying. *Emphasize the value of complementary therapies.		*Facilitate a peaceful, comfortable, and dignified death.	*Implement interventions in collaboration with members of the interdisciplinary team to address unrelieved symptoms and which may necessitate palliative/terminal sedation. *Identify situations of complicated mourning or acute spiritual distress and make appropriate referrals.	*Assign students to the care of the patient and family who is actively dying in an institutional, hospice, home-care, or long-term care setting. *Develop a plan of care for the patient and family who are actively dying using the nursing process.

Education Plan 12.1 *(continued)*

Knowledge	Attitude	Skills	Undergraduate Behavioral Outcome	Graduate Behavioral Outcomes	Teaching/Learning Strategies
					*Interview a family member regarding the death of a significant other, documenting the symptoms experienced in the last hours of life, spiritual perceptions, para-normal experiences, immediate family needs, and apparent signs of death.
				*Coordinate institutional and/or community resources in addressing cultural needs at the end of life.	*Develop a case study and plan of care for a dying person from a culture other than students'/nurses' own culture.
Culturally specific peri-death rituals and customs.	*Develop cultural awareness, sensitivity and responsiveness regarding peri-death rituals. *Accept cultural and spiritual diversity.		*Provide culturally competent care during the peri-death period.		

Education Plan 12.1 *(continued)*

Knowledge	Attitude	Skills	Undergraduate Behavioral Outcome	Graduate Behavioral Outcomes	Teaching/Learning Strategies
					*Interview a clergy member or community elder to discuss death rituals and customs specific to that culture. Report findings in post-conference or write a paper comparing and contrasting their findings with their own religion or culture.
Post-Death Nursing Care: Expected physiological changes and related nursing care. Care of the body. Family support. Pronouncing Death. Autopsy.	*Develop emotional and spiritual comfort in caring for the deceased and their family.	*Perform respectful post-mortem care.	*Administer respectful care of the deceased and support of the family	*Pronounce death and/or request an autopsy.	*Have senior staff nurses serve as preceptors in assisting students in the physical care of the deceased patient and support of the family.

Education Plan 12.1 *(continued)*

Knowledge	Attitude	Skills	Undergraduate Behavioral Outcome	Graduate Behavioral Outcomes	Teaching/Learning Strategies
					*Conduct a post-conference or seminar to explore feelings and fears related to care of the deceased and their family.
Funerals as Ceremonies of Death: —Components of funerals; —Therapeutic value; and —Personal grief in response to a patient's death.	*Appreciate the therapeutic value of ceremonies of death.		*Participate in death-related ceremonies or rituals.	*Coordinate and/or conduct bereavement rituals or support groups for colleagues.	*Visit a funeral home or invite a funeral director to class to discuss burial/cremation options, components of a funeral, and responsibilities of the funeral director as a member of the interdisciplinary team.

Education Plan 12.1 *(continued)*

Knowledge	Attitude	Skills	Undergraduate Behavioral Outcome	Graduate Behavioral Outcomes	Teaching/Learning Strategies
					Write a reaction paper that addresses students'/nurses' perceptions and experiences related to this experience. *During a post-conference or seminar have the students/nurses brainstorm strategies that would support health professionals in coping with a patients' death.

REFERENCES

Birchenall, J., & Streight, E. (1997). *Home care aide.* St. Louis, MO: Mosby.

Ferrell, B. R., Virani, R., & Grant, M. (1999). Analysis of end of life content in nursing textbooks. *Oncology Nursing Forum, 26*(5), 869–876.

Fields, M., & Cassell, C. (1997). *Approaching death: Improving care at the end of life.* Washington, DC: National Academy Press.

Gorman, L. M. (1998). In R. M. Carroll-Johnson, L. M. Gorman, & N. J. Bush (Eds.), *Psychosocial nursing care along the cancer continuum* (pp. 3–25). Pittsburgh, PA: Oncology Nursing Press.

Gates, R. A., & Fink, R. M. (1997). *Oncology nursing secrets.* St. Louis, MO: Mosby.

Green, J. (1989a). Death with Dignity: Baha'i Faith. *Nursing Times, 85*(10), 50–51.

Green, J. (1989b). Death with Dignity: Buddhism. *Nursing Times, 85*(9), 40–41.

Green, J. (1989c). Death with Dignity: Hinduism. *Nursing Times, 85*(6), 50–51.

Green, J. (1989d). Death with Dignity: Islam. *Nursing Times, 85*(5), 56–57.

Green, J. (1989e). Death with Dignity: Judaism. *Nursing Times, 85*(8), 65–65.

Horn, L. W. (1992). Terminal dyspnea: A hospice approach. *American Journal of Hospice and Palliative Care.* March/April, 24–32.

Iserson, K. V. (1994). *Death to dust: What happens to dead bodies?* Tucson, AZ: Galen Press, Ltd.

Kastenbaum, R., & Kastenbaum, B. (Eds.) (1989). *Encyclopedia of death.* Phoenix, AZ: Oryx Press.

Lynn, J., & Harrold, J. (1999). *Handbook for mortals: Guidance for people facing serious illness.* New York: Oxford University Press.

Miller, E. J. (1993). A Roman Catholic view of death. In K. Doka & J. D. Morgan (Eds.), *Death and spirituality* (pp. 33–50). Amityville, NY: Baywood Publishing.

Purnell, L. D., & Paulanka, B. J. (1998). *Transcultural heal care: A culturally competent approach.* Philadelphia, PA: Davis Co.

Raether, H. C. (1993). Rituals, beliefs, and grief. In K. Doka & J. D. Morgan (Eds.), *Death and spirituality* (pp. 207–216). Amityville, NY: Baywood Publishing.

Sorrentino, S. A. (1999). *Assisting with patient care.* St. Louis, MO: Mosby.

Strub, C. G., & Frederick, L. G. (1967). *The principles and practice of embalming.* Dallas, TX: Frederick.

Appendix 1

Symptom Relief Kit

(Reprinted with permission)

Health Care Provider Information Sheet

VNA Transitional Care and Hospice
1850 Elm Street
Manchester, NH 03104

- For signs/symptoms of **pain or dyspnea**: Morphine solution 0.25–.5-ml (20 mg./ml-solution) PO/SL q̄ 2 hours PRN May increase up to 1–2 ml q 1–2 h. prn as directed by the health care provider.
- For loud, **wet respirations or excessive secretions**: Hyoscyamine (Levsin) 0.125 mg. (1–2 tablets) PO/SL q̄ 6 hours PRN.
- For **unrelieved respiratory fluid accumulation**: Furosemide (Lasix) 40 mg. IV/IM/PO/SC. May repeat.
- For **nausea or vomiting**: Prochlorperazine 25 mg. suppository PR q̄ 8 hours PRN. If not effective, give ABH** Suppository PR q̄ 8 hours PRN.
- For severe agitation or restlessness:
  Determine if client is in pain and treat accordingly;
  Determine if client is constipated or having urinary retention, take appropriate action.

- If agitation persists, administer Pentobarbital suppository PR q̄ 6 hours PRN.

*Clients taking opiods for pain will need to increase their usual morphine dose (for breakthrough pain) for effective treatment of dyspnea.
**ABH Suppository = Ativan (Lorazepam), Benadryl (Diphenhydramine), and Haldol (Haloperidol). Reglan (Metochlopramide) may be added by the pharmacist for severe nausea/vomiting; this would become an ABHR Suppository.

Appendix 2

Symptom Relief Kit

(Reprinted with permission)

Information Sheet for Patients and Families

VNA Transitional Care and Hospice
1850 Elm Street
Manchester, NH 03104

The **Symptom Relief Kit** is designed to help you cope with physical problems that might unexpectedly arise. In the kit:

➤ **Liquid Morphine**: There are 4 syringes with caps for pain or difficulty breathing. It is given by mouth or can be inserted rectally.
➤ There are 4 kinds of suppositories in 4 differently labeled bags:

➤ **Prochlorperazine** (which is the active ingredient in **Compazine**). Use this for nausea with or without vomiting.
➤ **ABH** (this stands for Ativan, Benadryl, and Haldol). This is used for severe nausea and vomiting. They may also be used if the patient is very restless or anxious and may cause the patient to be very sleepy.
➤ **Pentobarbital** is used for severe agitation or seizures and will make the patient very sleepy.
➤ **Acetaminophen** is used for high fevers.

➤ **Levsin** tablets are used for noisy, wet, "gurgly" breathing sounds. They can help to dry up secretions.

➤ **Furosemide (Lasix)**: There are 2 syringes with caps and are used for severe difficulty breathing because of fluid buildup. The nurse will visit and give this medicine to the patient if you have not been taught how to give "shots."

If you feel that you need to use this kit, call the Hospice nurse first. You don't have to do this alone; we are here to help you. Take a moment for yourself, take a deep breath, and then call us.

Directions for Using the Contents of the Symptom Relief Kit

SYMPTOM	DRUG	HOW TO USE IT
➤Unrelieved Pain	Morphine Solution	1–2 ml in the mouth, under the tongue every 2 to 3 hours as needed.
➤ Unrelieved Short-ness of Breath	Morphine Solution	0.25–0.5 ml in the mouth, under the tongue every 2 hours as needed.
➤ Nausea & Vomiting	Prochlorperazine Suppository	One suppository inserted into the rectum every 8 hours as needed.
➤ Unrelieved Nau-sea & Vomiting or ➤ Restlessness & Anxiety	ABH Suppository	One suppository inserted into the rectum every 8 hours as needed.
➤ Severe Agitation & Restlessness	Pentobarbital Suppos-itory	One suppository inserted into the rectum every 4 to 6 hours as needed.
➤ Wet, "Gurgly" Breathing	Levsin Tablets	One or two in the mouth or under the tongue every 4 to 6 hours as needed.

Unrelieved Accumulation and Respiratory Distress	Furosemide Injection	Inject 40–80 mg as instructed by the nurse.
Fever	Acetaminophen Suppository	One suppository inserted into the rectum every 4 hours as needed.

Index